Tending Mothers and the Fruits of the Womb

Medizin, Gesellschaft und Geschichte

Jahrbuch
des Instituts für Geschichte der Medizin
der Robert Bosch Stiftung

herausgegeben von
Robert Jütte

Beiheft 64

Tending Mothers and the Fruits of the Womb

The Work of the Midwife in the Early Modern German City

by Gabrielle Robilliard

Franz Steiner Verlag Stuttgart
2017

Gedruckt mit freundlicher Unterstützung der Robert Bosch Stiftung GmbH

Coverabbildung:
Oil painting on canvas of midwife and woman tending a newborn. Marianne
Kürzinger, *In der Wöchnerinnenstube*, Munich, 1788 (Deutsches Historisches
Museum, Berlin / A. Psille).

Bibliografische Information der Deutschen Nationalbibliothek:
Die Deutsche Nationalbibliothek verzeichnet diese Publikation in der Deutschen
Nationalbibliografie; detaillierte bibliografische Daten sind im Internet über
<http://dnb.d-nb.de> abrufbar.

© Franz Steiner Verlag, Stuttgart 2017
Druck: Laupp & Göbel GmbH, Nehren
Gedruckt auf säurefreiem, alterungsbeständigem Papier.
Printed in Germany
ISBN 978-3-515-11668-8 (Print)
ISBN 978-3-515-11669-5 (E-Book)

Contents

List of Figures and Tables

Figures

Tables

Acknowledgements

This study is the lightly revised and updated version of the doctoral thesis accepted at the University of Warwick in 2011 for the Doctor of Philosophy in history. The original thesis would not have been possible without the four-year Doctoral Award I received from the Arts and Humanities Research Council, UK. Further thanks for financial assistance go to the former Max Planck Institute for History in Göttingen, Germany, where I commenced life as a doctoral student in 2005 supported by a Georg Christoph Lichtenberg Stipend from the State of Lower Saxony.

As is the case for any piece of research, many people have been involved in this project since I started out in 2005. My greatest thanks go to my supervisors Prof. Hilary Marland and Prof. Claudia Stein in the Department of History at the University of Warwick for their energetic enthusiasm for my project, their thought-provoking comments and wise suggestions, as well as their unfailing support both during my doctoral 'apprenticeship' and beyond. Further thanks go to my examiners, Prof. Beat Kümin (Warwick) and Dr. Adrian Wilson (Leeds), for their immensely constructive critiques and suggestions. To Prof. Dr. Jürgen Schlumbohm (Göttingen), my initial *Doktorvater* in Göttingen, I owe thanks in particular for the discussions about 'lay' midwives that undoubtedly helped to shape this project. I would also like to thank Sam Thomas for the stimulating email discussions on early modern midwifery that have likewise left their mark. And I also thank Prof. Dr. Rebekka von Mallinckrodt (Bremen) for encouraging me to get my thesis published.

My appreciation extends also to staff of the Stadtarchiv, the Kirchenarchiv and the Universitätsarchiv in Leipzig, who were so very helpful in assisting me navigate my way around their collections. Likewise to staff at the Sächsisches Staatsarchiv in Dresden and Leipzig.

Further thanks are due to the staff and doctoral students in both the History Department at the University of Warwick and the Max Planck Institute for History, who provided such insightful comments on my project, loads of encouragement and plenty of light relief along the way. Likewise, I am also indebted to the feedback my project received from countless fellow historians at conferences and workshops I have attended over the years.

I would also like to thank the editor of the Jahrbuch series of *Medizin, Gesellschaft und Geschichte*, Prof. Dr. phil. Robert Jütte, for accepting my manuscript into its publication series.

Revising the thesis for publication would have been impossible without the support of my parents-in-law Piet and Wiebke Witt, who spent many a weekend and most of the 2016 autumn school holidays looking after my children so that I could have the peace and quiet I needed to work. I am also eternally grateful to my mum and Liz Bodemer for proof-reading at various stages and reining in my comma abuses. All mistakes are, of course, my own.

My parents, Jacqueline and David Robilliard, have provided me with non-stop encouragement to do history since my captivation by the bling of the eighteenth century as an awestruck eight-year-old Antipodean at Schloss Schönbrunn in Vienna. They knew then that they had 'lost' me to Europe (and to History), but their support for my study and travels never wavered. For that I am eternally grateful.

For much of this project my husband Sönke has been ever patient with my 'creative' processes and my Excel- and Word-induced nervous breakdowns. Whilst writing up and revising the thesis, he and our sons Felix and Arved have been a source of unrelenting strength and welcome distraction: I thank all three for both.

Glossary of German and Medical Terms

Accoucheur
French term for physician or surgeon who practised obstetric surgery

Almosen Amt
Alms Office in Leipzig, a local municipal institution administering poor relief managed by the Leipzig Council

Amt (pl. Ämter)
district (jurisdiction of Saxon government)

Amtsphysicus
district physician (under jurisdiction of the Amt)

Beifrau (pl. Beifrauen)
apprentice midwife (under municipal oath)

craniotomy
crushing of the foetus' head in utero when obstruction has occurred to enable extraction of foetus

Gassenmagd
woman appointed by the Leipzig Council to serve a local neighbourhood

Gassenmeister
overseer of the local neighbourhood appointed by the Leipzig Council

Geburtshelfer
obstetrician (Term only began to be used at the close of the eighteenth century in Leipzig.)

gefallenes Mensch
a 'fallen' or unfortunate person (often refers to a woman)

geschwächte Weibesperson
'fallen' woman

Hebamme
midwife

Hebammenlehrer
municipal medical official responsible for teaching a city's midwives

Hebammenmeister
variant of *Hebammenlehrer*

hook extraction
Extraction of a foetus using a special obstetric hook. The foetus is first dismembered in utero and the hook then used to grip and extract the limbs, body and head piece by piece.

Kindermutter
midwife (terminology used in Leipzig)

Landtag
Saxon Diet

Lazarett
lazarette or general hospital in Leipzig catering to the local population

Leichenschreiberei
Corpse Registry Office

Lust	desire (used in midwife petitions in a non-sexual sense, e.g., to pursue a course of action)
medizinische Policey	medical police
mole	a false pregnancy; a growth
Sanitätskollegium	Board of Health
Schöppenstuhl	Court of Jurors
Sechswöchnerin	woman lying-in (*Sechswochen*: The six weeks between birth and churching in which new mothers were theoretically bound to the house and absolved from most household work.)
Stadt	intramural city
Stadtaccoucheur	doctor/surgeon employed by the Leipzig Council to oversee obstetric matters (*Accouchement*) in the city
Stadtgericht	Leipzig City Court (of Law)
Stadtphysicus	physician employed by the Leizpig Council to oversee medical matters in the city
Stadtrat	Leipzig City Council
Stadtrichter	judge of the City Court
Stand	estate
Ständegesellschaft	society of estates
Tor	city gate
version	Turning of the foetus in utero into the head-first position using the hands or specially designed ribbons. This technique did not necessarily lead to the death of the foetus.
Vorstadt	extramural neighbourhood(s)
Wehemutter	midwife
Wickelweib	literally 'swaddling woman', or a woman engaged informally by a midwife or Beifrau as an assistant
Willige Almosen	municipally run system of poor relief in Leipzig prior to 1704

Introduction

In 1799 an anonymous *Taschenwörterbuch* (pocket dictionary) of Leipzig for 'natives and foreigners' lamented the state of midwifery in the city:

> That one appoints women from the lowest estates as midwives might well be excused by the fact that no [women] from the middle estates enlist themselves. This surprises one all the more as the office of midwife is considered very lucrative. But there are also women of good reputation and impeccable performance in the lower estates: Should one not take this particularly into consideration?[1]

There is little known about the author, Moritz Cruciger, other than that he was critical of the political, social and economic culture of the *Ständegesellschaft* (society of estates). The power wielded by the guilds in defence of their economic territory was, according to Cruciger, the reason why manufacturing in Leipzig lagged so far behind other parts of Europe.[2] He was equally critical of that kind of economic protectionism perpetuated in other previously un- or ill-regulated occupations, and lambasted the Leipzig Council for attempting to make a 'privileged art' out of the barbers, which 'robs me of the power over my own beard!'[3] He also had a violent disrespect for learned medicine and mocked 'the doctors of this city', who each 'has his own way of carrying himself, behaving and speaking, yes even of treating illnesses'.[4] As a result 'the doctors' art' was 'innocent', so much so that 'no one should ever blame the doctor when an illness ends in death … least of all when a doctor's diploma gives him the exclusive right to populate the graveyard.'[5] Furthermore, the 'Medici' only had themselves to blame for the 'deep contempt' of the doctor's art; even those with means resorted to the medicine pedalled by quacks.[6]

Cruciger's intense criticism of the political and medical establishment informs his sympathetic commentary on the value of midwives, an attitude that had prevailed for much of the century. Around the middle of the eighteenth century, Zedler's encyclopaedia described the sworn midwife in positive terms as a 'careful, intelligent, experienced and God-fearing woman, who holds the good opinion of other people and commendation of her comportment … has borne children herself … has been present at births and helped the midwives, so that she has been able to acquire sufficient knowledge'.[7] Later eighteenth-century encyclopaedists and writers, however, were at times scathing of midwives' skill or, as they saw it, their lack thereof. In 1789, for example, Krünitz's encyclopaedia accounted for the existence of midwives as having

---

1 Originally published anonymously. Moritz Cruciger, *Leipzig im Profil. Ein Taschenwörterbuch* (Solothurn: Krüger und Weber, 1799), 18–19.
2 See ibid., 120–21.
3 Ibid., 29–30.
4 Ibid., 17.
5 Ibid., 18.
6 Ibid., 19.
7 Johann Heinrich Zedler, *Grosses vollständiges Universal-Lexicon aller Wissenschaften und Künste* (online version), (68 vols, Bayerische Staatsbibliothek: 1731–54), available at <http://www.zedler-lexikon.de/index.html>, accessed 26 October 2016, vol. 53, 993.

arisen from the 'shame of women', which had historically prevented men from practising the important duty of assisting human birth: 'people preferred to steal lives than to leave to a man this important office of holding onto the life of [mother] and the new burgher.'[8] This clash of rhetoric reflects the intense conflict between, on the one hand, the overwhelmingly positive value placed upon the office of midwife by both urban authorities and the community and, on the other, novel ideas about the superiority of male obstetrics, in particular during the second half of the eighteenth century.

The polarisation of the figure of the midwife was not merely a strategy deployed by an emerging group of obstetricians to carve out unchartered occupational territory. New economic and social forces were also reshaping social hierarchies, in particular within the 'middle estates', and this had direct implications for the provision of urban midwifery. We can glean from Cruciger's statement that, like many other types of female extra-domestic work, midwifery had undergone a process of social degradation over the course of the eighteenth century and was no longer a fitting task for women of social and economic means. Cruciger mocked the *nouveau* airs and graces of this emerging social group, whose women apparently deemed themselves too fine for midwifery, but whose households were still dependent upon earning a living. However, he did not consider this development as a reason for doing away with female midwives altogether. Rather, he argued that the traditional qualities sought in a midwife – a 'good reputation' and 'impeccable performance' – were also to be found in the masses of women still utterly dependent upon paid work. According to this deeply establishment-critical, late eighteenth-century observer, female midwives were both viable and necessary. As we shall see, this was a view shared by many in early modern Leipzig into the early nineteenth century and beyond; and it was the value the community placed upon the midwife together with social and economic custom that dictated the bounds of reforms to midwifery in this early modern city.

Midwifery in Leipzig

Leipzig, a large, bustling and commercially oriented city, felt acute anxieties over depopulation in the wake of the Thirty Years War and began to reform its established system of urban midwifery. It increased the number of midwives and, by the 1680s, the city had begun to employ at least one midwife-in-waiting to ensure that vacant midwife offices were quickly filled. In the early eighteenth century it appointed a special physician to oversee the city's sworn midwives and carry out operative obstetric procedures where necessary. Shortly thereafter the Leipzig Council formalised the system of midwife apprenticeship by creating the office of *Beifrau* (an apprentice midwife under municipal

---

8   Dr Johann Georg Krünitz, *Oekonomische Encyklopädie oder allgemeines System der Staats- Stadt- Haus- und Landwirthschaft* (242 vols, Berlin: 1789), available at <http://www.kruenitz1.uni-trier.de/>, accessed 27 October 2016, vol. 22(ii), 528.

oath) and in 1732 it appointed a *Stadtaccoucheur*, a physician/surgeon employed by the Council to preside over obstetric matters in the city, to supervise, examine and teach the city's sworn midwives and Beifrauen in anatomy and obstetrics. 1732 marked the last major 'reform' undertaken by the Leipzig Council for the rest of the century and, as Chapter Seven will demonstrate, the Leipzig Council spent much of the latter eighteenth century successfully resisting attempts by the Leipzig University and the Saxon government to build a maternity hospital for the purposes of training midwives and medical practitioners in a clinical setting.[9] Late seventeenth- and eighteenth-century reforms to midwifery in Leipzig were part of an earlier, localised attempt at combatting the problem of depopulation and reinstating an ideal social and religious status quo. These moves were influenced by the increasingly popular cameralist notion of population as the 'essential powerbase of the state' and the guiding hand of paternalism inspired by Reformation ideas about the family and procreation.[10]

As is evident from the chronology, all of these reforms preceded the era of *medizinische Policey* (medical police), the discourse of public health promulgated largely by academically trained medical practitioners throughout Germany from around the 1760s.[11] These developments were far from belonging to a progressive programme of medicalisation that began with midwives being placed under the supervision of the *Stadtphysicus* (municipal physician) and culminated in the introduction of clinical midwifery in the early nineteenth century. Although similar developments have been noted for a number of early modern cities, I argue here that the late seventeenth- and early eighteenth-century reforms to midwifery were local solutions to local problems that reflected and respected the political, social and economic status quo.[12] They occurred in fits and starts and implementation was sporadic and often lacklustre. As we shall see, it took some years for the Council to decide to make the office of Stadtaccoucheur a permanent fixture within the municipal medical hierarchy. Similarly, when the anatomical-obstetrical training of midwives ceased for several years under Stadtaccoucheur Johann Karl Gehler in

9   This was not unusual; as Gross notes, whenever the Saxon government encountered difficulties in implementing its plans, it was bound to seek compromise. Reiner Gross, *Geschichte Sachsens* (Leipzig: Edition Leipzig, 2001), 125.

10   Martin Dinges, 'Medicinische Policey zwischen Heilkundigen und "Patienten" (1750–1830)', in Karl Härter, ed., *Policey und frühneuzeitliche Gesellschaft* (Frankfurt am Main: Vittorio Klostermann, 2000), 268–69.

11   Caren Möller, *Medizinalpolizei. Die Theorie des staatlichen Gesundheitswesens im 18. und 19. Jahrhundert* (Frankfurt am Main: Vittorio Klostermann, 2005), 143–46. The political efficacy of medical Policey, however, has been severely overestimated for the period prior to 1830. See Dinges, 'Medicinische Policey', 294.

12   For example, a municipal midwife instructor was appointed in Lübeck in 1731. Christine Loytved, *Hebammen und ihre Lehrer. Wendepunkte in Ausbildung und Amt Lübecker Hebammen (1730–1850)* (Osnabrück: Universitäts-Verlag Rasch, 2002), 94–95. In contrast, the city of Braunschweig did not appoint a designated instructor but organised private training with one of the university professors. See Mary Lindemann, *Health and Healing in Eighteenth-Century Germany* (Baltimore, MD: Johns Hopkins University Press, 1996), 200.

the latter eighteenth century, there was no action taken to reinstate this institution. I will argue that these reforms altered midwifery practice in Leipzig very
little, not only because they were ineffectively implemented, but because they
worked within the traditional occupational structure and culture of midwifery,
which was grounded in a corporate understanding of the medical occupations.

Histories of midwifery

The 'Krünitz' view of midwifery long informed the motivation for examining
the historical trajectory of midwifery in Germany and elsewhere in Europe.
Many early studies concerned themselves with exploring the rise of obstetrics
in the eighteenth and nineteenth centuries as a triumph of medical Enlightenment.[13] In particular the institutional association of the history of medicine as
a sub-discipline of medicine – still the case today – served to hinder reflection
on this positivist narrative. These 'doctor-histories' of predominantly urban
midwifery concentrated largely on the process whereby academic medicine
conquered a female culture of midwifery practice fraught by un-reason, witchcraft and ignorance.[14] Interest from non-medical historians in midwifery was
less pronounced, although it is worth noting three works on midwifery ordinances and Elseluise Haberling's study, which was the first to examine midwifery from the perspective of women's work.[15] In the 1970s and 1980s feminist historians turned the tables on this interpretation of medical triumph,
situating midwives as innocent victims in a violent cultural battle between a
female culture of childbirth and male political and medical institutions.[16] This

13   For example, see H. Krauss, 'Zur Geschichte des Hebammenwesens im Fürstentum Ans-
     bach', *Archive für Geschichte der Medizin* 6 (1913): 64–71; Dr. F. C. Wille, 'Über Stand und
     Ausbildung der Hebammen im 17. und 18. Jahrhundert in Chur-Brandenburg', *Ab-
     handlungen zur Geschichte der Medizin und der Naturwissenschaften* Heft 4 (1934); Friedrich
     Baruch, 'Das Hebammenwesen im Reichsstädtischen Nürnberg' (Dissertation, Erlangen,
     1955).
14   The thesis linking midwifery to witchcraft and explaining regulation as modernisation
     was most famously expounded in Thomas Rogers Forbes, *The Midwife and the Witch* (New
     Haven, CT: Yale University Press, 1966). Forbes' thesis has been since laid to rest by
     David Harley. See David Harley, 'Historians as Demonologists: The Myth of the Mid-
     wife-Witch', *Society for the History of Medicine* 3 (1990): 1–26.
15   Georg Burkhard, *Die deutschen Hebammenordnungen von ihren ersten Anfängen bis auf die
     Neuzeit* (Leipzig, 1912); Johann Hub, 'Die Hebammenordnung des XVII. Jahrhunderts'
     (Dissertation, Würzburg, 1914); Alois Nöth, 'Die Hebammenordnungen des XVIII.
     Jahrhunderts' (Dissertation, Würzburg, 1931); Elseluise Haberling, *Beiträge zur Geschichte
     des Hebammenstandes I. Der Hebammenstand bis zum Dreißigjährigen Krieg* (Berlin, 1940).
16   In particular Barbara Ehrenreich and Deirdre English, *Witches, Midwives and Nurses: A
     History of Women Healers* (2nd edn, Old Westbury, NY: The Feminist Press, 1973); Gunnar
     Heinsohn and Otto Steiger, *Die Vernichtung der weisen Frauen. Beiträge zur Theorie und
     Geschichte von Bevölkerung und Kindheit* (2nd edn, Herbstein: März-Verlag, 1985). Both ac-
     counts have been widely discredited.

focus on the competition and conflict between midwives and the medical 'establishment' became a focus of later research.

Since the 1980s, the history of midwifery has cast off the polemics of both medical triumphalism and hard-line feminism, and has been incorporated as a serious field of study within the ever-growing corpus of the history of medicine as well as social and cultural history more generally. Much research on Germany has focused on the south and the fifteenth to the seventeenth centuries, largely because southwestern German cities were the first to produce midwifery ordinances; northern German cities did not tend to regulate via ordinance until the seventeenth century at the earliest.[17] Merry Wiesner's pioneering studies on midwifery as women's work throughout the sixteenth and seventeenth centuries paint a picture of midwifery as an occupational realm in which women enjoyed relative freedom to practise and were greatly valued by society.[18] This view of midwifery has been contrasted by studies concentrating on the official role midwives played in sanctioning illicit sexuality and illegitimacy in early modern communities.[19] Sybilla Flügge's work on the function of late medieval midwifery ordinances and their relationship to the concrete legal situation faced by women points to a richer understanding of how midwives (and women more generally) engaged in norm-setting before 1600.[20] Further regional studies have fleshed out this period considerably, although many have been concerned with the question of whether and to what degree midwives were controlled through regulation.[21]

---

17 Noted by Sibylla Flügge, *Hebammen und heilkundige Frauen. Recht und Rechtswirklichkeit im 15. und 16. Jahrhundert* (Frankfurt am Main: Stroemfeld, 1998), 15.

18 Merry Wiesner, 'Early Modern Midwifery: A Case Study', in Barbara A. Hanawalt, ed., *Women and Work in Preindustrial Europe* (Bloomington, IN: Indiana University Press, 1986); Merry E. Wiesner, *Working Women in Renaissance Germany* (New Brunswick, NJ: Rutgers University Press, 1986); Merry Wiesner, 'The Midwives of South Germany and the Public/Private Dichotomy', in Hilary Marland, ed., *The Art of Midwifery: Early Modern Midwives in Europe* (London: Routledge, 1993).

19 Ulinka Rublack, 'The Public Body: Policing Abortion in Early Modern Germany', in Lynn Abrams and Elizabeth Harvey, eds, *Gender Relations in German History: Power, Agency and Experience from the Sixteenth to the Twentieth Century* (London: UCL Press, 1996). For the eighteenth century, see also Ulrike Gleixner, 'Die "Gute" und die "Böse". Hebammen als Amtsfrauen auf dem Land (Altmark/Brandenburg, 18. Jahrhundert)', in Heide Wunder and Christina Vanja, eds, *Weiber, Menscher, Frauenzimmer. Frauen in der ländlichen Gesellschaft 1500–1800* (Göttingen: Vandenhoeck & Ruprecht, 1996).

20 Flügge, *Hebammen und heilkundige Frauen*.

21 Dagmar Birkelbach and Sabine Luecken, 'Zur Entwicklung des Hebammenwesens vom 14. bis zum 16. Jahrhundert am Beispiel der Regensburger Hebammenordnungen', *Beiträge zur feministischen Theorie und Praxis* 5 (1981): 83–98; Susanne Gabler, 'Das Hebammenwesen in Nördlingen des 16. Jahrhunderts' (Dissertation, Technical University Munich, 1985); Gabriela Signori, 'Defensivgemeinschaften. Kreißende, Hebammen und "Mitweiber" im Spiegel spätmittelalterlicher Geburtswunder', *Das Mittelalter. Perspektiven mediävistischer Forschung* 1: 2 (1996): 113–34. For the Renaissance through to the eighteenth century, see also Britta Schmitz, *Hebammen in Münster. Historische Entwicklung, Lebens- und Arbeitsumfeld, berufliches Selbstverständnis* (Münster: Waxmann, 1994); Claudia

Research on the seventeenth and eighteenth centuries, in part due to the richness of the available sources for that period, has yielded highly detailed results. Social historians of medicine have illuminated both the practice and the person of midwives as opposed to just regulation. Thus we now know a good deal about the obstetric input and practice of a handful of early modern midwives who either left behind diaries or published works.[22] Using archival sources, other historians have illuminated the practice of midwifery of 'normal' midwives in both urban and rural contexts and concentrate, for example, on occupational structures and occupational identity amongst midwives in northern Europe.[23] Others working on England, such as Doreen Evenden and Ann Hess, have concentrated more on the socio-economic situation of midwives and explored their social and occupational networks.[24] Within the German context, Eva Labouvie's historical-anthropological approach has proved most useful for exploring the everyday practice of rural midwives over a period of almost five hundred years and has provided great insight into the interplay between custom, collective and individual fields of action as well as established mentalities and practices. Her work illuminates in particular the magical and religious world of the midwife, as a pendant to the socio-eco-

Hilpert, *Wehemütter. Amtshebammen, Accoucheure und die Akademisierung der Geburtshilfe im kurfürstlichen Mainz, 1550–1800* (Frankfurt am Main: Peter Lang, 2000).

22   On the French midwives Louise Bourgeois and Madame du Coudray, see Wendy Perkins, *Midwifery and Medicine in Early Modern France: Louise Bourgeois* (Exeter: University of Exeter Press, 1996); Nina Rattner Gelbart, *The King's Midwife: A History and Mystery of Madame du Coudray* (Berkeley and Los Angeles: University of California Press, 1998). On the German midwife Justine Siegemund, see Waltraud Pulz, *"Nicht alles nach der Gelahrten Sinn geschrieben": Das Hebammenanleitungsbuch von Justina Siegemund. Zur Rekonstruktion geburtshilflichen Überlieferungswissens frühneuzeitlicher Hebammen und seiner Bedeutung bei der Herausbildung der modernen Geburtshilfe* (Munich: Münchner Vereinigung für Volkskunde, 1994); Justine Siegemund, *The Court Midwife. Justina Siegemund*, trans. Lynne Tatlock (Chicago, IL: The University of Chicago Press, 2005). See also Catharina Schrader, *"Mother and Child were Saved". The Memoirs (1693–1740) of the Frisian Midwife Catharina Schrader*, trans. Hilary Marland (Amsterdam: Rodopi, 1987); Laurel Thatcher-Ulrich, *A Midwife's Tale: The Life of Martha Ballard, Based on Her Diary, 1785–1812* (New York, NY: Vintage Books, 1991).

23   Lindemann, *Health*; 'Professionals? Sisters? Rivals? Midwives in Braunschweig 1750–1800', in Hilary Marland, ed., *The Art of Midwifery. Early Modern Midwives in Europe* (London: Routledge, 1993); Hilary Marland, '"Stately and dignified, kindly and God-fearing": midwives, age and status in the Netherlands in the eighteenth century', in Hilary Marland and Margaret Pelling, eds, *The Task of Healing: Medicine, Religion and Gender in England and the Netherlands, 1450–1800* (Rotterdam: Erasmus Publications, 1996); 'The "*burgerlijke*" midwife: the *stadsvroedvrouw* of eighteenth-century Holland', in Hilary Marland, ed., *The Art of Midwifery: Early Modern Midwives in Europe* (London: Routledge, 1993).

24   Doreen Evenden, *The Midwives of Seventeenth-Century London* (Cambridge: Cambridge University Press, 2000); Ann Giardina Hess, 'Community Case Studies of Midwives from England and New England c. 1650–1720' (PhD thesis, University of Cambridge, 1994); 'Midwifery Practice Among the Quakers in Southern Rural England in the Late Seventeenth Century', in Hilary Marland, ed., *The Art of Midwifery: Early Modern Midwives in Europe* (London: Routledge, 1993).

nomic 'world of work' approach mentioned above.[25] The history of childbirth has developed its own niche and, influenced in particular by cultural historical and anthropological approaches, it has provided a rich perspective on the vast array of 'non-medical' rituals and material culture deployed and communicated during childbirth.[26]

Competition between midwives and medical practitioners has also attracted the interest of historians, in particular those working on the late seventeenth and eighteenth centuries. Whereas historians of English midwifery have been preoccupied with explaining a shift amongst mothers in certain parts of England from using female midwives to calling for the man-midwife, in Germany, this occupational rivalry was largely of a textual or rhetorical nature.[27] Studies by Lynne Tatlock and Waltraud Pulz have drawn our attention to the way gender shaped obstetric discourse on what midwives could do and know about the female body and childbirth.[28] No widespread 'takeover' (whether reluctant or otherwise) ever took place in Germany; studies suggest that midwifery remained firmly in the hands of female practitioners throughout the eighteenth and well into the nineteenth centuries.[29]

The advent and effects of the maternity hospitals in the latter eighteenth and nineteenth centuries is a further theme attracting significant attention from historians, who have largely pursued a Foucauldian analysis of these institutions as a space in which the female body was standardized and disci-

---

25 Eva Labouvie, *Beistand in Kindsnöten. Hebammen und weibliche Kultur auf dem Land, 1550–1910* (Frankfurt am Main: Campus Verlag, 1999).

26 See, for example, Jacques Gélis, *History of Childbirth: Fertility, Pregnancy and Birth in Early Modern Europe*, trans. Rosemary Morris (Cambridge: Polity Press, 1991); Eva Labouvie, *Andere Umstände: Eine Kulturgeschichte der Geburt* (Cologne: Böhlau, 2000); Adrian Wilson, 'Participant or Patient? Seventeenth-Century Childbirth from the Mother's Point of View', in Roy Porter, ed., *Patients and Practitioners: Lay Perceptions of Medicine in Pre-Industrial Society* (Cambridge: Cambridge University Press, 2002). More recently Peter Murray Jones and Lea T. Olsan, 'Performative Rituals for Conception and Childbirth in England, 900–1500', *Bulletin of the History of Medicine* 89: 3 (2015): 406–33.

27 Adrian Wilson, *The Making of Man-Midwifery: Childbirth in England 1660–1770* (London: UCL Press, 1995); Lisa Forman Cody, *Birthing the Nation: Sex, Science, and the Conception of Eighteenth-Century Britons* (Oxford: Oxford University Press, 2005), 10–13.

28 Both focus on Justine Siegemund's midwifery manual. See Lynne Tatlock, 'Speculum Feminarum: Gendered Perspectives on Obstetrics and Gynaecology in Early Modern Germany', *Signs* 17: 4 (1992): 725–60; Pulz, *"Nicht alles"*; 'Gewaltsame Hilfsbereitschaft? Die Arbeit der Hebamme im Spiegel eines Gerichtskonflikts (1680–1685)', in Jürgen Schlumbohm et al., eds, *Rituale der Geburt. Eine Kulturgeschichte* (Munich: Verlag C. H. Beck, 1998).

29 See Hans-Christoph Seidel, *Eine neue Kultur des Gebärens. Die Medikalisierung von Geburt im 18. und 19. Jahrhundert in Deutschland* (Stuttgart: Steiner Verlag, 1998), 420. Noted also by Lindemann in Lindemann, *Health*, 194. Hampe suggests, for example, that surgeon men-midwives were simply beyond the means of most people. See Henrike Hampe, *Zwischen Tradition und Instruktion. Hebammen im 18. und 19. Jahrhundert in der Universitätstadt Göttingen* (Göttingen: Schmerse, 1998), 134.

plined.[30] Midwife education, on the other hand, has been largely neglected, with only two studies by historians Jürgen Schlumbohm and Christine Loytved plumbing this topic in any depth.[31] Of great importance – not least for reasons of comparison – to this study is Christine Loytved's work on 'traditional' midwife training in late eighteenth- and early nineteenth-century Lübeck, a commercially important, northern German town like Leipzig.[32] According to Loytved, 'traditional' midwife education remained largely intact until the first decade of the nineteenth century, when the selection and education of apprentice midwives came under the jurisdiction of the *Hebammenlehrer* (municipal midwife instructor). Up until this point, she argues, midwives enjoyed relative autonomy over their occupational affairs.[33] As we shall see in this study, there are certain parallels between the development of midwifery in Leipzig and Lübeck.

On a more recent, pan-European perspective, there has been renewed interest in the medico-legal activities of midwives and medico-legal knowledge of the female body.[34] Cathy McClive, Katherine Park and Silvia de Renzi have focused on the role of practitioners – including midwives – in early modern legal medicine in epistemological debates over the body as well as medico-legal evidence, thus providing new insights into the epistemological relationship between midwifery and other medical practitioners.[35]

All these studies combined provide a strong argument for the importance of midwifery and the importance accorded to midwives in early modern communities across Europe. This has broken the refrain of Enlightenment medical-political and academic medical rhetoric that denigrated the skills and the experience of eighteenth-century midwives. It is thus no longer necessary for historians to rehabilitate the early modern midwife – we have dismantled that

---

30 Jürgen Schlumbohm, *Lebendige Phantome: ein Entbindungshospital und seine Patientinnen 1751–1830* (Göttingen: Wallstein Verlag, 2012); Jürgen Schlumbohm, ed., *Die Entstehung der Geburtsklinik in Deutschland 1751–1850: Göttingen, Kassel, Braunschweig* (Göttingen: Wallstein, 2004); Marita Metz-Becker, *Der verwaltete Körper. Die Medikalisierung schwangerer Frauen in den Gebärhäusern des frühen 19. Jahrhunderts* (Frankfurt am Main: Campus Verlag, 1997). See also the collection of essays in Christine Loytved, ed., *Von der Wehemutter zur Hebamme. Die Gründung von Hebammenschulen mit Blick auf ihren politischen Stellenwert und ihren praktischen Nutzen* (Osnabrück: Universitäts-Verlag Rasch, 2001).

31 Schlumbohm's contribution concentrates on midwife training in the Göttingen maternity hospital. See Jürgen Schlumbohm, 'The Practice of Practical Education: Male Students and Female Apprentices in the Lying-In Hospital of Göttingen University, 1792–1815', *Medical History* 51: 1 (2007): 3–36.

32 Loytved, *Hebammen.*

33 Ibid., 281.

34 See for earlier, still fundamental work in this field Esther Fischer-Homberger, *Medizin vor Gericht. Gerichtsmedizin von der Renaissance bis zur Aufklärung* (Bern: H. Huber, 1983).

35 Cathy McClive, 'Blood and Expertise. The Trials of the Female Medical Expert in the Ancien-Régime Courtroom', *Bulletin of the History of Medicine* 82: 1 (2008): 86–108; Katharine Park, 'The Death of Isabella Della Volpe. Four Eyewitness Accounts of a Postmortem Caesarean Section in 1545', ibid.: 169–87; Silvia De Renzi, 'Medical Expertise, Bodies, and the Law in Early Modern Courts', *Isis* 98: 2 (2007): 315–22.

particular Enlightenment piety of the bumbling, inept and ignorant midwife.[36] We need instead to engage more critically in the relationship between midwifery, medicine, the community, the Church, the law and local and territorial governments in order to understand how their roles interlocked in the domain of childbirth and midwifery. The relationship between midwives, surgeon men-midwives and physicians is an area warranting particular attention. Understanding how midwifery functioned as an occupation within the city beyond the level of the ordinance or oath is likewise crucial to this endeavour. Despite the relative richness of research already mentioned here, few German studies have dealt with midwife–client relations and midwives' client networks during the seventeenth and eighteenth centuries in any great detail.[37] We have little knowledge of how the midwife–client relationship functioned in Germany, how it was demarcated and how midwives went about building up their client networks in urban spaces. Nor have many attempted to gauge the level of midwifery practice (in all its forms and varieties) that existed parallel to (and even within) the official municipally instituted midwife structures.[38] These are some areas that this thesis will examine in greater detail within the context of early modern Leipzig.

Even in urban centres such as Leipzig, midwives remained largely at the helm in the birthing room, not just because there was not a significant 'market' for male obstetricians, but also because local midwifery structures were actively maintained by government and community. As we shall see, the traditional occupational culture of midwifery – training via apprenticeship, informal channels of selection and a corporate notion of entitlement to practice – persisted into the early nineteenth century. This study explores the intricate dynamics of urban midwifery practice and the urban midwifery structure in the city of Leipzig between 1650 and 1810 and the tug-of-war between established customs/infrastructures and the somewhat novel ideas about the organisation of midwifery and training of midwives that emerged during this period.

36 As, for instance, portrayed in Johann Christoph Ettner von Eiteritz, *Des getreuen Eckharts Unvorsichige Heb-Amme* (Leipzig: Braun, 1715).

37 Perkins', Ulrich's and Thomas' studies are some of the few to deal with these themes in great detail. See Perkins, *Midwifery and Medicine*, 76–98; Thatcher-Ulrich, *Midwife's Tale*; Samuel Thomas, 'Midwifery and Society in Restoration York', *Social History of Medicine* 16: 1 (2003): 1–16. See also Doreen Evenden, 'Mothers and their midwives in seventeenth-century London', in Hilary Marland, ed., *The Art of Midwifery: Early Modern Midwives in Europe* (London: Routledge, 1993).

38 Hilpert, for example, mentions that unsworn midwives existed but excludes them from her analysis. Hilpert, *Wehemütter*, 138–41. Lindemann, by contrast, subsumes unofficial midwifery into the rubric of pre-official training. This was certainly the case in Leipzig, however, unsworn midwifery there was not merely part of a system of training but was a systemic aspect of urban midwifery. See Lindemann, *Health*, 204–5.

Midwifery and Enlightenment

The period under scrutiny here, dubbed 'the long eighteenth century', has been characterised in the history of medicine in particular as an era of great transformation. However, the focus of debates and the explanatory frameworks deployed have varied across national boundaries. In the English context historians have looked to the development of a culture of consumption and its impact on medical practices and cultures, reassessing the identity of the 'quack' and developing the concept of the 'medical marketplace'.[39] German scholarship has conversely focused on the tensions between the growing 'state' and traditional local structures and customs, in particular with reference to the development of medical Policey in the latter eighteenth and early nineteenth centuries. In this narrative, medicalisation and professionalisation form the key processes in the development of the state, on the one hand, and the 'rise' of academic medicine and the 'demi-gods in white', on the other.[40] Many historians now agree that prior to the nineteenth century, 'medicine' was an eclectic, largely unregulated, overwhelmingly domestic and female domain.[41] This medical world, so the theory goes, was altered by the process of 'medicalisation'; the process whereby the state came to control the health of its subjects, not just by eradicating the plethora of irregular and unlicensed healers and forcing people to use state-sanctioned and (state-)trained practitioners, but also by 'civilising' and controlling the body via the inculcation of norms about body health and hygiene.[42] Ute Frevert's and Claudia Huerkamp's studies of

39   See Roy Porter, *Health for Sale: Quackery in England, 1660–1850* (Manchester: Manchester University Press, 1986). More recently the collection of essays in Mark S.R. Jenner and Patrick Wallis, eds, *Medicine and the Market in England and Its Colonies c.1450–c.1850* (Basingstoke: Palgrave Macmillan, 2007).

40   As coined by Claudia Huerkamp. Claudia Huerkamp, *Der Aufstieg der Ärzte im 19. Jahrhundert: Vom gelehrten Stand zum professionellen Experten. Das Beispiel Preußens* (Göttingen: Vandenhoeck & Ruprecht, 1985), 9.

41   See Robert Jütte, '"Wo kein Weib ist, da seufzet der Kranke" – Familie und Krankheit im 16. Jahrhundert', in Robert Jütte, ed., *Medizin, Gesellschaft, und Geschichte. Jahrbuch des Instituts für Geschichte der Medizin der Robert Bosch Stiftung* 7 (Stuttgart: F. Steiner, 1989), 7; Annemarie Kinzelbach, 'Konstruktion und konkretes Handeln. Heilkundige Frauen im oberdeutschen Raum, 1450–1700', *Historische Anthropologie: Kultur, Gesellschaft, Alltag* 7: 2 (1999): 165–90, 188–89. Healing also involved spiritual healers, of which many were also women. See Gianna Pomata, '"Practising between Earth and Heaven": Women Healers in Early Modern Bologna', *Dynamis* 19 (1999): 119–43, 121–22; Hans de Waardt, 'Chasing Demons and Curing Mortals: The Medical Practice of Clerics in the Netherlands', in Hilary Marland and Margaret Pelling, eds, *The Task of Healing: Medicine, Religion and Gender in England and the Netherlands, 1450–1800* (Rotterdam: Erasmus Publications, 1996), 194.

42   The concept of medicalisation in German scholarship is largely based on Gerhard Oestreich's and Max Weber's theories of 'social discipline', which locate the source of power in this process within the state. Hence, medicalisation is a repressive process. Michel Foucault's notion of medicalisation, meanwhile, decentralises this process and situates it in an array of spaces, for example the clinic, the prison and the school. Foucault's medicalisation process is all about inculcating norms so that the modern individ-

Prussia identify physicians as the key actors in this process: eager to professionalise as well as increase their power and status in the late eighteenth and early nineteenth centuries, this group of medical men put itself in the service of a state whose policy it was to increase population by improving public health.[43] Accordingly, the developments in the regulation of medical matters, in particular of official medical personnel and practitioners more generally, were part of an unfolding project of the developing Prussian state that specifically targeted public health.[44]

Historians have since questioned the applicability of the Prussian narrative to other parts of the Germanies. Indeed they have gone even further and critiqued the idea that the processes of medicalisation and professionalisation were a 'project' of Enlightenment. Both Frevert and Huerkamp acknowledge that the implementation of this public health project was severely hampered by the lack of an effective state-controlled medical-administrative infrastructure and, as Sabine Sander has shown, by the fractured sources of political power that characterised early modern society.[45] However, Frevert's and Huerkamp's critics do not merely dispute the efficacy of the Enlightenment project. Mary Lindemann finds little evidence to suggest that the ducal government in eighteenth-century Braunschweig Wolfenbüttel operated with a long-term vision for medically modernising cultures and practices of health. The 'state' and 'state policy', Lindemann claims, 'represent little more than an imprecise shorthand for an extraordinarily complex mélange of the ideas, the ambitions, and the self-promotion of individuals and groups – here, of physici, Amtmänner, members of the privy council and Collegium medicum, local communities (who in themselves were not, of course, monolithic in their wants and desires), with the occasional strong influence of miscellaneous others.'[46] Eighteenth-century lawmakers had no intention of jettisoning older conventions, practices and 'administrative pathways' for the sake of introducing rational, enlightened practices.[47] The pursuit of *Pfuscher* (quacks), for example, was not the result of this clash between the old and the new, but was instead part

ual is constantly censuring his or her own body and health, rendering repression from a particular body redundant. See Stefan Breuer, 'Sozialdisziplinierung. Probleme und Problemverlagerungen eines Konzepts bei Max Weber, Gerhard Oestreich und Michel Foucault', in Christoph Sachße and Florian Tennstedt, eds, *Soziale Sicherheit und soziale Disziplinierung. Beiträge zu einer historischen Theorie der Sozialpolitik* (Frankfurt am Main: Suhrkamp, 1986), 52–60.

43   Ute Frevert, *Krankheit als politisches Problem 1770–1880: Soziale Unterschichten in Preußen zwischen medizinischer Polizei und staatlicher Sozialversicherung* (Göttingen: Vandenhoeck & Ruprecht, 1984), 43–44; Huerkamp, *Aufstieg*, 20–21.

44   Frevert, *Krankheit*, 27.

45   Ibid., 36–44; Huerkamp, *Aufstieg*, 42–43; Sabine Sander, 'Die Bürokratisierung des Gesundheitswesens. Zur Problematik der "Modernisierung"', *Jahrbuch des Instituts für Geschichte der Medizin der Robert Bosch Stiftung* 6 (1987): 185–218, 186–96.

46   Lindemann, *Health*, 139.

47   Ibid., 139–40.

of a broader occupational culture of entitlement grounded in the practices and structures of the guilds.[48]

In her study of Baden, Franziska Loetz has likewise asserted that state initiatives in health provision were too varied, too chaotic and too disparate for us to comprehend the eighteenth- and early nineteenth-century state as an institution that sought to systematically discipline its population with the assistance of academic medicine.[49] The problem with the concepts of medicalisation and professionalisation is, according to Thomas Broman, that they are anachronisms projected onto Enlightenment discourses. When historians see medicalisation and professionalisation as the 'basis and purpose of these discourses', it becomes difficult to conceive of Enlightenment other than as a 'part of a modernisation process'.[50] And more recent research on the lingering entanglement of Enlightenment and religion into the nineteenth century teaches us to be very wary of pitting the one against the other, urging us instead to appreciate 'the diversity and complexity of the Enlightenment with respect to medicine'.[51]

Midwifery has been neatly woven into these narratives of medicalisation and professionalisation. Historians have interpreted the changes to midwifery in the eighteenth century, in particular in the quantity of regulation, as evidence of the creeping state and the loss of a 'golden age' of midwifery characterised by female autonomy over the female body and childbirth.[52] It is cru-

---

48   Ibid., 166–71. Work on quackery in England strongly suggests that quacks were defined on the basis of their *non*-membership of a medical corporation, that is, in economic-occupational terms rather than on the basis of knowledge. See Margaret Pelling, *Medical Conflicts in Early Modern London: Patronage, Physicians and Irregular Practitioners 1540–1640* (Oxford: Oxford University Press, 2003), 136–88. The division between 'regular' and 'irregular' practitioners was not something that necessarily shaped the medical choices of patients in the eighteenth century. See Mary Fissell, *Patients, Power and the Poor in Eighteenth-Century Bristol* (Cambridge: Cambridge University Press, 1991), 63.

49   Francisca Loetz, *Vom Kranken zum Patienten: 'Medikalisierung' und medizinische Vergesellschaftung am Beispiel Badens 1750–1850* (Stuttgart: Franz Steiner, 1993), 157.

50   Thomas Broman, 'Zwischen Staat und Konsumgesellschaft: Aufklärung und die Entwicklung des deutschen Medizinalwesens im 18. Jahrhundert', in Bettina Wahrig-Schmidt and Werner Sohn, eds, *Zwischen Aufklärung, Policey und Verwaltung. Zur Genese des Medizinalwesens 1750–1850* (Wiesbaden: Harrossowitz Verlag, 2003), 93. Broman attributes the eventual achievement of hegemonic power of academic medical practitioners in the nineteenth century to the development of the press and the practice of criticism, which provided medical practitioners with a platform for objectifying their knowledge in a literary domain and presenting themselves as representatives of that knowledge. See ibid., 105–7.

51   Andrew Cunningham, 'Introduction: "Where there are three physicians, there are two atheists"', in Ole Peter Grell and Andrew Cunningham, eds, *Medicine and Religion in Enlightenment Europe* (Aldershot and Burlington, VT: Ashgate, 2007), 4. This volume surveys both Catholic and Protestant Europe.

52   Labouvie, for example, describes rural midwifery as 'women's business' that took place within a female public sphere of midwife, married and widowed relatives and neighbours. See Eva Labouvie, 'Sofia Weinranck, Hebamme von St. Johann. Städtische Geburtshilfe und die Entrechtung der Bürgerinnen im 18. Jahrhundert', in Annette Kein-

cial, however, to remember that most women in Germany (and indeed throughout Europe) would continue to give birth at home, often under the care of a midwife, until the early twentieth century. Much research has focused on the rupture of traditional childbirth and traditional midwifery through the newly established maternity hospitals in the eighteenth and early nineteenth centuries.[53] I suggest here, however, that this development predominantly affected the setting and culture of midwife training for rural midwives and has thus been overrated in the narrative of eighteenth-century urban midwifery. Maternity hospitals or midwife training institutes existed for several decades parallel and even in opposition to the more traditional form of midwife training: in Leipzig, for example, the apprenticeship and anatomical instruction at the hands of the local Stadtphysicus or Stadtaccoucheur. There is even some evidence to suggest that smaller towns and cities appear to have resorted to maternity hospitals to train their midwives sooner than the major cities.[54]

Thus, we need to rethink the underlying assumption evident in many studies that clinical midwifery was significant for urban midwifery and formed a natural and inevitable progression from older professionalised and regulated structures of urban midwifery. Firstly, the eighteenth-century German maternity hospitals were almost universally university institutions, not part of urban health and welfare provision. Moreover, the early aim of the maternity hospitals was to train midwives in readiness for deployment in rural regions. Secondly, midwifery in seventeenth- and eighteenth-century urban centres had its own occupational culture shaped by local institutions, local norms, and the quirks of the local urban economy and community. It is the peculiarities of these urban cultures of midwifery that this thesis will explore.

In the German historiography, the regulation of midwives has been construed as an overwhelmingly negative phenomenon, measurable by the degree to which midwifery had been placed under the control of municipal councils and male medical practitioners, and/or the degree to which lay women steered the selection process of local midwives.[55] The spectacular clashes between rural communities and the women trained in the maternity

horst and Petra Messinger, eds, *Die Saarbrückerinnen. Beiträge zur Stadtgeschichte* (St Ingbert: Röhrig Universitätsverlag, 1998), 225. Cody notes that in England birth was a 'secret, private affair, left to the management of women alone'. Women were considered to be the 'natural authorities over birth' because knowledge about the body could only be derived through experience. See Cody, *Birthing the Nation*, 31–32.

53   For example, see Jürgen Schlumbohm, '"The Pregnant Women Are Here for the Sake of the Teaching Institution": The Lying-In Hospital of Göttingen University', *Social History of Medicine* 14: 1 (2001): 59–78; Metz-Becker, *Der verwaltete Körper*, Loytved, ed., *Von der Wehemutter*.

54   For example, in the small town of Hannoversch Münden in Lower Saxony, town midwives received their training in the nearby Göttingen maternity hospital from 1780. See Lena Irene Steilen, 'Zwischen Vertrauen und Kontrolle. Hebammen im Münden des 19. Jahrhunderts' (MA thesis, Göttingen, 2003), 33.

55   See Birkelbach and Luecken, 'Zur Entwicklung des Hebammenwesens'. See also Labouvie, 'Sofia Weinranck', 242; Schmitz, *Hebammen in Münster*, 23–29.

hospitals and then sent out by late eighteenth-century states to rural outposts have, I argue, overshadowed the dynamics of the urban experience.[56] In accounts of rural midwifery, the sudden attempts at regulation at the end of the eighteenth century assumed a repressive form and were synonymous with disempowerment and, eventually, the extinction of the local (female) community and culture of neighbourly assistance.[57] However, as Christine Loytved's recent study of midwife training in Lübeck has suggested, urban midwives demonstrated little in the way of resistance (at best passive resistance) to either the introduction of the municipal midwife instructor or formalised anatomical and obstetric training.[58] The changes to urban midwifery were not as seismic as one might like to think; I am therefore interested in examining the extent to which eighteenth-century reforms actually altered the occupational culture of midwifery, that is, the structures, norms and practices that guided urban midwives in their daily work.

In contrast to the pessimistic view of regulation, Merry Wiesner argues that regulation and control afforded sixteenth-century midwives higher status than any other group of women in urban centres. The fact that midwives were entrusted with additional functions where their 'opinions and judgements were taken seriously' by municipal governments, such as arranging baptism and providing medico-legal testimony, served to 'underline their importance in the early modern city'.[59] Historians working on other European urban centres have similarly argued that regulation there was often beneficial to midwives. Hilary Marland and Christina Romlid suggest that regulation actually shored up, even increased the status enjoyed by urban midwives in Holland and Sweden.[60] Historians of English midwifery argue that it was precisely this lack of regulation and the cessation of ecclesiastical licensing that contributed to the decline of midwifery in many parts of England, in particular London, during the middle and latter eighteenth century.[61]

---

56   Labouvie, *Beistand*; 'Selbstverwaltete Geburt. Landhebammen zwischen Macht und Reglementierung (17.–19. Jahrhundert)', *Geschichte und Gesellschaft* 18 (1992): 477–506; Gunda Barth-Scalmani, '"Freundschaftlicher Zuruf eines Arztes an das Salzburgische Landvolk". Staatliche Hebammenausbildung und medizinische Volksaufklärung am Ende des 18. Jahrhunderts', in Jürgen Schlumbohm et al., eds, *Rituale der Geburt. Eine Kulturgeschichte* (Munich: Verlag C. H. Beck, 1998).

57   Labouvie, 'Selbstverwaltete Geburt', 505–6.

58   Loytved, *Hebammen*, 286.

59   Wiesner, *Working Women*, 81.

60   Marland, '"Stately and dignified"', 276–78, 296. Romlid argues that the regulation and relatively strong position of midwives in Sweden was directly related to the perceived need to produce more soldiers for the Swedish army. See Christina Romlid, 'Swedish midwives and their instruments in the eighteenth and nineteenth centuries', in Hilary Marland and Anne Marie Rafferty, eds, *Midwives, Society and Childbirth: Debates and Controversies in the Modern Period* (London: Routledge, 1997), 54–55.

61   Evenden, *Midwives*, 174–75; Jean Donnison, *Midwives and Medical Men: A History of Inter-Professional Rivalries and Women's Rights* (2nd edn, London: Heinemann Educational, 1988), 41.

A history of midwifery, I argue, needs to move beyond the question of whether regulation was positive or negative for midwives as an occupational group, or whether midwives demonstrated resistance to or acceptance of new training or organisational strategies. The story is far more complicated than a label of 'good'/'bad' for regulation and a 'yes'/'no' to resistance. This study avoids, as far as possible, this paradigm of regulation as a force that stripped midwives of their autonomy (if that ever really existed) and deflated their social value, a paradigm which has so strongly shaped the history of German midwifery thus far. To do this, it is necessary to reassess the genesis and function of regulation; I have therefore drawn on recent research in the area of early modern legislative techniques and processes that re-conceptualises eighteenth-century police ordinances (known as *gute Policey*) as a 'process of learning ... in which the norm-setters, the norm-implementers and those addressed by these norms participate equally.'[62] The demand for Policey came to a great extent from the subjects, not just territorial rulers.[63] The practice of petitioning or seeking grace was thus not so much an act of resistance, but a formalised channel for the flow of information between subject and ruler; norms were negotiated on an individual basis between the ruling and the ruled. On a microlevel, this kind of legislative practice was also what characterised the political process in Leipzig. Midwives and mothers were part of the process of norm-setting because they participated actively in the process of petitioning. As Chapter Four will demonstrate, because they so ardently defended their entitlement to practice and appealed to older traditional boundaries of occupational corporatism, sworn midwives and sworn Beifrauen actually demanded sharper contours of practice when it suited their own individual situations.[64] Hence, this persistent reiteration of the boundaries of practice was productive. As Mary Fissell has noted, the 'cultural work' of a particular group to demarcate their medical practice from other healers around them might 'create, invoke, and break boundaries', and thereby actually structure health care.[65]

Time and place: Leipzig, 1650–1810

This study focuses on the development of midwifery in a single city – Leipzig – in the late seventeenth and 'long' eighteenth centuries. My research is framed chronologically by two events. The first, the end of the Thirty Years War in 1648, marks the beginning of large-scale organisational changes to midwifery provision in the city. Saxony, like no other German territory, had

62 Martin Dinges, '"Policeyforschung" statt "Sozialdisziplinierung"?', *Zeitschrift für Neuere Rechtsgeschichte* 24: 3/4 (2002): 327–44, 344.
63 Ibid.
64 See also Lindemann, *Health*, 194–205.
65 Mary Fissell, 'Introduction: Women, Health and Healing in Early Modern Europe', *Bulletin for the History of Medicine* 82 (2008): 1–17, 7–8.

suffered grand-scale devastation and sustained massive loss of life in the final decade of the war. In the ensuing decades, anxieties about depopulation – there were few years in which fertility outnumbered mortality – transmuted into a greater interest in infant and maternal mortality which, in turn, spurned on reform. Yet the impetus for reforming urban midwifery provision was also born out of optimism about the future. Thanks to its international fair, Leipzig's economic recovery was relatively speedy and thus ensured the city's status as the financial and commercial powerhouse of Saxony. In 1688 the Leipzig Council was in a position to regain its fiscal autonomy, which it had been forced to cede to the Electoral Commission of Finance after being bankrupted eighty years previously. The last decades of the seventeenth century marked a period in which Leipzig blossomed as a politically more independent and powerful element within Saxony. This was the period in which the Council established the Court for Trade, the Leipzig Stock Exchange and the Trade Deputation, all institutions designed to support the Leipzig trade fairs.[66]

The second event, the establishment of the *Hebammeninstitut* (Midwife Institute) within the Faculty of Medicine of the Leipzig University in 1810, marks only the 'beginning of the end' of midwifery provision as it had been organised and practised in the centuries before. In the short term, the clinical training of midwives did not replace the traditional method of knowledge and skill transfer based upon the apprenticeship and lessons from the Stadtaccoucheur; it was not until 1818 that the Saxon government decreed all midwives train in the midwifery institutes in Leipzig or Dresden.[67] When this did take place, however, it established a rival system of midwifery training that lay beyond the reach of the municipal authority.

My rationale for selecting a case study format is both pragmatic and conceptual. Not only does a local approach permit more extensive use of archival records; the organisation of early modern medical provision, indeed politics itself, was an intensely local phenomenon, especially in the larger, politically powerful urban centres. Many of the major cities had been conferred *Stadtrecht* (the right of a town to form its own jurisdiction) in the late Middle Ages and enjoyed either partial or full political autonomy until the political administrative reforms of the early nineteenth century.[68] The relationship between Leipzig and the Saxon Elector was complex. On the one hand, the Leipzig Council was, for example, entrusted with assisting centralised state collection of the *Landsteuer* (tax). The city was also the location for many state legal, ecclesiastical and administrative state authorities such as the *Leipziger Schöppenstuhl* (Court of Jurors) and the Consistorium. As in most other cities, the Saxon

66   Karl Czok, *Leipzig. Geschichte der Stadt in Wort und Bild* (Berlin GDR: VEB Deutscher Verlag der Wissenschaften, 1978), 25–26.

67   StadtAL, Tit. (F) XLIV.A.18a, 'Churfürstliche Mandate (1768–1816)', 104–6, 'Mandat, die Erlernung und Ausübung der Geburtshülfe in hiesigen Landen betreffend', 2 April 1818.

68   For an overview of the literature on the development of the early modern city, in particular its relationship to territorial states, see Heinz Schilling, *Die Stadt in der frühen Neuzeit* (2nd edn, Munich: R. Oldenbourg Verlag, 2004), 72–78.

Elector was represented by the *Amt* (district office, here the Leipzig Amt), which was largely responsible for collecting taxes owed to the Elector, implementing the justice system and carrying out police but not, however, for the day-to-day running of municipal affairs.[69] On the other hand, although subject to allegiance to the Saxon crown, Leipzig was to a very great degree politically and economically independent and wielded considerable political power as head of all the cities in the Saxon *Landtag* (Saxon Diet). It is this dependent/ independent relationship with the territorial government that makes Leipzig an ideal vehicle for examining the interaction between the local and the territorial on matters medico-social.

Leipzig was a major urban centre in seventeenth- and eighteenth-century Saxony, second only in size to the electoral residence Dresden. At the end of the Thirty Years War (1618–48), the city's population numbered around 14,000. Strong migration levels from the countryside into the cities during the following decades ensured that Leipzig's population grew substantially to roughly 21,000 in 1700 and rose to 35,000 in 1750.[70] Since the sixteenth century the Leipzig trade fairs shaped the local economy more than any other single trade or proto-industry. As the major trade routes through southern Germany shifted eastwards and northwards, Leipzig was poised to take its place as Europe's premier marketplace. It had the infrastructure and sophisticated administrative and financial transaction systems, such as a stock exchange, a commercial court and a wholesalers' directorate, that enabled the city to support a large volume of trade.[71] The trade fairs took place three times a year after New Year, Easter and Michaelis and lasted between two and three weeks. During the fairs both local and foreign wealthy merchants traded from residences, shops or vaults, whereas less wealthy traders and hawkers, frequently drawn from the surrounding countryside, would populate every corner of the city with their stalls.[72] The 'trade fair economy' created a lot of short-term employment for both those involved in the fairs directly, such as

---

69　Karlheinz Blaschke, 'Zur Behördengeschichte der kursächsischen Lokalverwaltung', in Staatliche Archivverwaltung im Staatssekretariat für innere Angelegenheiten, ed., *Archivar und Historiker. Studien zur Archiv- und Geschichtswissenschaft* (Berlin: Rütten & Loening, 1956), 345. The Leipzig Amt, with its office in the city of Leipzig, was established in the fourteenth century. By 1827 its jurisdiction covered 5 cities and 134 villages.

70　For population statistics, see Robert Beachy, *The Soul of Commerce: Credit, Property and Politics in Leipzig, 1750–1840* (Leiden: Brill, 2005), 22–23; Karlheinz Blaschke, *Bevölkerungsgeschichte von Sachsen bis zur industriellen Revolution* (Weimar: Hermann Böhlaus Nachfolger, 1967), 140. On the centrality of country-to-city mobility for urban Saxony during this period, see Uwe Schirmer, 'Wirtschaftspolitik und Bevölkerungsentwicklung in Kursachsen (1648–1756)', *Neues Archiv für sächsische Geschichte* 68 (1997): 125–55, 154; Volkmar Weiss, 'Bevölkerungsentwicklung und Mobilität in Sachsen von 1550 bis 1880', ibid. 64 (1993): 53–60, 56–57.

71　Beachy, *Soul of Commerce*, 32.

72　Susanne Schötz, 'Von Kauffrauen und Kuchenweibern. Weibliche Handelstätigkeit auf Leipzigs Messen im 18. und 19. Jahrhundert', in Günter Bentele et al., eds, *Leipzigs Messen 1497–1997. Gestaltwandel – Umbrüche – Neubeginn, Teilband 1: 1497–1914* (2 vols, Cologne: Böhlau, 1999), vol. 1, 388, 393, 401.

market helpers and hawkers, and indigenous businesses, which housed, fed, clothed, preened and entertained incoming merchants and their entourages. There was also a downside to the fairs; they ensured that the population in Leipzig was transient, thus eroding the traditional barriers to civic member-ship. The demographic pressures stemming from its peculiarly commercial economy make Leipzig an equally interesting test case for exploring how bur-geoning population and trade impacted on a city's medical infrastructure.

Unlike most other larger cities in Saxony (including Dresden), the Leipzig citizenry was dominated numerically by burghers without property, so-called *unangesessenen Bürger*, who made up around 60 per cent of the citizenry. This suggests that the commercial spin-off from the trade fairs had a profound ef-fect on extricating property from burgher status and producing a wealth of employment opportunities not dependent upon property ownership.[73] The socio-economic spread of the population was not even across the urban space, which in economic as well as jurisdictional terms consisted of both the intra-mural city (*Stadt*) and the extramural neighbourhoods nestled around the city gates (*Vorstadt*) (see Figure 1). Both the Stadt and the Vorstadt were divided into quarters for both customary and administrative reasons. The Stadt had four quarters: the Grimmaisches Viertel, which included the city's main politi-cal institutions and the University; the Hallisches Viertel to the north; the Rannisches Viertel to the west; and the Petersviertel to the south. The Pleißen-burg, the city garrison located near the Peterstor, belonged to the Grimmai-sches Viertel. The Vorstadt also had four districts, each corresponding to one of the city gates (*Tor*): the Grimmaisches Tor, the Hallisches Tor, the Rann-städter Tor and the Peterstor.

In the mid- to late sixteenth century the Vorstadt contained almost half the city's dwellings and, although not exclusively a space inhabited by the poor, it tended to house the lower end of the socio-economic spectrum. It was also home to many of Leipzig's 'dirty' forms of production: the tanneries, slaughterhouses, dairies, grain mills and tile kilns that formed a major part of the urban and regional economy.[74] Indoor medical provision also belonged to the Vorstadt landscape. The *Lazarett* (lazarette), which had formerly housed pilgrims, orphans, the poor and the sick, was located at the Rannstädter Tor.

---

73 According to the *General-Konsumtionsakzise* records from 1697, the number of burghers (i. e., male heads of households) without property but who carried out a trade or had their own business outnumbered propertied burghers by a staggering 1,520 to 1,031. Middle-sized cities such as Chemnitz or Pirna generally had significantly more proper-tied burghers. In Dresden burghers without property made up only 42 % of the citizenry. Note these statistics do not include non-burgher heads of household. See Blaschke, *Bevölkerungsgeschichte*, 178.

74 Christian Ronnefeldt, 'Zur Gewerbe- und Sozialtopographie in der Grimmaischen Vor-stadt in Leipzig vom 15. Jahrhundert bis zur 1. Hälfte des 17. Jahrhunderts', *Leipziger Kalender* (2004): 73–94, 76.

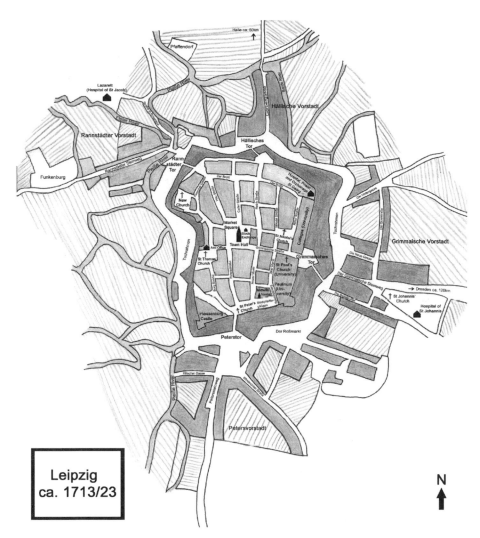

Figure 1 Map of Leipzig 1713/23

Sources: Leipzig, eine florisante, auch befestigte Handels-Stadt und weitberühmte Universitaet in dem Ober-Saexischen Craiß (M. Seutter: Augsburg, 1723), in Pro Leipzig/Th. Nabert, ed., *Leipziger Stadtpläne: Verzeichnis der in Leipziger Institutionen verfügbaren Karten und Pläne* (2 edn, Leipzig: Passage-Verlag, 1994); Hans August Nienborg, *Description über die Grund-Legung und in richtigen Abriß gebrachte berühmte Handels-Stadt Leipzig* [Nienborgscher Atlas] (Leipzig, 1710), facsimilie of original (Berlin: Akademie-Verlag, 1997); Ernst Müller, *Häuserbuch zum Nienborgschen Atlas* (Berlin: Akademie-Verlag 1997), 132.

The Hospital of St Johannis, erected to house the city's lepers in 1300, stood just outside the Grimmaisches Tor on the road to Dresden.[75]

The Stadt, on the other hand, was the institutional, commercial, cultural and political heart of Leipzig. The focus of political life, the baroque *Rathaus* (Town Hall), stood at the centre of the city, flanked on either side by the main town market square and, from 1679 onwards, the *Börse* (stock exchange). The Town Hall was home to the *Leipziger Stadtrat* (Leipzig Council) and the *Stadtgericht* (Leipzig City Court). By the eighteenth century Leipzig was a city ruled by a porous patriciate of jurists and merchants, more politically akin to the Hanseatic city-states than other territorial cities.[76] The Leipzig Council, although sensitive to the demands of commerce, was 'a conservative body that understood its own authority in very traditional terms'.[77] The Council consisted of three groups of twelve councillors, which rotated every three years. The *Ratsenge*, or the group of councillors in active service, was headed up by one of three *Bürgermeister* (burgomasters), who were rotated once a year before Easter. The Leipzig Council was responsible for making political decisions on issues within Leipzig as well as external diplomatic matters, recruiting new councillors and large expenditures.[78] The burgomaster also assumed the role of *Stadtrichter* (judge of the City Court) in the Leipzig City Court, which tried both petty and capital crimes committed within the city's jurisdiction. The day-to-day running of the city and its administrative, police and welfare institutions was carried out by a large number of council employees: gatekeepers and scribes manned the city's fortifications and kept tabs on those leaving and entering the city; doctors, nurses and servants ran the municipal hospitals; scribes registered burials and handled quarantine measures in the *Leichenschreiberei* (the Corpse Registry Office); and a city regiment defended Leipzig against invasion and generally kept the peace.

The Stadt was also the main centre of religious life in the city. Baptisms, marriages and funerals – the major sacramental and festive points in Lutheran life – were held in the two main churches in the Stadt, St Thomas in the Petersviertel (where Johann Sebastian Bach lived and worked as cantor from 1723 to 1750) and St Nikolai in the Grimmaisches Viertel. The other churches in the city, the New Church in the Rannisches Viertel and St Peter's, were reopened in 1699 and 1713 respectively in response to larger numbers of parishioners and higher levels of participation in church life. However, they were

---

75   Czok notes that medieval hospitals were located outside the city walls for logistical reasons (closer to pilgrims) or quarantine reasons, but also because the hospitals were largely self-sustaining institutions requiring farming land. Karl Czok, *Vorstädte. Zu ihrer Entstehung, Wirtschaft und Sozialentwicklung in der älteren deutschen Stadtgeschichte* (Berlin: Akademie-Verlag 1979), 20–21.

76   Beachy, *Soul of Commerce*, 23–24.

77   Beachy refers here to the Council's promotion of the 1750 electoral sumptuary code (*Kleiderordnung*) which, despite protest from the city's merchants, revealed the Council's commitment to old regime corporatism. Ibid., 25.

78   Ibid., 45–46.

used only to administer mass.[79] Although the Leipzig clergy had its own corporation, called the *Stadtministerium* (City Ministry), ecclesiastical matters were still very much the business of the Leipzig Council. Clerics, for example, were appointed by the Leipzig Council directly, much in the same way as with secular municipal offices.[80]

The traditionalist and staunchly Lutheran University, founded in 1409, formed its own legal jurisdiction within the walls of the Stadt and presided over its own *Universitätsgericht* (University Court). The *Paulinum,* a former monastery housing the University Church of St Paul, and the *große* and *kleine Fürstenkollegien* (Large and Small Prince's Colleges), wedged in between the Ritter Straße and the city wall in the Grimmaisches Viertel, made up the main University precinct. Like most early modern universities, the Leipzig faculties participated in legal, medical and theological debates on both a territorial and local municipal level: the Medical Faculty provided medico-legal opinions in criminal trials, the Law Faculty provided legal opinions and recommendations, and the Theological Faculty could be consulted on religious questions. There was also considerable personnel cross-over between the University and local and territorial institutions, for example, law professors were often also jurors on the Leipziger Schöppenstuhl, which had been a territorial institution since 1574, or in the Saxon *Obergericht* (High Court) also located in Leipzig.[81] Not least, the University was a breeding ground for municipal, ecclesiastical and state officials. Many of Leipzig's councillors, and a vast majority of the city's and the state's higher office holders were alumni of Leipzig or Wittenberg Universities.[82] Both the geographical and the social proximity – one might even call it entanglement – between the University and Leipzig's local government makes the city a particularly interesting case study for the enmeshment of local and territorial power in eighteenth-century institutions.

As in many other German cities, medical and charitable provision lay in the hands of the Leipzig Council and the local parishes rather than with territorial princes.[83] Medical relief, like poor relief, was largely outdoor (or domiciliary), reflecting a culture of tending the sick and elderly within the household space that dominated the early modern period. As well as running the

79　Tanya Kervorkian, 'Laien und die Leipziger religiöse Öffentlichkeit 1685–1725', *Leipziger Kalender* (1996), 88. Kervorkian notes that many residents in the Vorstadt attended mass in the chapel located in the Hospital of St Johannis. See ibid., 93.

80　Tanya Kervorkian, 'Clerics and their Career Paths in Early Modern Leipzig', in Heide Wunder, ed., *Jedem das Seine. Abgrenzungen und Grenüberschreitungen im Leipzig des 17. und 18. Jahrhunderts* (Frankfurt am Main: Klostermann, 2000), 301–2.

81　Notker Hammerstein, 'Die Universität Leipzig im Zeichen der frühen Aufklärung', in Wolfgang Martens, ed., *Zentren der Aufklärung III: Leipzig. Aufklärung und Bürgerlichkeit* (Heidelberg: Verlag Lambert Schneider, 1990), 129.

82　See, for example, Blaschke, 'Zur Behördengeschichte', 350.

83　This was the case in large cities like Frankfurt as well as smaller ones like Überlingen. See Robert Jütte, *Obrigkeitliche Armenfürsorge in deutschen Reichsstädten der frühen Neuzeit. Städtisches Armenwesen in Frankfurt am Main und Köln* (Cologne: Böhlau, 1984), 118–20, 129–31; Annemarie Kinzelbach, 'Heilkundige und Gesellschaft in der frühneuzeitlichen Reichsstadt Überlingen', *Medizin, Gesellschaft und Geschichte* 8 (1989): 119–49, 120–26.

city's hospitals and its poor relief (*Willige Almosen*), the Council also employed a number of medical personnel as advisors providing medical treatment to the poor during epidemics. The political strength of the Council meant that it retained complete control over its municipal medical structure until the early nineteenth century.[84] As this study will demonstrate, the trajectory of urban midwifery in Leipzig was intimately tied to local structures, in particular individuals and local socio-economic circumstances.

Leipzig's political and commercial strength meant that it was not a typical middle-sized city. In smaller cities such as Göttingen, where the influence and power of the territorial government and the resident university was greater, the switch to clinical midwife training at the expense of the traditional apprenticeship system appears to have occurred earlier and was actively encouraged by the municipal government.[85] In a large royal residence like Berlin, the state could also be ever-present; the training of Berlin midwives in the Charité hospital began in 1751.[86] In both Göttingen and Berlin the introduction of clinical midwifery training was not completely successful. However, this had more to do with the inefficiency of the infrastructure than political unwillingness.[87] Leipzig, as we shall see, actively protected its political sovereignty over its municipal infrastructure and its ability to self-govern. At times the city's interests coincided with those of the Saxon state and the University; at others they did not.

Sources

Given the fact that midwifery was largely a municipal matter during this period, the conspicuous near total absence of documents relating to midwifery in Leipzig in the State Archive of Saxony hardly surprises.[88] The sources I have drawn upon most heavily here are the administrative and legal records of the Leipzig Council, located in the Municipal Archive (Stadtarchiv) in

84   This was the case even during the reign of August the Strong (1670–1733), noted as a period of major growth in the state administration. See Gross, *Geschichte*, 125–26, 131–34.

85   Henrike Hampe, 'Hebammen und Geburtshelfer im Göttingen des 18. Jahrhunderts. Das Jahr 1751 und seine Folgen', in Christine Loytved, ed., *Von der Wehemutter zur Hebamme: Die Gründung von Hebammenschulen mit Blick auf ihren politischen Stellenwert und praktischen Nutzen* (Osnabrück: Universitäts-Verlag Rasch, 2001), 59–60.

86   Christine Loytved, 'Zur Gründung der Hebammenschule an der Berliner Charité 1751', ibid., 68–72.

87   It was not until 1791, when the new, larger maternity hospital was built, that Göttingen midwives routinely trained in a clinical setting and the apprenticeship system finally disintegrated. See Hampe, 'Hebammen', 60. Loytved also notes that the apprenticeship system endured in Berlin beyond this time. See Loytved, 'Zur Gründung', 76–77.

88   When the Board of Health surveyed midwifery provision in larger Saxon towns and cities such as Plauen, Freiberg, Dresden and Zwickau in 1768–70, Leipzig appears not to have been included. See, for example, SächsHSADD, Loc. 11609, Bd. I, 83–147, 53–62, 'Die Einrichtung und Verbesserung des Hebammenwesens betr.', 1769–1782. See also UAL, Med. Fak. A01/52, Bd. 1, Medizinal Polizei, 25 etc.

Leipzig. It appears that the Council began to collect and archive its documentation relating to midwifery separately when it first employed a midwife-in-waiting in 1673. Prior to this it appears that any documents relating to appointments, petitions or internal conflicts (if still extant) were subsumed into general collections and are thus difficult to recover. Aside from the decades following the Thirty Years War, there is no overarching gap in the council midwifery records. Documentation prior to the 1690s is, however, comparatively thin. Court cases tried in the Leipzig Stadtgericht are extant for the entire period. In addition to the council records, I have also drawn upon the collection of letters and reports located in the Leipzig University Archive relating to the proposed midwifery institute, all of which circulated between the University, the Saxon government and the Leipzig Council.

Oaths (*Eide*), instructions (*Instruktionen* – quasi-licenses) and medical ordinances (*Medizinalordnungen*) make up one subset of sources I have used. These 'normative' documents emanated largely from the Leipzig Council and span the early sixteenth to the early nineteenth centuries. An extensive collection of petitions for appointment and reports compiled by council administrators on individual women comprise another major source genre. These documents were produced during the recruitment process for midwives, which, by the late seventeenth century at least, followed a formal procedure. When a midwife office became vacant, prospective candidates expressed their interest in the position in the form of a formal supplication addressed to the Leipzig Council. Candidates either wrote these themselves or drew on the assistance of husbands, family members or scribes. Women from outside of Leipzig were also required to submit references from their home council, the local *Stadt-* or *Landphysicus* (rural district physician), the local pastor and honourable women they had attended.[89] The Council then collected information on each candidate's reputation in the community, often by sending out a council officer to visit the women in their homes and speak to the neighbourhood women.[90] The Council also instructed a physician, usually the Stadtphysicus or later the Stadtaccoucheur, to submit the women to an oral examination in the art of midwifery and provide the Council with a written report and recommendation. With the inauguration of the role of Stadtaccoucheur in 1731, these tasks were assigned completely to this new office. Some twenty-one appointments extant for the period 1705–89 together with one petition from 1680 provide the source base for many of the following chapters. Many of these sources include several individual petitions from candidates as well as records of recommendations and reports filed by the Council and the Stadtaccoucheur. Al-

89   See StadtAL, Tit. (F) XLIV.D.1, 'Kindermütter bey hiesiger Stadt betr. ingl. die angenommene Bey Weiber betr. 1673–1756', 16–43, 'Midwife appointment (Catharina Ehrlich)', 10 January–24 July 1713, 16–21. See documentation for Anna Catharina Streller in Tit. (F) XLIV.D.5, 1–12, 'Kindermütter Attestata', 1727–28, 1–7.

90   This appears to have been the case in 1713, where the *Oberleichenschreiber* (senior death registry official) composed the reports on candidates, however, it is not certain exactly who carried out these visits. See Tit. (F) XLIV.D.1, 16–43, 'Appointment (Ehrlich)', 10 January–24 July 1713, 22–25.

though I doubt that these particular sources cover all appointment procedures during this period, with the exception of a large gap between 1740 and 1760, most of the period is represented.[91] Nine of these appointments occurred in the first thirty-five years of the period (1705–40) and the other twelve took place between 1760 and 1789. Given that the number of offices increased sharply after the introduction of Beifrauen in 1715, this small difference is insignificant.

Another large collection of petitions, used in particular in Chapter Four, relates to conflicts between midwives, Beifrauen and other unsworn women working as midwives during the period. The 'complaint' petitions were almost universally initiated by the sworn midwives and Beifrauen themselves and reflect tensions in the midwifery structure from the perspective of women working within it. These sources range from single petitions to collections of several petitions, counter-petitions and, in some instances, reports and investigations undertaken by the Stadtphysicus, Stadtaccoucheur and the Leipzig Council. They cover a period spanning 1680 to 1789. Some such sources for the period after 1789 are extant but were not included in this study. A smaller collection of complaints from midwives, Stadtphysici, Stadtaccoucheurs and burghers that sparked council investigations into matters of quackery or negligence amongst midwives or women working within the midwifery landscape constitute another source category. These most often relate to incorrect baptism or the suspicious death of a mother.

I have also drawn upon the reports on midwifery that the physician in charge of supervising the midwives (the Stadt- and Amtsphysici and later the Stadtaccoucheur) submitted to the Leipzig Council. From around 1716 onwards, these reports became a regular communicative feature of the Stadtaccoucheur's office and were generally submitted twice a year to the Council for scrutiny. The chronological coverage of these reports is patchy; for certain office holders we have an almost complete series, for others nothing at all or, at best, one or two reports. The format of the reports varied greatly, however, they generally included details about the level and success of instruction (sometimes also manuals used or lesson content), major disputes between the midwives or other problems as well as the number of difficult deliveries carried out by the Stadtaccoucheur.

A further set of sources used here comprises criminal trial records (*Strafakten*) produced by the City Court. These trial records contain reports of crimes, witness statements, suspect depositions and confessions, expert witness reports and the interim and final verdicts handed down by the Leipziger

---

91 I am unable to account for this gap in its entirety and it appears to be peculiar to this particular set of records. It is possible that some documentation was destroyed in the fire at the *Amtshaus* (Amt Office) in 1747. The general chaos of the Seven Years War (1756–63) and the ensuing breakdown of Council procedures might explain the latter part of this gap. However, it is puzzling that the earlier part of this gap corresponds to the period following the second Silesian War (1744–45), which was one of remarkable peace and prosperity for Leipzig.

Schöppenstuhl.[92] Involvement of a midwife as either witness or suspect formed the basis for selecting the criminal trial records consulted. Most of the trial records I use here relate to crimes such as infanticide, illegitimate sexual activity or infant abandonment, all matters in which the law directed courts to confer with sworn midwives in the examination of the infant corpse or the body of a woman suspected of one of these crimes. Records of nineteen such trials exist for the period 1647–1800.

As this study focuses on concrete midwifery practice, I wanted to find out as much as I could about the life stories of individual midwives. To achieve this, I mined all of these administrative sources for every skerrick of information on midwives' person, familial situation, career, etc. and collated the details in a database. As a result I have data (with varying degrees of detail) on almost all office-bearing midwives working in Leipzig during the eighteenth century and many more women otherwise involved in the midwifery landscape. As well as the data gleaned from the midwifery records on individual midwives and women working in midwifery, I also turned to the baptismal and marriage registers of the churches of St Nikolai and St Thomas held in the Church Archive in Leipzig, and to the *Leichenbücher* (Corpse Registers) in the Leipzig Municipal Archive, all of which are preserved for the entire period in question. A handful of wills and testaments of midwives in the Leipzig Municipal Archive provided further valuable biographical and socio-economic information on individual women and their families. The resulting prosopographies form an important counterpoint to the normative oaths, instructions and legislation, for they provide us with hard data on factors such as age, marital status, number of children, etc. They also offer an insight into the diversity of individual experience.

Due to the highly variable spelling of names throughout the different sources, the reader should note that the spelling I have chosen to use here may not always correspond exactly to the spelling used in archival source titles.

There is no doubt that these types of administrative sources force the historian to view his or her historical subjects through a particular lens and many historians working on midwifery have sagaciously warned of the pitfalls of relying on normative sources such as these.[93] Ordinances, so it has been argued, might only help us ascertain the intentions or anxieties of political bodies and society more generally because they project an elite discourse onto the culture and mentality of the common people. The Leipzig petitions, in particular those penned by professional scribes, often adhered to formulaic prose and

---

92   Although the procedure of gathering witness statements and interrogating suspects was the responsibility of the Leipzig City Court, it was obliged to submit its records to the state legal body (the Leipziger Schöppenstuhl) for instructions on how suspects should be interrogated and tortured and, of course, for the final judgement. Although a state organisation, three of the Schöppenstuhl's seven members were selected by the Leipzig Council, thus ensuring the Council's influence in this important legal body. See Beachy, *Soul of Commerce*, 38.

93   Labouvie, *Beistand*, 15–22; Flügge, *Hebammen und heilkundige Frauen*, 16–18.

style, however, the greater the supplicant's need or outrage, the more person-
alised and colloquial the petitions of appointment and complaint tended to
be.[94] And yet, convention and formality were less present in other kinds of
documents. Court records, protocols of investigations and petition letters are
often blissfully, albeit at times confusingly, idiosyncratic in both form and language. The frequently illogical trains of testimony, sometimes seemingly recorded near verbatim, suggest the urgency, anger and distress of their testi-
fiers. My translations of these sources attempt to preserve the disjointedness of
the voices, but have at times been amended for the purposes of clarity. These
narratives were certainly less censored in the eighteenth century than critics of
such sources might claim. Moreover, midwives were participants, not powerless bystanders, in the process of defining and staking out their occupational
space. Their interactions with the Council suggest that midwives spoke the
same language and appealed to the same set of ideals about occupational propriety that both ruling groups and wider society held dear.[95]

Overview

The structure of this study is thematic rather than chronological. Not every
chapter reflects the chosen period in its entirety because the sources utilised
in each topic do not always permit this. At a few places I incorporate data
from the late sixteenth and early seventeenth centuries for the purposes of
comparison. The first chapter analyses the intersection of local and state governance in the area of midwifery and health provision more broadly. It focuses on the genesis of reforms to midwifery – the introduction of sworn apprentice midwives, the Stadtaccoucheur and formal midwifery instruction – all of
which took place prior to the 1730s.

The second and third chapters turn to the worlds of the women working
as midwives in early modern Leipzig in order to comprehend the lived structure of midwifery in the city. Although the Leipzig Council employed a corps
of sworn midwives to provide assistance to all burghers and residents in the
city, these sworn office holders were only one group amongst many women
working as midwives in the city. Chapter Two examines what I will call the
'midwifery landscape' and traces the various ways that women participated in
midwifery throughout the late seventeenth and eighteenth centuries. In Chapter Three I pursue the questions of why women became midwives and how
midwifery fitted into the family oeconomy by exploring the relationship be-

---

94   There appears to be strong parallels in the authoring of petitions with the process of
     co-authorship between supplicant (as the primary author) and the scribe and sometimes
     lawyer (as the secondary authors) as described by Natalie Zemon Davis for sixteenth-cen-
     tury French letters of remission. See Natalie Zemon Davis, *Fiction in the Archives: Pardon
     Tales and Their Tellers in Sixteenth-Century France* (Cambridge: Polity Press, 1987), 15–25.
95   Lindemann notes this for Braunschweig-Wolfenbüttel. See Lindemann, *Health*, 204–5.

tween midwifery appointments, life-cycle and socio-economic status as well as the social meaning of midwifery held by contemporaries.

Chapters Four, Five and Six concentrate on the occupational culture of midwifery. In Chapter Four I explore how the older concept of livelihood remained central to ideas of occupational propriety and how the problem of livelihood continued to generate intra-occupational conflict between women working within the midwifery landscape throughout the period. Livelihood was also central to the concepts midwives deployed to shape and define the contours of their occupation. Chapter Five examines the central role played by trust in midwives' client patterns and client-building practices. Chapter Six explores the way in which midwives, physicians and lay people demarcated the sphere of midwifery, and investigates the way in which midwifery instruction reinforced the older divisions of labour between midwives and male medical practitioners on the basis of a division between natural and unnatural births. Chapter Seven returns once more to the relationship between the city and the state by exploring the 'difficult birth' of clinical midwifery in Leipzig during the second half of the eighteenth century.

Chapter One

Midwifery, the City and the State Between Tradition and Reform

In the late seventeenth and early eighteenth centuries the task of improving midwifery provision within the city became a priority for Leipzig's municipal government. Rather than increasing the number of sworn midwives working in the city, a measure it had undertaken during the sixteenth and early seventeenth centuries, the Leipzig Council and its medical officials focused on midwife education. The Council initially set about formalising the relationship between midwives and apprentice midwives. It then later appointed a designated municipal medical practitioner to supervise and instruct the city's corps of sworn midwives. Although the 'improvements' altered the channels and sources of knowledge open to midwives, they had only a modest impact on the day-to-day practice and working organisation of midwifery in Leipzig; there was no seismic clash between 'traditional' midwifery and public health reforms as documented in some rural, small-town, or regional midwifery settings in the late eighteenth century.[1]

This chapter examines the political scaffolding – that it, the roles of the Leipzig Council, the Saxon state and medical officials – surrounding midwifery in Leipzig between 1650 and 1800, in particular before 1750, and its impact on local urban midwifery structures and practices. The first section outlines the types of formal regulation (ordinances, oaths, etc.) affecting midwifery in Leipzig from the late Middle Ages through to around 1800 on both a communal and territorial level. The second section ties these 'normative' texts to the practice of reform by exploring the genesis of concrete reforms to midwifery and their effect on the provision of official midwifery in the city.

Regulating midwifery from the Middle Ages to the Reformation

Women working as midwives in urban Germany had been subject to some kind of external control since the late Middle Ages. The earliest source of regulation was ecclesiastical. Since the Synods of Mainz (1233) and Trier (1277), the Church had entrusted midwives with the responsibility for baptising sickly infants and giving the last rites to dying mothers. Midwives were instructed how to confer these sacraments by the local parish priest, following which they swore an oath to the Church to live as devout Christians, to treat the poor as they would the rich, and to eschew magic, superstition and the use of abortifacients.[2] Medieval midwives also assumed a moral-policing function

---

1   See, for example, Labouvie, *Beistand*; Barth-Scalmani, '"Freundschaftlicher Zuruf"'.
2   Flügge, *Hebammen und heilkundige Frauen*, 132–34.

and were required to report suspected cases of infanticide or illegitimacy to the Church authorities.[3]

Ecclesiastical regulation began to disintegrate during the fourteenth century as the political importance of the cities increased. Blossoming political self-confidence and economic success prompted many important towns to seek greater independence from local and territorial rulers. Autonomy over charitable and medical institutions, including midwifery, was a vital aspect of this burgeoning burgher consciousness. Many of the large free imperial cities in southern Germany such as Nuremberg and Constance had appointed midwives under oath by the early fifteenth century, although in smaller cities such as Nördlingen, midwifery remained under ecclesiastical control until the sixteenth century.[4] After spending much of the twelfth century procuring legal, political and economic autonomy from the city's feudal lords, Leipzig's newly formed burgher Council (Leipziger Rat) began acquiring control of key institutions and establishing its own fledgling bureaucracy to deal with communal needs. By 1300 Leipzig was a thriving commercial centre presiding over a relatively autonomous administration and a wealth of feudal privileges.[5]

As in many northern German cities, medical care and poor relief in Leipzig were tightly interwoven.[6] Even before the Reformation, the Council had begun to assume responsibility for medical infrastructure in the city, taking control of the Hospital of St Johannis in 1391 and purchasing the hospital of St Georg in 1439.[7] A municipally run system of alms, initiated and funded by

3   For Germany, see Eva Labouvie, 'Frauenberuf ohne Vorbildung? Hebammen in den Städten und auf dem Land', in Elke Kleinau and Claudia Opitz, eds, *Geschichte der Mädchen- und Frauenbildung: Bd. 1 Vom Mittelalter bis zur Aufklärung* (2 vols, Frankfurt am Main: Campus Verlag, 1996), vol. 1, 218–19. For the Low Countries, see Myriam Greilshammer, 'The Midwife, the Priest, and the Physician: The Subjugation of Midwives in the Low Countries at the End of the Middle Ages', *Journal of Medieval and Renaissance Studies* 21: 2 (1991): 285–329, 312–19. On ecclesiastical licensing in France, see Tiffany D. Vann Sprecher and Ruth Mazo Karras, 'The Midwife and the Church. Ecclesiastical Regulation of Midwives in Brie, 1499–1504', *Bulletin of the History of Medicine* 85: 2 (2011): 171–92.

4   In Nuremberg since 1417. See Baruch, 'Das Hebammenwesen', 9; Wiesner, 'Early Modern Midwifery', 96. In Constance since 1379. See Britta-Juliane Kruse, *Verborgene Heilkünste: Geschichte der Frauenmedizin im Spätmittelalter* (Berlin: W. de Gruyter, 1996), 133. On Nördlingen, see Gabler, 'Hebammenwesen', 32.

5   In 1261 Dietrich von Landsberg conferred autonomous legal status onto the city, which permitted the establishment of two markers of late medieval self-governance: a council and a city court of jurors (*Schöffengericht*). See Ottto Künnemann and Martina Güldemann, *Geschichte der Stadt Leipzig* (Gudensberg-Gleichen: Wartberg Verlag, 2000), 12–17.

6   Robert Jütte, 'Health care provision and poor relief in early modern Hanseatic towns: Hamburg, Bremen and Lübeck', in Andrew Cunningham and Ole Peter Grell, eds, *Health Care and Poor Relief in Protestant Europe, 1500–1700* (London: Routledge, 1997), 112–13.

7   The Council used St Johannis to house persons suffering from the French disease from around 1500 and to house the elderly after c. 1550. St Georg functioned as a hospice for the elderly, a hospital for the sick and a lazarette during epidemics until it burnt down in 1661. When rebuilt in 1671, it functioned as a hospice for the mad, disorderly and poor

wealthy burghers, had been in place in the city since 1463. However, it was not until 1616 that the Willige Almosen part-funded a doctor to work in the Hospital of St Johannis and the Georg Hospital.[8] A particularly virulent epidemic of plague, war and the burning down of the Georg Hospital in 1631 lead the Council to direct the Willige Almosen to administer and fund emergency medical care for the poor. Soon thereafter the Council assumed direct responsibility not only for the sick poor, but also for the city's sick more generally. To do so, it redirected Church collections that had previously flowed into the Willige Almosen.[9] In response to an electoral decree, the Council established the Almosenamt (Office of Alms) in 1704, with direct medical care of poor relief recipients falling to the so-called *Almosenchirurg*, a surgeon appointed by the Office of Alms who treated patients in their homes.[10] In the 1550s the Council founded a dedicated plague hospital, known as the lazarette, which in the latter eighteenth century also admitted destitute pregnant women. It was headed up by the lazarette surgeon who, by the beginning of the eighteenth century, was an academically trained physician with surgical expertise.[11] The first municipal medical post created by the city fathers in 1480 was that of sworn midwife.[12] The contents of this sworn midwife's oath was similar to that of many ecclesiastical oaths, however, her allegiance was now to the Leipzig Council.[13] It was not until 1512 that the Council appointed a *Stadtarzt* (city doctor).[14]

Political self-realisation, however, was only one aspect of the trend towards civic regulation of midwifery, medical and poor relief. Dramatic changes to the socio-structural conditions in the cities during the fourteenth and fifteenth centuries likewise served as a catalyst for municipal midwife licensing. These bustling late medieval urban centres enjoyed high population growth courtesy

orphans before it too began to admit the general poor. See Elisabeth Dietzmann, *Die Leipziger Einrichtungen der Armenpflege bis zur Übernahme der Armenverwaltung durch die Stadt 1881* (Leipzig: Steiger, 1932), 11–20.

8   The Leipzig Willige Almosen, supervised by the Leipzig Council, was the first of its kind in the German territories. It provided 24 persons selected by the Council with bread and vegetables on a fortnightly basis. By 1475 it was also distributing monetary alms. See ibid., 7–11.

9   Ibid., 10–11.

10   Ibid., 29–30.

11   The Council appointed Dr Etmüller as *Lazarettmedicus* in 1706 and sought to appoint Dr Benjamin Benedict Petermann to the Hospital of St Georg in 1718. See StadtAL, Tit. (F) VIII Nr. 53, 'Protokoll zum Drey Rathen', 18, 94–95. The lazarette was managed by a husband-and-wife team. Care of the patients was carried out by a staff of women. See Elke Schlenkrich, *Von Leuten auf dem Sterbestroh. Sozialgeschichte obersächsischer Lazarette in der frühen Neuzeit* (Beucha: Sax-Verlag, 2002), 74–84.

12   Horst Thieme and Sigrid Gerlach, eds, *Das Leipziger Eidbuch von 1590* (Leipzig: VEB Fachbuchverlag, 1986), 149.

13   Flügge, *Hebammen und heilkundige Frauen*, 132–34.

14   A *Ratsdienerarzt* (barber-surgeon) had been in the employ of the Council since 1469, however, his responsibility was restricted to treating the councillors only. See Beate Berger et al., *Vom Aderlass zum Gesundheitspass. Zeittafel zur Geschichte des öffentlichen Gesundheitswesens in Leipzig* (Leipzig: Leipziger Universitätsverlag, 2000), 5–6.

of in-migration. Plenty of permanent and seasonal job opportunities meant that amongst parvenus and seasonal workers, the well-groomed social networks that underpinned midwifery as a form of reciprocal neighbourly and familial assistance in rural communities were either fragmentary or non-existent.[15] A substantial population, estimated at approximately 6,500 in the 1480s, coupled with a market-fair-based economy made the social structure in Leipzig particularly porous.[16] Those new to the city – domestic servants, day labourers, fair workers and prostitutes as well as the wives of artisans, merchants and healers – might, in the case of a birth, be forced to call upon the services of a stranger for assistance. Likewise, large populations in the cities necessitated a number of midwives working simultaneously who competed with each other for work. The oath as a regulative instrument was only deployed in this particular demographic situation; small towns, in which the number of women earning a living from midwifery was negligible, rarely bothered to license or regulate their midwives.[17]

Midwifery in larger cities thus began to assume a commercial character. In the fifteenth century cities struggled to keep enough sworn midwives working within their walls and many councils were forced to offer a variety of financial and material incentives such as a salary and/or naturalia, the right to reside and practice in the city or the much sought-after and costly status of burgher.[18] Some councils also looked to training as a means of ensuring the supply of competent midwives and obligated their sworn midwives (who were often unwilling to educate their future competitors) to teach younger women the craft in return for remuneration.[19]

From oath to instruction: midwifery regulation in Leipzig

The earliest extant midwife oath for the city of Leipzig dates from 1590 and is located in the Council's *Eidbuch* (Book of Oaths). Until 1609 councillors recorded the names of midwives and the date they were sworn in on the page beneath the oath.[20] A number of factors, including recurrent episodes of the plague between 1610 and 1613 and regulations about managing the plague, compelled the Council to revise the midwife oath just twenty-three years later in 1613.[21] Although the 1590 oath had been amended to incorporate specific instructions for midwives to attend inmates of the plague hospital or women

---

15   See Flügge, *Hebammen und heilkundige Frauen*, 149–50.
16   Ingolf Bergfeld, *Leipzig. Eine kleine Stadtgeschichte* (Erfurt: Sutton, 2002), 19–21.
17   Flügge, *Hebammen und heilkundige Frauen*, 172.
18   As Flügge finds in Nuremberg and Constance. Ibid., 150–51.
19   For example, in Nuremberg in 1516. Ibid., 151.
20   StadtAL, Ohne Sig., 'Eidbücher des Leipziger Rates', 'Der Kindermuetter oder Hebammen Aidt', 1590, 28.
21   Between 1610 and 1617 the city was besieged every summer by the plague. See Anhang 94 and Anhang 95 on the epidemic years in Leipzig, 1350–1542 and 1700–1892 in Berger et al., *Vom Aderlass*.

confined to households under quarantine, by 1613 this measure had proven inadequate. The Council formulated a separate oath for so-called 'plague midwives', women appointed specifically for the term of an epidemic to attend infected and/or quarantined mothers.[22] These plague midwives held temporary offices and did not preside over the full range of duties and obligations usually accorded to the city's sworn midwives, such as attendance at medico-legal examinations.[23] The amended oath of 1613 also formalised the use of midwives as medico-legal experts as set out in the *Constitutio Criminalis Carolina*, the first Germany-wide written criminal penal code of 1532. The Carolina obliged midwives to examine infants and women on behalf of the city or territorial court of law.

The oath was amended again in 1689, this time to include the matter of emergency baptism. Although customarily one of the midwife's duties, the Leipzig Council had never deemed it necessary to elucidate precisely how and when a midwife should perform the sacrament. This was instead the preserve of the Church which, after Lutheranism was proclaimed the state religion in Saxony in 1539, published a church ordinance for the whole of Saxony. The 1624 edition of the Saxon Church Ordinance suggests that by the early seventeenth century, the ability of midwives to carry out emergency baptism had become a point of heated discussion. The Saxon Church nonetheless continued to permit midwives to perform emergency baptism:

> Because a laudable and well-established custom has been maintained, that all Christian persons, and in particular the midwives, in that respect that women too be heirs to Christ's Realm, (and emergency is not subject to the common ordinance and rule), have baptised the little children in the absence of men in times of emergency, we do not wish to abolish this [custom], but rather leave it in place.[24]

Of greatest concern was the problem of double baptism – forbidden by Lutheran doctrine – which the ordinance decreed could be countered by adequate training through the local parish priests. Despite the religious peace of 1648, baptism (in particular emergency baptism) persisted as a matter of great doctrinal and cultural divergence between the three Christian confessions well into the eighteenth century. Furthermore, as research into baptismal practices has shown, the divide between the practice and doctrine of baptism persisted in Catholic, Calvinist and Lutheran communities well beyond this time.[25]

---

22 StadtAL, Ohne Sig., 'Eidbücher des Leipziger Rates', 51r–51v, 'Der Kindermuetter oder Hebeammen Aidt', 1613.

23 Ohne Sig., 'Eidbücher des Leipziger Rates 1613', 51v, 'Der Kindermütter Eidt, so auff die Inficirten Personen bestellet', 1613.

24 Section entitled 'Von der Nothtauffe' in *Agenda, das ist: Kirchenordnung / Wie sich die Pfarrherrn vnd Seelsorger in ihren Ampten und Diensten halten sollen / Für die Diener der Kirchen in Hertzog Heinrichen zu Sachsen V. G. H. Fürstenthumb gestellet*, (Leipzig: Henning Großen des Altern, 1624), x–xiv.

25 In Catholic regions, for example, parents feared that unbaptised infants would haunt the family, and went to great lengths to circumvent doctrine that forbade them from burying their unbaptised infants on sacred ground. This included undertaking pilgrimages with the dead child in order to 'revive' it and have it baptised. See Marion Kobelt-Groch,

Whereas Catholics and Lutherans agreed that an emergency baptism sufficed for the salvation of a child, Calvinists were intent on eradicating the practice. For Catholics baptism in utero was unproblematic. For Lutherans and Calvinists, a child could only be baptised once it had been fully born. And whilst in Catholic doctrine the emergency baptism was a matter for midwives and the circle of women involved in the birth, many Lutherans began calling for restrictions on midwives carrying out emergency baptism, fearing that they would only perform a so-called *Scheintaufe* (an improper baptism that necessitated a second baptism through a pastor).[26]

Double baptism was problematic for Lutherans precisely because of a fundamental doctrinal shift in the concept of the state of the infant soul. Both Luther and Bugenhagen had propagated the idea that unbaptised children were no longer damned because God had the power to ensure their salvation.[27] Recent research on funeral sermons has illuminated the rhetorical practices underpinning this new idea in the late sixteenth and seventeenth centuries as well as parents' need to reiterate this new concept. Parents deployed a variety of techniques in funeral sermons in order to do so, such as: employing biblical references to God's intention that all infants are innocent, narrating their intention to have the child baptised as a demonstration of doctrinal compliance, and alluding to the idea that the child was already communicating with God in utero and thus already possessed a soul prior to the birth.[28] Underpinning this new voice on baptism was the concept of parental love in the seventeenth century modelled on God's love: Children were 'entrusted' to their parents by God for a period of time and it was the duty of both children and parents to prove themselves worthy of God's trust. The death of a child was thus an act of God's love, akin to a resurrection, and parents could console themselves in the knowledge that for the infant, death was beneficial as it could assume its place in paradise next to God all the sooner.[29]

Although it emerged as a theme in the Leipzig midwife oath comparatively late, emergency baptism had featured in the ordinances and/or oaths of many other large cities in the Germanies since the fifteenth and sixteenth

'Selig auch ohne Taufe? Gedruckte lutherische Leichenpredigten für ungetauft verstorbene Kinder des 16. und 17. Jahrhunderts', in Marion Kobelt-Groch and Cornelia Niekus Moore, eds, *Tod und Jenseits in der Schriftkultur der Frühen Neuzeit* (Wiesbaden: Harrassowitz Verlag, 2008), 66–67. On Catholic regions, see also Eva Labouvie, '"Sanctuaires à répit". Zur Wiedererweckung toter Neugeborener, zur Erinnerungskultur und zur Jenseitsvorstellung im katholischen Milieu', ibid.

26 For an overview of these various doctrinal differences, see 'Zur Wiedererweckung', 81.

27 Kobelt-Groch, 'Selig', 68, 70–72; Susan C. Karant-Nunn, 'Babies, Baptism, Bodies, Burials, and Bliss: Ghost Stories and their Rejection in the Late Sixteenth Century', in Marion Kobelt-Groch and Cornelia Niekus Moore, eds, *Tod und Jenseits in der Schriftkultur der Frühen Neuzeit* (Wiesbaden: Harrassowitz Verlag, 2008), 21.

28 Kobelt-Groch, 'Selig', 70–72.

29 Claudia Jarzebowski, 'Loss and Emotion in Funeral Works on Children in Seventeenth-Century Germany', in Lynne Tatlock, ed., *Enduring Loss in Early Modern Germany: Cross Disciplinary Perspectives* (Leiden: Brill, 2010), 197, 212–13.

centuries.[30] The Leipzig Council, however, only felt it necessary to incorporate explicit instructions for emergency baptism in the 1689 revision of the midwife oath, in which midwives were reminded to baptise according to the Saxon Church Ordinance 'with nothing other than water and not sooner than when … [the child] is fully born to the world'.[31] Notably, neither of these aspects – props and timing – were mentioned in the section governing emergency baptism in the Saxon Church Ordinance, which remained valid (unamended) from 1624 to 1748. The mid-eighteenth-century oath contained more detailed instructions on how to baptise infants and instructed midwives to refrain from performing emergency baptism save 'in the greatest emergency of the child's weakness' and to fetch a 'servant of the Church or other Christian man' to carry out the baptism.[32] Should this prove impossible, the oath instructed the midwives to gather together two or three people, recite the Lord's Prayer, give the child its name, and then to baptise the child with water.[33] For all the Lutheran doctrine, the Saxon Church Ordinance took a relatively relaxed, indeed pragmatic, view of double baptism. If, upon the pastor's questioning, the persons bringing the child to baptism say that:

> They do not know / what they thought / much less what they said or did in such great emergency (as is want to be the case in such situations) so one should not dispute the matter too much / but rather take the child as unbaptised and baptise it / just as one does an unbaptised child.[34]

This may help account for the very small number of cases relating to emergency baptisms in which the midwife was accused of negligence.[35] The legislative treatment of baptism in Leipzig thus demonstrates a trend towards more

---

30 Wiesner, 'Public/Private', 85. The Leipzig Council's baptismal ordinance (1669) only regulated sumptuary matters, for example, the number of guests, permissible gifts, etc. according to the estate of the family. Detailed in Johann Jakob Vogel, *Leipzigisches Geschichts-Buch oder Annales, das ist: Jahr- und Tagebücher der weltberühmten Königl. und Churfürstlichen Sächsischen Kauff= und Handels=Stadt Leipzig … von Anno 1661 … bis in das 1714 Jahr* (Leipzig: Friedrich Lanckischens sel. Erben, 1714), 737. For the Leipzig Council's proposal for the 1669 ordinance, see StadtAL, Tit. LX.B (F) Nr. 7, 'Verordnungen und Patente des Rates', 250, 'Baptismal ordinance (proposal)', 1669.

31 Presumably referring to the Saxon church ordinance from 1681. Ohne Sig., 'Eidbücher des Leipziger Rates 1689', 67v, 'Midwife oath', 1689.

32 See the oath in Ratsstu Tit. LV B (F) Nr. 8, 483–84, 'Hebammen= oder Kinder=Mutter Eyd, Specification', undated, in use by 1728.

33 Ibid.

34 *Sächs. Kirchenordnung,* XIV(v).

35 Only four such cases are extant for the period 1728–74. See II. Sekt. W (F) Nr. 332, 'Die inn: und vor der Stadt wohnende Wehmütter: und Beÿweiber, auch deren Amt und Verrichtung betr. (1717–1737)', 70–73, 'Leipzig Council reprimands midwives about emergency baptisms', 28 June 1728; II. Sekt. R (F) Nr. 442, 1–14, 'Hebamme. Anna Maria Rein unterlässt eine Nottaufe', 23 December 1733–8 January 1734; II. Sekt. M (F) Nr. 760, Bd. I, 'Hebammen. Verschiedenes über die Kindermütter, Wehemütter und Beifrauen', 1–22, 'Acta, Die Wehmutter Regina Elizabeth Mendin betr.', 15 March 1742–13 May 1743; II. Sekt. S (F) Nr. 2013, 'Acta, Das von Elenoren Wilhelminen Stahlin erzeugte, unter falschen Nahmen zur Tauffe gebrachte Kind betr.', 25 January–5 March 1774.

regulatory involvement on the part of the Council over the course of the latter seventeenth and first half of the eighteenth century. By treating religious matters in the municipal oath, the Leipzig Council was augmenting its purview of governance to an area of midwifery normally regulated on a territorial-ecclesiastical level.

With the Reformation came a shift in many cities across Germany from a midwife oath to a midwife ordinance. Whereas oaths were aimed at regulating midwifery to ensure adequate provision for the community, in the religious and social tumult of the Reformation ordinances marked an attempt to (re-)define ideal norms for the occupation of midwife as an aspect of *gute Policey* (the practice of the well-ordered state).[36] The Frankfurter ordinance of 1573, composed by Stadtphysicus Adam Lonicerus, *Reformation / oder Ordnung für die Hebammen*, for example, recast the practice of midwifery, and indeed the subject of procreation, within Lutheran orthodoxies: it subordinated women to men and curbed female sexuality by outlawing extramarital sex, circumscribing intramarital sexual practices and promulgating the idea of procreation as an aspect of the worldly 'common good' rather than a mere means of ensuring spiritual salvation.[37] Partly through the ideas of the Reformation, town elders were beginning to understand their function as that of an *Obrigkeit* (governing authority) whose responsibility it was to regulate the public sphere and ensure the 'common good'. Governance by ordinance was not exclusive to midwifery but extended to many aspects of early modern life from clothing to protocol during epidemics.

Despite their size and commercial importance, neither Leipzig nor the royal residence Dresden regulated midwifery per ordinance until the latter eighteenth century. Even then, only Dresden produced one in 1764.[38] This ordinance was amended in 1818 and was promulgated as the first Saxon midwifery ordinance.[39] Unlike in Frankfurt, where lengthy ordinances had taken over as the normal form of regulation by 1600, Leipzig's midwives were regulated solely by a page-long oath. It was not until the early eighteenth century that this oath was augmented by the so-called 'instruction', of which the earliest extant document dates from 1715. This instruction regulated in great detail the occupational activities of midwife-apprentices (Beifrauen); the first midwife instruction extant is from 1758. Whereas an ordinance was a piece of quasi 'legislation', the instruction was a document designed specifically for the

---

36 Flügge, *Hebammen und heilkundige Frauen*, 186–88.
37 See especially Chapter Nine of ibid., 463–91; Heide Wunder, 'Überlegungen zum Wandel der Geschlechterbeziehungen im 15. und 16. Jahrhundert aus sozialgeschichtlicher Sicht', in Heide Wunder and Christina Vanja, eds, *Wandel der Geschlechterbeziehungen zu Beginn der Neuzeit* (Frankfurt am Main: Suhrkamp, 1991), 13–26, esp. 14–15.
38 For further details, see Arlett Mielisch, *Wie die Hebamme ihren Meister fand. Der lange Weg zur ersten Dresdner Hebammenordnung von 1764* (Technische Universität Dresden: 2014/15), available at <https://tu-dresden.de/gsw/phil/ige/fnz/ressourcen/dateien/studium/dat_praes/plakmiel?lang=de>, accessed 15 November 2016.
39 Tit. (F) XLIV.A.18a, 104–6, 'Mandat Geburtshülfe', 2 April 1818.

office bearer.[40] Unlike an ordinance, which was usually printed, the instruction was copied by a scribe for each new office-holder and could thus be easily amended to incorporate particular duties whenever necessary. This was the case when, in the 1790s, the midwife at the Rannstädter Tor had her instruction amended to include the duty of attending destitute pregnant women in the city's lazarette.[41] Possession of this document conferred upon the holder the status of sworn midwife and the instruction was intended as a kind of reference work of occupational comportment for sworn midwives.

The midwife instruction dating from 1758 remained in use, albeit undergoing various amendments, until at least 1818. It was a lengthy, ten-page document covering twenty-four items relating to all aspects of the midwife's occupation: from when to call the 'Herrn Accoucheur' and how to behave towards women, to the relationship between midwives and their apprentices.[42] Besides a supplementary, printed *Specification* listing the herbs and medications midwives were permitted to use by the Stadtphysici, the instruction did not touch on the medical aspects of midwifery, for example, how to deliver a child or the accessories of which a midwife should avail herself (for example, a birthing stool).[43] The Council's focus on medicinal treatments is indicative of where it considered its regulatory responsibility to lie, as the matter of who held the right to prescribe and apply internal medicines had been a bone of contention within the Leipzig medical community since at least the mid-seventeenth century. Indeed the problem of *Pfuscherei* (quackery) in the area of health and healing was the main reason why the Leipzig Council attended to medical matters per ordinance in the city at all.[44] The Council did not consider itself responsible for regulating the medical detail of midwifery beyond those aspects of the occupation that disrupted the propriety of the occupational structures of official medicine. Internal medicines, traditionally the preserve of the physician, was one such sticking point that required careful legislation.

Midwifery and the state

The Collegium Medicum of 1710 and the Ämter

The Saxon state was a relatively minor player in matters relating to everyday health and well-being up until the early nineteenth century. Its attempts at

40   Ordinances promulgated by the Leipzig Council on medical matters tended to address matters of immediate concern, for example, quackery, rather than matters considered part of the status quo.
41   StadtAL, Tit. (F) X Nr. 23b, Bd. XIII, 'Instruktionen (1676–nach 1800)', 58r–69v, 'Instruktion vor die Kinder Mutter N. N.', 14 July 1758, 67v.
42   See Items 8, 9, 16 and 18 in ibid.
43   See the 'Specification' appended to the 1758 instruction. According to a postscript, this specification was removed from the instruction sometime after c. 1770s. See ibid.
44   In the repetorium of ordinances and patents issued by the Leipzig Council, most of the medically related ordinances dealt with quackery.

legislating on the health of its population were intermittent and reactive, and it rarely had the bureaucratic mechanisms in place to facilitate implementation and enforcement. It was not until yet another outbreak of plague in 1710 that the Saxon government established the first territorial public health institution, the Collegium Medicum.[45] Comprising the ordinary professors of the medical faculties in Leipzig and Wittenberg, the royal physicians and the municipal physicians in Dresden, the College tabled a number of reforms, including equipping its *Ämter* (designated territorial administrative districts within Electoral Saxony, of which Leipzig and its immediate surrounds was one) with an *Amtsphysicus* (district physician in the employ of the territorial government).[46]

During the early modern period, the Saxon territorial government had transformed the Ämter, which had grown rather haphazardly out of the medieval margrave Vogtei, into its direct administrative representatives. The Ämter were responsible for collecting territorial taxes, executing justice within their jurisdictions and taking care of general matters of Policey, such as maintaining thoroughfares and managing outbreaks of contagion. The Amt Leipzig, which had its headquarters in the former Pleißenburg palace in Leipzig, consisted of 5 cities and 134 villages. These did not include, however, the city of Leipzig – governed by the Leipzig Council – or the Leipzig University, both of which were jurisdictions unto themselves and subject to territorial rule directly.[47] Furthermore, the relationship between the city of Leipzig and the Saxon government was complex, characterised by both autonomy and reciprocity. As the head of the *Städteausschuss* (Committee of Cities) in the Landtag, Leipzig played a leading political role in territorial politics and its position as an economic powerhouse and location for territorial educational and cultural institutions cultivated territorial interest.[48] At the same time, as Karlheinz Blaschke argues, with its burgher culture and economic savvy, Leipzig was in a position to shape territorial political developments like no other political actor in eighteenth-century Saxony. Many of the movers and shakers in Dresden, in particular those involved in the 1760s Saxon Rétablissement, hailed from the Leipzig burgher estate and Leipzig was thus able to mediate political decisions, often to its advantage.[49] After being forced into administration by the territorial government in 1625 following bankruptcy, the city endured almost sixty years of financial oversight from Dresden. The Council managed to purchase its political independence from the Saxon crown in 1688, and had since

---

45 Volker Klimpel, *Das Dresdner Collegium Medico-Chirurgicum* (Frankfurt am Main: Peter Lang, 1995), 70.

46 W.J. Kleemann, 'Die gerichtliche Medizin an der medizinischen Fakultät vor der Gründung des Institutes', in A. Graefe et al., eds, *100 Jahre forensische Toxikologie im Institut für Rechtsmedizin in Leipzig* (Leipzig: MOLINApress, 2004), 4–5 (online pagination).

47 Beachy, *Soul of Commerce*, 60–61; Blaschke, 'Zur Behördengeschichte', 343–45.

48 According to Karlheinz Blaschke, 'Die kursächsische Politik und Leipzig im 18. Jahrhundert', in Wolfgang Martens, ed., *Leipzig. Aufklärung und Bürgerlichkeit* (Heidelberg: Verlag Lambert Schneider, 1990), 29–31.

49 Ibid., 33–37. The Rétablissement will be discussed in the next section.

vigorously asserted its right to self-rule. In 1689 this independence was sealed with the *Senatus consultum*, a municipal constitution liberating the city government from interference from territorial officials, in particular in matters of a financial nature.[50] As a dispute between the Leipzig Council and the Lutheran Church / territorial government over the secularisation of a suicide burial lasting from 1702 to 1704 shows, the city did not always prevail.[51] However, at least officially, the everyday running of the city continued to be largely a matter for the Leipzig Council, despite the Amt's physical presence in the city. The territorial government signalised its interest in midwifery in 1723 by ordering the visitation of the pharmacists and midwives in the Ämter, however, the city of Leipzig was not subject to this legislation.[52] Medical provision and everyday medical practice in Leipzig remained largely a matter for the Council, on one level, and individual practitioners and families, on the other.

The Collegium Medico-Chirurgicum of 1748

The perceived inefficacy of the Collegium Medicum prompted the Saxon government to found a second territorial body to oversee matters of public health. This time, the territorial government's sights were set on more than just epidemics and a network of medical officials: professional medical standards were the order of the day. In 1748 the Saxon government founded the Collegium Medico-Chirurgicum (College of Medical Surgeons, CM) in the royal residence of Dresden and charged it with the task of training, examining and licensing both military and civil surgeons throughout Saxony. At the same time, realising that its network of Amtsphysici was sparse and feeble, it passed additional legislation demanding the appointment of an Amtsphysicus in each Amt and ordering all Amtsphysici to provide the Collegium Medicum with regular reports on epidemics and other health matters in their districts.[53]

At the time of the CM's establishment, the court surgeon and *Hebammen-meister* (midwife master) in Dresden, August Friedrich Langbein, had been agitating for a midwifery school in the royal residence without success. Financially wasted after the Seven Years War, the government was not in a position to heed Langbein's suggestions and it was not until 1775 that a privately run midwifery school began providing formal instruction to midwives in Dresden.

---

50 Beachy, *Soul of Commerce*, 46.
51 The Leipzig Council had sought to retain its de facto administrative control over suicide burial in the city, which it had already secularised, but the Church and the Saxon government won the battle to incorporate suicide burials into Church jurisdiction. See Craig Koslofsky, 'Suicide and the Secularization of the Body in Early Modern Saxony', *Continuity and Change* 16 (2001): 45–70, 56–62.
52 Joachim Richter, 'Zur Geschichte des Öffentlichen Gesundheitsdienstes in Sachsen', *Ärzteblatt Sachsen* 11 (2001): 518–21, 518.
53 This legislation was the 'Verordnung über die Errichtung eines Sanitäts-Collegii zur Verbesserung des Medicinal-Wesens' from 18 September 1748. See ibid. On the origins of the CM, see Klimpel, *Das Dresdner CM*, 53–55.

The territorial government soon realised the midwifery school's value and turned it into a state-run institution. It opened its doors in 1784 as a territorial midwifery school for obstetricians, students of surgery, midwives and military surgeons from the surrounding region.[54] Although the Dresden midwifery school appears to have had an influence beyond Dresden, there is no evidence that midwives recruited in Leipzig ever attended this school. Nor did the Leipzig Council make a point of preferencing women who had received training there (or indeed in any other midwifery school) in its appointments. This points to the limited reach of this kind of midwifery training in cities in which the local midwifery infrastructure was strong, enjoyed a lengthy tradition and was supported by the local municipal government.

The Sanitätskollegium of 1768

The Seven Years War (1756–63) bequeathed Saxony a heavy burden. Aside from the usual by-products of war – many of the large cities had sustained serious damage, the population had shrunk by around eight per cent, epidemics raged and agricultural production had stagnated – the government had accumulated an astronomical debt.[55] In Leipzig, manufacturing was flagging, with many producers decamping to more convivial territory, causing the Leipzig trade fairs to take on 'the appearance of modest country markets'.[56] Even before the official peace treaty of February 1762, the Saxon government had its sights set high on the matter of rebuilding the territory: the Saxon Rétablissement was to be no mere mop-up, but rather a program of renewal and reform touching almost every aspect of life from agriculture and religious freedom to internal governance and foreign relations.[57] The road to reform, however, was paved with compromise with the variously powerful limbs of the body politic. The political organ assembled for the task, the Restoration Commission, was, for example, unable to persuade the Leipzig Council on the benefits of introducing civil emancipation for non-Lutheran Christians because the Council wanted to protect the interests of its own Lutheran mercantile elite. The non-noble burgher establishment in Leipzig continued to be a force unto itself.[58]

In this gush of renewal, matters medical were to be dealt with by a new state public health body, the *Sanitätskollegium* (Board of Health), which commenced operations on 13 September 1768. The Sanitätskollegium was made

---

54 *Das Dresdner CM*, 96–97.
55 The Saxon government had to use roughly 65% of its annual income from taxes in order to repay capital and interest on its war debt according to Gross, *Geschichte*, 152–53, 160. Beachy estimates that Leipzig shouldered around 20% of the reparations paid to the Prussians. See Beachy, *Soul of Commerce*, 79.
56 *Soul of Commerce*, 78.
57 Plans for the Rétablissement were drawn up by the Restoration Commission 1762–63. See Gross, *Geschichte*, 160–61.
58 Beachy, *Soul of Commerce*, 94–96.

up of three discrete political entities: the Saxon territorial government, Leipzig University and Wittenberg University.[59] This triage of interests was reflected in the structure of the Sanitätskollegium, which divided the Saxon Ämter into three groups, each assigned administratively to the Sanitätskollegium in Dresden, the Medical Faculty in Leipzig or the Medical Faculty in Wittenberg. The city of Leipzig and its environs fell under the jurisdiction of the Leipzig Medical Faculty.[60]

Although intended as the highest instance of medical bureaucracy within Saxony, the Sanitätskollegium had to work very hard to build an aura of authority on medical matters, for in eighteenth-century Saxony, health and well-being were first and foremost a personal matter. Corporate and guild institutions, city and district governments and, not least, the medical faculties in Leipzig and Wittenberg, which provided medical attests to institutions as well as private individuals for a variety of legal purposes, were involved in a largely reactive capacity.[61] Thus in the first year of the Sanitätskollegium, the Leipzig Medical Faculty lamented that even those physicians 'who want to do something, do not have enough authority and the lower authorities do not support them as they should, so that the deficiencies of the medical system were able to be remedied only very little, or not at all'.[62] Yet trouble also came from within the ranks of the Sanitätskollegium itself. The relationship between the Leipzig Medical Faculty and the Dresden arm of the Sanitätskollegium had been fractious from the outset, with the Medical Faculty, for example, not shy about canvassing for revision of the planned territorial medical ordinance or insisting on its right to admit practitioners without the approval of the Saxon government.[63]

From a technical and organisational perspective, the Sanitätskollegium brought negligible change to midwifery in Leipzig; its purpose was neither medical-technical innovation nor a major reshuffle of organisational responsibilities amongst either office holders or the incorporated medical professions. It sought instead to clamp down on patchy practices of medical licensing: its

---

59   The Saxon territorial government was represented by the *Generalstabsmedicus* (head military physician), the teacher of anatomy in the Dresden Collegium Medico-Chirurgicum, and the royal physicians to the Elector-King in Dresden. Leipzig University and Wittenberg University were each represented by the dean of their respective medical faculties.

60   See Item 3 of StadtAL, Tit. (F) LX.A.18a, 'Churfürstliche Mandate (1768–1816)', 35–40, 'Mandat wegen Errichtung eines Sanitaets-Collegii zur Verbesserung des Medicinal-Wesens (Friedrich August)', 13 September 1768, 37.

61   The Leipzig Medical Faculty acted as a medico-legal authority for all civil courts in Saxony. Faculty members also exerted significant influence on a political level, with many also holding posts as municipal or royal medical officials. See Kleemann, 'Die gerichtliche Medizin', 1–2.

62   UAL, Med. Fak. A01/52, Bd. 01–03, Medizinal Polizei (Film Nr. 1285), 'Medizinal Polizei', 221–23, 'Eines Schreiben von der Medicinischen Facultat zu Leipzig an das Collegium Sanitatis [re: the Physici]', 4 August 1769, 222. Lindemann notes that a similar net of (mal-)relations, poor co-operation and weak authority existed in the Duchy of Braunschweig-Wolfenbüttel. See Lindemann, *Health*, 49–65.

63   Klimpel, *Das Dresdner CM*, 135.

charter was restorative. Midwifery warranted an entire section in the *Mandat* of 1768, which largely dealt with the matter of examination. Midwives 'both in the cities, as well as in the countryside of every locality' were to be 'thoroughly examined' and instructed on 'how they are to behave in all situations' by a Land-, Amts- or Stadtphysicus within six weeks of the mandate's publication.[64] Although prefaced by a disapproving paragraph on the 'abuses' of the territorial ordinances, which 'have not been followed everywhere', the Sanitätskollegium's primary concern lay in the rural shadowlands of midwifery, where examination and instruction through a medical official was at best rudimentary and on the whole non-existent.[65] The midwifery structure already in place in cities such as Leipzig posed as the model to be rolled out in the darkest and most recalcitrant corners of the realm. For this reason there was little attempt to change the tried and tested provision of midwifery in the cities until the Leipzig Medical Faculty, with the support of the Saxon government and the Sanitätskollegium, began planning a midwifery school in Leipzig in the 1780s – a project only realised some thirty years later following a very 'difficult birth'.[66]

Policey, cameralism and early modern governance

One of the chief tools of the cameralists was the *Policeyordnung* (police ordinance). More recent research on cameralism and Policey has fundamentally reconfigured the way we grasp the aims, function and reach of civic and territorial legislation prior to 1800 and Marc Raeff's now phrasal concept of the 'well-ordered police state', in which cameralist-designed Policey aimed to 'transform and guide' society, has sustained substantial revision.[67] This concept of Policey as 'social discipline' is indebted to German sociological and philosophical theories about the teleological nature of Enlightenment developed by Max Weber (discipline as the key to modernisation), Theodor Adorno and Max Horkheimer (dialectic of Enlightenment). All three are united by a fundamental belief that Enlightenment was a process of inevitable modernisation and rationalisation that resulted in a rational social order.[68] Drawing in

---

64 See Item 14 of Tit. (F) LX.A.18a, 35–40, 'Mandat Sanitäts-Collegium', 13 September 1768, 40.

65 'Mandat wegen Errichtung eines Sanitäts=Collegii zur Verbesserung des Medicinalwesens vom 13. September 1768', *Handbuch der im Königreich Sachsen geltenden Medicinal= Polizeigesetze, sämmtliche Gesetze enthaltend, welche der unterm 30. Juli 1836 erschienene, allgemeinen Instruction der Bezirksärzte, Gerichtsärzte und Amtschirurgen zum Grunde liegen* (Leipzig: Ch. S. Kayser'sche Buchhandlung (F. Beyer), 1837), 1.

66 See Chapter Seven of this volume.

67 Marc Raeff, *The Well-Ordered Police State: Social and Institutional Change through Law in the Germanies and Russia 1600–1800* (New Haven, CT: Yale University Press, 1983), 44–46.

68 For an overview of these theories, see Martin Dinges, 'The Reception of Michel Foucault's Ideas on Social Discipline, Mental Asylums, Hospitals and the Medical Profession in German Historiography', in Colin Jones and Roy Porter, eds, *Reassessing Foucault:*

particular on Weber's notion of the inevitable modernisation of society through discipline emanating from territorial rulers, Gerhard Oestreich's account of the early modern state with its concept of 'social discipline' has been particularly influential in German historiography. Oestreich argued that the absolutist monarch disciplined society starting with the army, the bureaucracy and the priesthood and later the general population. He discerned two phases in this process: Between 1450 and 1650 it was the cities that produced and played around with laws and regulation. From 1650 onwards territorial governments shouldered responsibility for legislative activity and – crucially – enforcement.[69]

Perhaps no single intellectual has succeeded in denting the armoury of this modernisation theory as has Michel Foucault. From the margins of the discipline, Foucault directed all his energies towards the question of power and the way in which it is exercised through discourse. His aim was to reveal the 'deep structures of discourse', or the structures of thought and practice (epistemes/discourses) to which the individual was always subject and which a society understood as an ahistorical given.[70] For Foucault, the emergence of rationality (so-called 'modernisation') did not challenge power. The collusion of knowledge and power that produced the institutions of the modern, rational state in which disciplining took place served instead to legitimise power in a softer, more subtle manner.[71] Thus according to Foucault, power is a productive force that brings forth, for example, the discursive encounter between doctor and patient. And it is not 'up there' in the Oestreichian/Weberian sense but is instead ubiquitous and permanent through the new mechanisms of power (institutions), even amongst the seemingly powerless.[72]

Responding in part to the challenge posed by Foucault that discipline is not only diffuse but also non-teleological, a number of historians have begun questioning the Oestreichian model of early modern governance and norm-setting, generating fruitful results for the field of Policey research. Some critics reject outright the idea that cameralism was a reflection of actual administrative practice, labelling it variously as a scholarly discourse (not penned by those doing the administrating) or a discursive career strategy for the ambitious and politically cunning intent on securing positions in territorial governments and German universities.[73] However, a number of German historians

---

Power, medicine, and the body (London: Routledge, 1994), 186–87. On Weber's concept of discipline, see Breuer, 'Sozialdisziplinierung', 45–52.

69 'Sozialdisziplinierung', 52–56; Dinges, 'Foucault's Reception', 187.

70 For a brilliant summary of Foucault's theories and their application in the history of medicine, see Colin Jones and Roy Porter, 'Introduction', in Colin Jones and Roy Porter, eds, *Reassessing Foucault: Power, medicine, and the body* (London: Routledge, 1994), here esp. 1, 9.

71 Jones and Porter use the metaphor of the 'velvet glove'. See ibid., 1–2.

72 Breuer, 'Sozialdisziplinierung', 56–57; Jones and Porter, 'Introduction', 9.

73 Keith Tribe quoted in Andre Wakefield, 'Books, Bureaus, and the Historiography of Cameralism', *European Journal of Law and Economics* 19 (2005): 311–20, 315–16; *The Disordered Police State: German Cameralism as Science and Practice* (Chicago: University of Chicago Press, 2009), 137–38.

have not been content to throw the baby out with the bath water, preferring instead to reassess the reception and use of ordinances – that is, the practice of Policey – in very concrete cases.[74]

A major bone of contention has centred on the matter of (in-)efficacy, for as Jürgen Schlumbohm urged in 1997, the 'strange miscellany of the balance sheet of success must confound us'.[75] The gargantuan number of Policey ordinances recorded for the early modern period, estimated by Michael Stolleis to number some two to five million individual 'norm-setting documents', contrasts with a paltry level of implementation as evidenced by manifold repetition and complaints about non-compliance.[76] Stolleis, however, claims that measuring the efficacy of ordinances before 1800 using such a formula is to retro-project a nineteenth- and twentieth-century construction of a 'perfectly functioning territorial state, which received impulses from the top and conveyed these without frictional loss to the bottom [of society]'.[77] Accordingly, the early modern state was certainly chaotic, but even more importantly, its legislative efforts were mere intentions – persuasive and chiding at once but without the threat of enforcement.[78] André Holenstein offers such a framework for understanding the intention and outcome of early modern Policey. The practice of dispensation and court practices, he argues, demonstrate that legislation was effective in that it functioned as guidance for decisions made by authorities and subjects that always revolved around the individual situation of the person, community or matter at stake, which he coins a 'theory of circumstances' ('Theorie der Umstände').[79]

This new way of thinking about Policey has broader implications for agency. In rejecting the notion of the territorial ruler as the sole generator of early modern legislation, historians have also begun reassessing the matter of who produced early modern legislation and in what constellation. Policey, according to Stolleis, was the product of a much tighter dialogue between the authorities and the Stände, and the implementation of norms combined a complicated interplay of social forces emanating from all levels of society.[80] Martin Dinges concurs that not only was the state unable to promulgate and enforce its police ordinances, administrative practice was only ever guided by

---

74   The collection of papers in the following volume remains one of the most comprehensive overviews of research in this area. Karl Härter, ed., *Policey und frühneuzeitliche Gesellschaft* (Frankfurt am Main: Vittorio Klostermann, 2000).

75   Jürgen Schlumbohm, 'Gesetze, die nicht durchgesetzt werden – ein Strukturmerkmal des frühneuzeitlichen Staates?', *Geschichte und Gesellschaft* 23 (1997): 647–63, 655.

76   Michael Stolleis, 'Was bedeutet "Normdurchsetzung" bei Policeyordnungen der frühen Neuzeit?', in Peter Landau and R. H. Helmholz, eds, *Grundlagen des Rechts: Festschrift für Peter Landau zum 65. Geburtstag* (Paderborn: F. Schöningh, 2000), 741, 745.

77   Ibid., 745.

78   Ibid., 748–51.

79   See André Holenstein, 'Die Umstände der Normen – die Normen der Umstände. Policeyordnungen im kommunikativen Handeln von Verwaltung und lokaler Gesellschaft im Ancien Regime', in Karl Härter, ed., *Policey und frühneuzeitliche Gesellschaft* (Frankfurt am Main: Vittorio Klostermann, 2000), 38–39.

80   Stolleis, 'Was bedeutet "Normdurchsetzung"', 753–55.

ordinances to a minor degree. Medical ordinances were not hard and fast laws but instead 'merely orientations for the prospective negotiations with the local population and its representatives'.[81]

Achim Landwehr's critique of traditional evaluations of Policey pushes the barrow even further. Instead of trying to explain how those 'down there' accepted laws using the 'antagonistic pair of terms norm and practice' and searching for evidence of compliance or non-compliance, historians ought to comprehend 'norm' and 'practice' as 'components of a circular process in which not the difference between normative expectation and actual (non-)compliance is of interest, but rather the manner in which various social groups negotiate norms and for what reason.'[82] By teasing out three groups that interacted in the production of Policey – norm-givers, norm-receivers and norm-implementers – Landwehr demonstrates the 'field of power' in which Policey was generated and the normatively defined 'corridor' that it laid out for subjects. Instead of a simple dialectic between the governing and the governed, the practice of Policey was an ever-continuing 'polylectic' between these three groups.[83]

What this all boils down to is that we can no longer think about norm-setting documents, such as midwife ordinances and instructions, as a measure of the power of early modern governing institutions – no more than we can regard them as a measure of the regulation of early modern subjects. They were one aspect of a complex, communicative practice of norm-setting and they need, therefore, to be embedded in the early modern practices of governance as well as everyday practices.

Reforming midwifery in Leipzig, c. 1650–1740

The major reforms to midwifery in Leipzig took place during the latter seventeenth and early eighteenth centuries, well before the medico-political discourse emerging in the 1760s co-opted (at least on a rhetorical level) medicine and health into the service of state-building. This chronological glitch alone ought to make us cautious when considering the degree of influence we accord the territorial state as the initiator of change. As we have seen here, for all its attempts at regulating medical matters in Electoral Saxony, the territorial government's arm was both short and weak for the best part of the eighteenth century. It was only one institutional player in a complex web of governance in which communal authorities in cities such as Leipzig enjoyed a good deal of legal and practical autonomy. The relationship between the state and

---

81 Dinges, 'Medicinische Policey', 277–82, 294.
82 Achim Landwehr, 'Policey vor Ort. Die Implementation von Policeyordnungen in der ländlichen Gesellschaft der frühen Neuzeit', in Peter Landau and R. H. Helmholz, eds, *Grundlagen des Rechts: Festschrift für Peter Landau zum 65. Geburtstag* (Paderborn: F. Schöningh, 2000), 48–50.
83 Ibid., 69–70.

the commune was not simply one of opposition; the Leipzig Council cooperated on state directives and used its position to secure favourable conditions for the city. As will also become apparent from the following discussion, the circulation of medical personnel between municipal office, territorial office and university was considerable, providing ample opportunity for the conduit of ideas and practices about how midwifery ought to be organised from one sphere of governance to another.

In Leipzig, operational knowledge of midwifery appears to have flowed from communal to territorial sphere where it informed later territorial ordinances. This begs the question: How disparate was the practice of governance and the ideas and mentalities that produced it between these spheres? To what extent must we conceive the early modern state (and indeed all players in the early modern web of governance) as 'a product of society, dependent upon it and saturated by the beliefs prevalent in that society'?[84] Nevertheless, reforming midwifery in Leipzig meant finding largely local solutions to local problems. If a directive came from the territorial government, it was relatively roughshod and it was left up to the Council and its medical officials to sort out the details.

The late seventeenth- and early eighteenth-century reforms to midwifery were motivated to a great extent by an anxiety about depopulation, a theme that continued to concern policy-makers – on both a communal and territorial level – as well as scholars well into the early nineteenth century. As Jacques Gélis has argued for France, anxiety about depopulation was central to the development of midwifery in the eighteenth century and beyond, although ideas about the properties of population (as well as the origins of its fluctuations) underwent a major transformation over this period. Prior to the 1740s, concepts of population were guided by the principle of a static equilibrium that reflected the religious doctrine in which birth and death were the will of God. The fear of depopulation and the related fear of degeneration stemmed from the idea that a period of equilibrium was at an end. Around the mid-eighteenth century, however, population came to be understood as a living organism subject to laws of behaviour, rendering population explicable and arithmetically describable.[85] In France, as Gélis argues, campaigns against midwives were accordingly sporadic and local up until 1730, increasing only after 1750 when practically all of Europe began to address, in one form or another, midwife education.[86]

Viewing midwifery reform on a macro European scale, as done by Gélis, has been useful for revealing grand trends, however, it overlooks the relationship between earlier local developments taking place in cities such as Leipzig and the more (or less) systematic political agenda of latter eighteenth-century territorial governments in the area of health. In Leipzig a connection between

84   Michael Stolleis, 'Was bedeutet "Normdurchsetzung"', 757.
85   Jacques Gélis, *La sage-femme ou le médecin: une nouvelle conception de la vie* (Paris: Fayard, 1988), 69–73.
86   Ibid., 102–9.

depopulation and midwifery had already been drawn at a political level in the mid-seventeenth century. Not reproduction, which was commonly thought to be a static phenomenon at this time, but infant and maternal mortality were considered by contemporaries as the bugbears of society.[87] Although in Leipzig medical officials only began to enumerate – initially in a very crude fashion – infant and maternal mortality in the 1710s, they were conscious of their mal-effect half a century earlier. As we shall see, this linkage prompted a number of reforms in the city of Leipzig that specifically addressed both midwife provision and midwife training and education. As will become apparent, many of the developments to the midwifery infrastructure in late seventeenth- and early eighteenth-century Leipzig conceptually anticipated the measures proposed, for example, by the 1768 Sanitätskollegium.

The resulting preoccupation with maternal and, in particular, infant mortality that we witness in the communications between Council and its medical personnel was not per se the product of a set of progressive ideas and ideals that we have come to term 'Enlightenment' and which sparked off a trajectory of medical modernisation to which we today are heir. The anxiety about depopulation and the desire to do something about it sprang chiefly from prevailing religious concepts of procreation as God's will and the duty of Lutheran Protestants to go forth and multiply. And whilst many of the reforms aimed to improve both the knowledge of midwives and midwifery provision within the city, reformers did not charge forth onto paths untrodden in a crusade of modernisation. They sought instead to reinstate an ideal form of provision that contemporaries felt had fallen by the wayside. Late seventeenth- and early eighteenth-century states, communal governments and the medical colleges were concerned with the equilibrium of the world around them, often content to merely tinker around with existing structures and practices in order to improve the status quo. The concerns that moved the Leipzig Council to regulate and re-regulate – anxieties about depopulation and, more specifically, infant and maternal mortality – were merely echoed in the late eighteenth-century territorial ordinances. Measures undertaken to combat the problems in midwifery – principally targeting examination and training – might have been cribbed from Leipzig's own regulatory documents. The normative discourse of midwifery regulation in Leipzig functioned as a kind of 'best-practice' scenario for late eighteenth-century territorial midwifery ordinances and decrees.

---

87   Seventeenth-century authors on population generally favoured reducing mortality as the key to population growth. See Lisa Forman Cody, 'The Body in Birth and Death', in Carol Reeves, ed., *A Cultural History of the Human Body in the Age of the Enlightenment* (6 vols, Oxford: Berg, 2010), vol. 4, 16.

Midwife instruction and the conduit of medical knowledge

In 1659 the Saxon state passed an electoral decree placing responsibility for overseeing midwifery in the cities into the hands of the Stadtphysici.[88] In Leipzig the Stadtphysicus appointed in that same year by the Leipzig Council was Gottfried Welsch, professor of anatomy and surgery at the University of Leipzig.[89] Welsch, who had worked as a military doctor in Sweden before returning to Leipzig to take his Doctor of Medicine in 1644, also had obstetric form: in 1652 he had published a German translation of Mercurio Scipione's well-known 1596 midwifery treatise *La Commare dell Scipione Mercurio*, reprinted in 1653 and 1671.[90] Midwifery was only one of Stadtphysicus Welsch's areas of medical responsibility. His letter of appointment lists six discrete tasks, the second of which was to 'inspect the midwives and their apprentices, to examine them before their appointment, and to inform them of any necessary items [of knowledge] whether anatomical or other, to give them good advice and to assist them in difficult cases and difficult births'.[91]

Welsch was the first to introduce some kind of semi-formal instruction for the city's midwives, however, he did not seek to revolutionise midwife education. His approach relied instead on the traditional channels of learning and hierarchies of knowledge and seniority between the midwives and their apprentices: he 'instructed' the two eldest midwives in 'various difficult cases [and] in many areas how to handle this and that [situation]', intending his obstetric knowledge to trickle down through the hierarchy of midwives from the most senior and experienced through the middling ranks right down to the apprentices.[92] Read in conjunction with his *Commare* translation – which he nicknamed his 'midwife' – it becomes clear that Welsch desired to introduce (new) knowledge of obstetric matters through the medium of print without bypassing the traditional occupational structure of midwifery. Whilst the book was to function as a 'midwife' (i. e., as a source of information for both apprentice midwives and the general public), it was intended to complement rather than replace traditional training.[93]

88 The city of Leipzig had retained a *Stadtarzt* (municipal doctor) since 1512.
89 Welsch was appointed extraordinary professor of anatomy and assessor to the Medical Faculty in Leipzig in 1644, ordinary professor of anatomy and surgery in 1654, and in 1668 to the highest chair in the Medical Faculty (therapy), see Kleemann, 'Die gerichtliche Medizin', 4–5 (online pagination).
90 Mercurio Scipione, *La Commare dell Scipione Mercurio. Kindermutter. Oder Hebammen Buch*, trans. Gottfried Welsch (Leipzig: Timothei Ritzschens, 1652). For biographical details, see entry for 'Welsch, Gottfried' in Julius Leopold Pagel, (1896), available at <https://www.deutsche-biographie.de/gnd117345814.html#adbcontent>, accessed 6 September 2016, vol. 41, 681 [online version].
91 StadtAL, Tit. (F) XLIV.A.1a, 2r–6v, 'Stadtphysicus appointment (Dr. Gottfried Welsch)', 27 January 1659.
92 Tit. (F) XLIV.A.1a, 'Bestallungen zum Stadt Physicat ingl. wegen derer kreisenden Weiber', 14r–16r, 'Stadtphysicus Gottfried Welsch petitions the Leipzig Council re: earnings', Undated (post 1659).
93 See the introduction 'An den Leser' of Scipione, *Commare*, b–b4.

By the early eighteenth century, women aspiring to midwife office in Leipzig had begun to actively seek out instruction from both municipal and university physicians/surgeons and deploy this information in their bids for office. In her supplication of 1713, Johanna Sabina Netzold claimed to have commenced lessons in obstetrics with Dr Johann Christian Schamberg, professor of anatomy and surgery at the University, who had studied medicine in Leiden and subsequently made a name for himself in obstetrics.[94] Another prospective midwife, Christina Lorend, who was apprenticed to her mother (a sworn midwife), had attended lessons with Dr Benjamin Benedict Petermann (then Amtsphysicus in the Leipzig environs, later responsible for the city's midwives) for six months 'in order to become more skilled [in midwifery]'.[95] The midwife eventually appointed over both these candidates also claimed to have been given instruction by 'a medico in fundamentis artis'.[96]

Of course it would be naïve to think that midwives before Welsch had never had encounters with textual knowledge. Studies of book ownership and readership suggest that literacy levels increased dramatically over the sixteenth and early seventeenth centuries in many regions of Germany due in part to widespread educational reforms in the 1530s and 1540s.[97] According to Michael Hackenberg, book ownership was significantly higher in northern Germany, even amongst artisans and day labourers.[98] The sixteenth and early seventeenth centuries had witnessed an explosion of relatively cheap do-it-yourself literature, in particular in medicine and other areas of interest to women.[99] Midwifery was a particular best-seller. Eucharius Rößlin's legendary 1513 midwifery manual *Der schwangeren Frauen und Hebammen Rosengarten* enjoyed a stupendous European career, undergoing seventeen editions (with one hundred re-prints) in German, translations into Dutch, Danish, Czech and Latin, the latter which was then translated into French, Spanish, English and Italian.[100] Most midwives never soared to the literary heights of Louise Bour-

---

94 See the Council's shortlist of midwife candidates from 28 January 1713 in Tit. (F) XLIV.D.1, 16–43, 'Appointment (Ehrlich)', 10 January–24 July 1713, 22–25.

95 Ibid.

96 Ibid.

97 Rolf Engelsing, *Analphabetentum und Lektüre. Zur Sozialgeschichte des Lesens in Deutschland zwischen feudaler und industrieller Gesellschaft* (Stuttgart: J. B. Metzler, 1973), 38–39; Michael R. Hackenberg, 'Books in Artisan Homes of Sixteenth-Century Germany', *Journal of Library History* 21 (1986): 72–91, 72–73.

98 'Books in Artisan Homes', 75–76.

99 Tebeaux finds that the increase in technical writing for women was related to increasing female literacy. See Elizabeth Tebeaux, 'Women and Technical Writing, 1475–1700: Technology, Literacy, and Development of a Genre', in Lynette Hunter and Sarah Hutton, eds, *Women, Science and Medicine 1500–1700: Mothers and Sisters of the Royal Society* (Stroud: Sutton Publishing, 1997), 29–32.

100 Gundolf Keil, *Neue Deutsche Biographie* (2003), available at <https://www.deutsche-biographie.de/gnd104156686.html#ndbcontent>, accessed 27 September 2016, vol. 21, 752–53 [online version]. On the English career of the *Rosengarten*, see Chapter One of Mary E. Fissell, *Vernacular Bodies: The Politics of Reproduction in Early Modern England* (Oxford: Oxford University Press, 2004), 14–52.

geois (1563–1636), Justine Siegemund (1636–1705) and Sarah Stone (active 1701–1737), all shining examples of highly literate and, in particular, medically literate, midwives.[101] But it seems that many, in particular in the cities, could read and write to varying degrees and would have had the capacity to avail themselves of certain vernacular and popular medical literature.

Thus Welsch's improvement did not necessarily introduce midwives to 'book knowledge', but it did launch a new way of communicating this knowledge. What had commenced under Welsch as a semi-formal, trickle-down instruction had, by 1713, become a well-established, albeit informal, practice amongst aspirant midwives marking a watershed moment for the transmission of obstetric knowledge: it opened up new conduits for obstetric knowledge between women aspiring to midwife office and male medical practitioners. The formalisation of this kind of instruction would not take place, however, until some twenty years later.

Formalising the apprenticeship

Once in office Welsch suggested a further improvement relating to midwife training – the formalisation of apprentice midwives through the creation of the office of Beifrau (apprentice midwives under municipal oath). In the wake of the Reformation, which heralded a particular alignment of medical provision with poor relief, the Council expanded its corps of sworn midwives so that by 1600 they numbered seven, supervised by the most senior midwife in office (known as the *Inspectrix* or *Oberkindermutter*), and superintended by a group of lay sworn wives (*geschworene Frauen*).[102] The apprenticeship, however, remained below the radar of the Leipzig Council until the late seventeenth century.

As in many large European cities, in Leipzig the apprenticeship was the sole means of training available to aspiring midwives at this point in time. Women seeking the office of midwife were required to apprentice themselves to an experienced midwife for anywhere between six months and four years, a practice which also appears to have been widespread throughout other parts of Europe.[103] In Dutch towns, the cost of training in such an apprenticeship

---

101 On Bourgeois, see Perkins, *Midwifery and Medicine*. On Siegemund, see Siegemund, *Court Midwife*. On Stone, see Isobel Grundy, 'Sarah Stone: Enlightenment Midwife', *Clio Medica* 29 (1995): 128–44.

102 On health care and poor relief, see Jütte, 'Health care', 124. On Leipzig, see Thieme and Gerlach, eds, *Leipziger Eidbuch*, 153. The organisation of midwifery in Leipzig will be dealt with in detail in Chapter 2.

103 In London, midwives served as 'deputies' for seven years, although in the early eighteenth century just three years might suffice for obtaining a licence. See Evenden, *Midwives*, 55. In sixteenth-century Nuremberg, the apprenticeship lasted four years. See Wiesner, 'Early Modern Midwifery'. For Germany, see also Labouvie, 'Frauenberuf', vol. 1, 22. In Paris, the apprenticeship was often three years. See Rattner Gelbart, *The King's Midwife*, 45.

was very high and the length of apprenticeship long (between three and ten years), which Hilary Marland associates with a sharp decline in the number of midwives in offices between 1668 and the mid-eighteenth century.[104] In some larger cities in southwest Germany the period of apprenticeship was codified in municipal midwife ordinances in the sixteenth century.[105] Further evidence of contracts between midwives and their apprentices suggests a variety of arrangements. Christine Loytved discovered a brief contract of services from 1685 amongst the Lübeck council records, however, this document only codified the obligation struck between midwife and apprentice rather than any financial details.[106] Eighteenth-century Parisian midwives and apprentices, on the other hand, drew up very detailed formal contracts that set out the terms of remuneration, board and victuals (should the apprentice live-in with the midwife) as well as precisely what and how the midwife was going to instruct her apprentice.[107] The major precondition for becoming a midwife was a woman's own experience of giving birth. Some ordinances even went so far as to stipulate that only women who had borne two or three children should be taken on by midwives as apprentices.[108] In seventeenth- and early eighteenth-century Lübeck only women who had undergone such an apprenticeship were actually appointed as midwives, and apprentices were required to wait until their teacher died before taking over the office.[109] Apprenticeships thus functioned both as a means of transmitting knowledge and skills and of maintaining broader social order within the profession in a society unfamiliar with our modern concept of meritocracy, of which Welsch and his successor must have been keenly aware.

In Leipzig the training of apprentices was left up to the midwives entirely, a situation Welsch felt no longer tenable. In a worried letter to the Leipzig Council in December 1673, Welsch advised that 'One currently has grave concerns', as one of the city's midwives had died and it was proving impossible to find a 'skilled, and diligent person' to take her place.[110] Welsch was clearly concerned that a shortage of midwives might compromise Leipzig's families and the city's population, but the problem also revolved around civic status and political representation, for capable and skilled midwives were something that 'one should certainly have in such a noble, and world-famous

104 Marland, "'Stately and dignified'", 291.
105 For example, in Nuremberg. See Flügge, *Hebammen und heilkundige Frauen*, 395–98.
106 Loytved, *Hebammen*, 71–72.
107 Likely due to the highly commercial nature of midwifery in Paris and the relatively good earnings a midwife and her apprentice could expect. See Rattner Gelbart, *The King's Midwife*, 45–58.
108 Labouvie, 'Frauenberuf', 21.
109 Loytved, *Hebammen*, 71–72.
110 See Welsch's letter to the Leipzig Council from 8 December 1673 in StadtAL, Tit. (F) XLIV.D.1, 'Kindermütter bey hiesiger Stadt betr. ingl. die angenommene Bey Weiber betr. 1673–1756', 1–6, 'Letters from Stadtphysicus Gottfried Welsch to Leipzig Council re: introduction of Beifrauen', 8–16 December 1673, 1.

city'.[111] For Welsch, midwifery – indeed medical infrastructure as a whole – was part of the fabric of urbanity, something that differentiated a great city from a rural backwater. Welsch was not explicitly concerned with infant mortality or demographic statistics, but saw midwives as the key to the integrity of the family/household – the fundamental building block of urban society – as a procreative unit. 'Good' midwives were indispensable to the urban burgher classes, whose honourable status rested upon marriage, household, and children: 'It is at first unnecessary to mention, what and how much value the general city and all honourable married couples place on an expert, skilful, and experienced midwife'.[112] Welsch's solution to the problem was qualitative and pragmatic: He advised the Council to enlarge the status quo within the city walls, which consisted of a *Beÿ=Kindermutter* (a fourth midwife-in-waiting) employed at a lower salary than the three ordinary sworn midwives. In a subsequent letter he suggested remedying the lack of experienced and suitable midwife candidates by forcing each sworn midwife to take on a Beifrau apprentice who, like the midwives, would be sworn into office and receive some kind of remuneration.[113]

What provoked Welsch and the Council to act when they did? We might like to account for this preoccupation with depopulation by offering explanations hinging on extremely high mortality through war and epidemic. Certainly, as some historians have claimed, the 250 years prior to 1648 were an exceptionally war-, famine- and epidemic-prone period which, coupled with the feverish tone of religious zealotry in the wake of the religious schism, produced an 'apocalyptic age' in which all natural and social events were turned into signs and portents of the final coming.[114] But what about Leipzig? Politically Lutheran from the outset, Leipzig's experience of the Counter-Reformation was at an arm's length. It had endured a number of epidemics, not just plague, over the second half of the seventeenth century, however, nothing out of the ordinary.[115] The devastation of the Thirty Years War, the last ten years of which had reduced large swathes of Saxony to wasteland and decimated the population, also played its part in providing a vivid and concrete example of how depopulation could disrupt urban and rural economies.[116] Although

111 Tit. (F) XLIV.D.1, 1–6, 'Welsch to LC re: Beifrauen', 8–16 December 1673, 1. On the value system in the early modern city and the rhetoric of the chroniclers, see Helmut Bräuer, *Stadtchronistik und städtische Gesellschaft. Über die Widerspiegelung sozialer Strukturen in der obersächsisch-lausitzischen Stadtchronistik der frühen Neuzeit* (Leipzig: Leipziger Universitätsverlag GmbH, 2009), 253–59.

112 Tit. (F) XLIV.D.1, 1–6, 'Welsch to LC re: Beifrauen', 8–16 December 1673, 2.

113 Ibid.

114 Andrew Cunningham and Ole Peter Grell, *The Four Horsemen of the Apocalypse: Religion, War, Famine, and Death in Reformation Europe* (Cambridge and New York, NY: Cambridge University Press, 2000), 322–23.

115 According to the summary of epidemics collated in Berger et al., *Vom Aderlass*, 92.

116 Blaschke estimates that at the end of the Thirty Years War the population of Leipzig and its environs had shrunk to one third of its pre-war size. See Blaschke, *Bevölkerungsgeschichte*, 94–97; Beachy, *Soul of Commerce*, 22–23.

Leipzig recovered relatively quickly, trade in the city had suffered woefully, with the income from the Leipziger Waage (weighing and customs house) down from 21,000 Gulden in 1629 to just 6,000 in 1645.[117] Rural areas suffered more long-term ruin: of the eighty farms that existed in four villages near Leipzig, thirty-eight had still not been rebuilt in 1661. Yet war and biblical-scale epidemics were no newcomers to Europe. Scrutiny of baptism already discussed here reflected heightened concerns about the religious, social and political role played by midwives. However, also of importance were novel ideas formenting in the late seventeenth century about political economy and the role of the population therein.

Cameralism, or the theory of statecraft, was the burgeoning political-economic theory in late seventeenth- and eighteenth-century Germany. For the cameralists, stimulating population growth constituted the pivotal mechanism for ensuring the wealth and *Glückseligkeit* (happiness) of the state's subjects.[118] Cameralists aimed therefore to harness the state's population and promote its growth. As the state discovered its strength in the quantity and quality of its population, it recognised the need for regulating the social life of its subjects; areas of everyday life that had previously been private and/or ecclesiastical-moral issues came under the direct scrutiny of the state.[119] Thus reproduction, obstetrics and child rearing became targets of a late eighteenth-century Policey discourse targeting depopulation, known as 'medical police'.[120] In the late eighteenth century cameralists encouraged procreation by lifting the bans on marriage, attempting to rein in infant and child mortality by improving midwifery provision, relaxing legal and social sanctions against illegitimacy and encouraging women to breastfeed their own babies rather than entrusting them to the dubious and dangerous care of a wet nurse.[121] Yet all this discursive 'action' was a feature of the latter eighteenth century.

Early cameralism, as theorised in Germany, was perceived by contemporaries more as a means of restoring the 'essential harmony' of society through economic strategies; these ideas were supposed to function within old tradi-

---

117 Figures not taking into account inflation. Rainer Aurig, 'Betrachtungen zur wirtschaftlich-sozialen Situation in Sachsen im Gefolge des Dreißigjährigen Krieges', *Sächsische Heimatblätter* 6 (1995): 343–51, 348.

118 Martin Fuhrmann, *Volksvermehrung als Staatsaufgabe? Bevölkerungs- und Ehepolitik in der deutschen politischen und ökonomischen Theorie des 18. und 19. Jahrhunderts* (Paderborn: Ferdinand Schöningh, 2002), 413.

119 Fuhrmann concedes that this new-found control was largely theoretical. See ibid., 413–14.

120 The term 'medizinische Policey' was first coined in 1764 by the Ulm Stadtphysicus Wolfgang Thomas Rau in his work *Gedanken von dem Nutzen und der Nothwendigkeit einer medicinischen Policeyordnung in einem Staat* (Ulm: Gaum, 1764). For a genealogy of the term and the discourse of medical police, see Möller, *Medizinalpolizei*, 15–55.

121 On marriage politics, see Fuhrmann, *Volksvermehrung*, 72–107. On midwifery and reproduction, see Möller, *Medizinalpolizei*, 75–80. On how breastfeeding one's own child came to be a patriotic virtue, see Sabine Toppe, *Die Erziehung zur guten Mutter. Medizinisch-pädagogische Anleitungen zur Mutterschaft im 18. Jahrhundert* (Oldenburg: BIS Universität Oldenburg, 1993), 184–89.

tions and respect different local customs.[122] The cameralist state was modelled on the (whole) household: the relationship between ruler and subject mimicked that of the *Hausvater* (master of the house) and his children.[123] 'A Hausvater', wrote the cameralist Wilhelm von Schröder, 'has to plough and manure his fields if he wishes to reap a harvest … Thus a ruler first has to assist his subjects in attaining a sufficient livelihood if he wishes to take something from them.'[124] Cameralism, in particular early cameralism, was therefore all about good management and maintaining the status quo. By 'economic order', cameralists understood maintaining equilibrium through the good management of both the land and its people, rather than the modern state's aim of economic growth and the accumulation of wealth.[125] Welsch's suggestions for midwifery in Leipzig reflected this desire to restore order by ameliorating the population deficit. With the exception of instructing the midwives, nothing he proposed broke with established practices or revolutionised the structure of midwifery within the city.

Pundits writing in the late eighteenth-century were still concerned about Leipzig's high mortality, despite the fact that the population increased by almost one-third between 1750 and 1843.[126] The Leipzig professor of economics Friedrich Gottlob Leonhardi, for example, proclaimed in his 1799 description of Leipzig that the city had consistently experienced an 'extraordinary mortality'. Buttressing his claim with an arsenal of statistics on infant and child mortality, Leonhardi argued that Leipzig's population problem was attributable to the 'poor nutrition and care which the children of the lower burgher classes … and the illegitimate children in particular enjoy'.[127] Popular texts similarly played on the theme of depopulation. In his originally anonymous satirical dictionary of life in Leipzig, Moritz Cruciger stated bluntly that 'the number of deaths exceeds that of births to such a degree that one would like to believe that the city is in danger of dying out in the near future'.[128] Only high levels of migration into the city, he claimed, enabled the city to grow.[129] However, the idea that a city such as Leipzig was particularly prone to mortality was not new and Leonhardi was at pains to point out that medical men before him had grasped the particularly high mortality in the city. As early as 1725, Leonhardi pointed out, the physician Christian Michael Adolphi (1676–1753) had spoken of Leipzig's high mortality as a curse, albeit one

122 Mack Walker, *German Home Towns. Community, State and General Estate, 1648–1871* (Ithaca, NY: Cornell University Press, 1971), 147.

123 Keith Tribe, *Governing Economy. The Reformation of German Economic Discourse 1750–1840* (Cambridge: Cambridge University Press, 1988), 26.

124 Wilhelm von Schröder, *Fürstliche Schatz- und Rentenkammer* (edn unknown, Königsberg: 1752), originally published in 1686. Quoted in Tribe, *Governing Economy*, 19.

125 Ibid., 27; Walker, *German Home Towns*, 147.

126 According to Blaschke, *Bevölkerungsgeschichte*, 140.

127 Friedrich Gottlieb Leonhardi, *Geschichte und Beschreibung der Kreis- und Handelsstadt Leipzig nebst der umliegenden Gegend* (Leipzig: Beygang, 1799), 258–59.

128 Cruciger, *Leipzig*, 186.

129 Ibid.

with geographic origins: impure and unhealthy air as well as its flood-prone, low-lying geography.[130]

Late seventeenth-century depopulation anxieties were not, however, the sole preserve of learned circles; they also loomed large in the consciousness of Leipzig's political and social elite. In 1680, during the city's last major but particularly brutal plague epidemic, burghers in the city founded a number of friendly societies designed to offer mutual assistance amidst death and dearth.[131] One such association, consisting of sixteen Leipzig merchants, was Die Vertrauten (The Trusted), which was inaugurated in 1680 when a group of friends met to enjoy food, wine and a pipe to ward off the plague.[132] The society endured the epidemic and in 1686, at the suggestion of one of its members, turned into the 'Vermehrende Gesellschaft' (a society for procreation) named 'Kind=Tauffen=Kränzgen'.[133] Although over the course of the eighteenth century the society also functioned as a 'bank' to its members, raising considerable funds to spend on charitable purposes in Leipzig, according to its constitution, its central focus was the business of begetting children.[134] Members swore to bear a child every three years or hold a costly and representative feast as a penalty. Particular attention was paid to the well-being of the infant by inventing a new ritual at baptism, in which the wet nurse was given a financial incentive or reward of eight Groschen.[135]

It would be premature to link these associations directly to a coherent, economically motivated political agenda, first and foremost because these burghers saw their procreative activities as fulfilling God's will. Welsch, for example, was concerned about good management, but this goal was infused with religious motivation. Protestantism, which exulted the married state, attached particular importance to the biblical calling to 'go forth and multi-

---

130 Leonhardi, *Geschichte und Beschreibung*, 258.
131 The epidemic lasted over five months, killing around one tenth of the population. Two such associations were the Albertsche Gesellschaft and the Union und Gesellschaft (also known as the XVIer Gesellschaft). See Herbert Helbig with Joachim Gontard, *Die Vertrauten, 1680–1980: eine Vereinigung Leipziger Kaufleute: Beiträge zur Sozialfürsorge und zum bürgerlichen Gemeinsinn einer kaufmännischen Führungsschicht* (Stuttgart: Anton Hiersemann Verlag, 1980), 18–19.
132 Ibid., 21.
133 Literally 'child baptismal wreath'. The reference to a 'well-scented wreath to refresh life that is in danger, And whose smell heals better than an expensive amulet' likened the society to one of the many chattels used to ward off the plague. See the preamble of the society's constitution as transcribed in ibid., 13.
134 Items III and IV of the preamble to the first portrait volume of the society Die Vertrauten, as transcribed in the following. The society also kept exact records of births and genealogical tables. It began functioning as a creditor to its own members in 1695 and, by 1700, it had accumulated around 640 Taler in capital, of which some was given to charitable institutions in the city. See ibid., 15, 25.
135 Ibid., 15; Katharina Middell, 'Leipziger Sozietäten im 18. Jahrhundert. Die Bedeutung der Soziabilität für die kulturelle Integration von Minderheiten', *Neues Archiv für sächsische Geschichte* 69 (1998): 126–57, 136–37; Heide Wunder, *"Er ist die Sonn', sie ist der Mond". Frauen in der frühen Neuzeit* (Munich: Verlag C. H. Beck, 1992), 37–38.

ply'.[136] However, we can see that generation and the imperative to ensure the lineage was an issue on a local level in the politics of the Leipzig Council *and* in the social sphere of the burghers long before it rose to be a matter for medical police in the late eighteenth century. We therefore need to understand the midwifery reforms of the latter seventeenth and early eighteenth centuries as a manifestation of this very diffuse social concern about depopulation grounded in the idea of generation – the 'preservation of our families and progeny' – as a religious rather than strictly medico-political imperative.[137] As Tanya Kervorkian has demonstrated in her study of the combined poor-, workhouse and orphanage of St Georg, built by the Leipzig Council between 1700 and 1704, religion was the guiding principle informing all of the Council's actions in the area of providing for the poor, the destitute and the 'wicked'. So too did it inform the reform of midwifery.[138] Welsch's invocation of an urban utopia in which knowledgeable and skilled midwives were a salient feature, played to a concept of urban governance in which the physical and the spiritual well-being of a city's inhabitants were one, and the protection of the weak and the ill a matter for the common weal.[139] Hence his suggestion to instigate a regular payment for the midwives to boost their meagre income, which he recommended be funded by voluntary contributions from the entire population. For as he claimed, there was no household in the city where the Hausvater and *Hausmutter* (mistress of the house) were not still having children or expecting grandchildren.[140]

---

136 On this and the belief in God's physical involvement in the development of the foetus, see Kathleen Crowther-Heyck, '"Be Fruitful and Multiply": Genesis and Generation in Reformation Germany', *Renaissance Quarterly* 55: 3 (2002): 904–35, 908–15.

137 Quoted from the preamble of the 'Vertrauten': 'Die gantze werthe Gesellschafft / hat durch göttliche Güte mit den Ihreigen d.Leben als ein Beute davon bracht. … Zu dem Ende soll unter uns ferner fortgesetzet werden / Die angefangene Vertraulichkeit, / Doch nicht wie vormahls unter Furcht des Todes, … Sondern unter den Gesegneten, / In einer Ehrliebenden und durch Göttlichen Seegen fruchtbringenden Gesellschaft, / Zur Ehre GOTTES / In Preisung Seiner Herrlichen Güte, / Bey der Fortpflanzung des Menschlichen Geschlechts, / Insonderheit aber in Erhaltung unserer Familien und Nachkommen.' Transcribed in Helbig with Gontard, *Die Vertrauten*, 13.

138 Tanya Kervorkian, 'The Rise of the Poor, Weak, and Wicked: Poor Care, Punishment, and Religion in Leipzig, 1700–1730', *Journal of Social History* 34 (2000): 163–81, 165–68, 77–78. Of course, as a recent collection of essays suggests, religion continued to be a major force in the construction and practice of 'Enlightenment' medicine. See contributions in Ole Peter Grell and Andrew Cunningham, *Medicine and Religion in Enlightenment Europe* (Aldershot and Burlington, VT: Ashgate, 2007).

139 Kervorkian, 'The Rise of the Poor', 166. This late seventeenth-century concept of (sick) poor relief differed in many ways from the concept of poverty prevalent around one century later, which comprehended poverty as a structural phenomenon of mercantile and proto-industrial economies. See Mary Lindemann, 'Urban Charity and the Relief of the Sick Poor in Northern Germany, 1750–1850', in Ole Peter Grell and Andrew Cunningham, eds, *Health Care and Poor Relief in Eighteenth- and Nineteenth-Century Northern Europe* (Aldershot: Ashgate Publishing Limited, 2002), 138–39.

140 Letter from Welsch to Council, 16 December 1673. Tit. (F) XLIV.D.1, 1–6, 'Welsch to LC re: Beifrauen', 8–16 December 1673, 2–5.

The Council did not implement Welsch's ideas immediately and the dearth of administrative records during the office of his successor Stadtphysicus Andreas Petermann, who held the post from 1690 until his death in 1703, makes it difficult to pinpoint dates or assess the individual contribution of Petermann to Leipzig's midwifery infrastructure. Andreas Petermann (1649–1703) was appointed Stadtphysicus in Leipzig following his 'heroic' involvement in the city's plague epidemic of 1680–81. He then settled in Leipzig and continued to practise as a physician with an active interest in obstetric matters until, in 1691, he was appointed ordinary professor of anatomy and surgery to the Medical Faculty in Leipzig.[141] It was in this capacity that Petermann published his 1692 critique of Justina Siegemund's midwifery manual, which the Medical Faculty in Frankfurt an der Oder had vetted and approved. Midwife Siegemund's response was to publish a counter-publication adding to the tension between the Faculty and Petermann.[142]

Petermann's term of office coincided with increased activity on the part of the Council in the area of poor relief in the city. As mentioned above, 1704 saw the inauguration of the city's rebuilt hospital of St Georg (a combined workhouse and orphanage) as well as the formation of a new poor law (*Almosenordnung*) and the establishment of an office (*Almosenamt*) to replace the city's centuries-old Willige Almosen. Plagued by the problem of beggary over the last decades of the seventeenth century, the city had devised its new system of poor relief to distinguish more sharply between beggars and the poor, and to delegate the day-to-day running of the city's poor relief to an administrative unit of municipal officials. According to Helmut Bräuer, the strategy of the new ordinance differed little from that of previous regulations so that the major development was the devolvement of duties to a quasi-professional team of poor relief officials.[143] The new poor law had nothing to say about midwifery, however, as an element of the city's poor relief, we need to view any changes to the status quo within the context of this more widespread concern with organising and distributing poor relief (including medical relief for the poor) in Leipzig.[144] By 1715 the city had in place a formalised system of midwifery apprenticeship consisting of three free-floating apprentices on call to the seven midwives servicing the intra- and extramural city. Soon thereafter the Council began implementing Welsch's recommendations, assigning these Beifrauen to individual midwives and thus formalising the midwife–apprentice

---

141 On Petermann, see August Hirsch, ed., *Biographisches Lexikon hervorragender Ärzte aller Zeiten und aller Völker vor 1880* (6 vols, Vienna: Urban & Schwarzenberg, 1886), vol. 4, 566.

142 On the dispute between Siegemund and Petermann, see Pulz, *"Nicht alles"*.

143 Helmut Bräuer, *Der Leipziger Rat und die Bettler: Quellen und Analysen zu Bettlern und Bettelwesen in der Messestadt bis ins 18. Jahrhundert* (Leipzig: Universitätsverlag, 1997), 62–63. In 1715 the Council increased the number of poor relief officials (*Armenvögte*) from four to seven in order to deal with the city's beggars.

144 'Leipziger Almosenordnung. 1704', transcribed in Helmut Bräuer, ed., *Der Leipziger Rat und die Bettler: Quellen und Analysen zu Bettlern und Bettelwesen in der Messestadt bis ins 18. Jahrhundert* (Leipzig: Universitätsverlag), 133–44.

relationship. Once again, it was the educational infrastructure of midwifery that most concerned the Council.

A 'certain medicum' for midwifery: Benjamin Benedict Petermann

By the early eighteenth century the Leipzig Council deemed it necessary to extricate midwifery from the set of general medical responsibilities usually accorded to the Stadtphysicus and, in 1715, it appointed physician Benjamin Benedict Petermann (1680–1724) as a 'certain medicum' responsible both for the city's pregnant women and overseeing the city's midwives. Benjamin B. Petermann was no stranger to medical officialdom. Having occupied the office of Amtsphysicus of the Amt Leipzig (which excluded the city of Leipzig in its jurisdiction) since 1708, he had amassed a reputation for particular skill in handling difficult births in the Leipzig environs.[145] Like Gottfried Welsch before him, Petermann had published (his father's medico-legal case books, which contained much information on cases of infanticide) and was similarly a keen performer of autopsies and dissections.[146] As the son of former Stadtphysicus Andreas Petermann and brother of the royal physician to the Saxon Elector-King, Benjamin B. Petermann also had medical-obstetric pedigree.[147]

The city of Nuremberg pursued a similar strategy to Leipzig, appointing a physician whose responsibilities included the instruction of midwives in 1715.[148] Other cities followed suit much later; Lübeck, for example, appointed its first salaried *Hebammenlehrer* (municipal midwife instructor) in 1731.[149] Although Strasbourg's Hebammenmeister Jakob Fried was associated with the private maternity hospital that opened in the city in 1728, most of the men appointed to such offices provided largely outdoor care to the community. In comparison to the increasingly large body of studies on the interaction between midwives and male obstetric practitioners within the maternity hospitals, relatively little attention has been paid to the 'birth' of these municipal medical offices charged with responsibility for overseeing midwifery in the early eighteenth century.[150] Christine Loytved's study of Lübeck suggests that

---

145 See also SächsSAL, Loc. 20009, Nr. 3891, 'Anstellung von Dr. Benjamin Benedix Petermann Beim Kreisamt und Landphysicus', 1708–23.

146 Andreas Petermann, *Casuum medico-legalium decas II* (2 vols, Leipzig: Benjamin B. Petermann, 1709), vol. 2. In 1718 he was appointed physician in the hospital of St Georg 'where he could carry out his dissections and instruct the midwives'. See the entry from 24 October 1718 in Tit. (F) VIII Nr. 53, 'Protokoll zum Drey Rathen', 94–95.

147 Another brother, Ludwig Moritz, was a lawyer who had occupied the office of *Landschreiber* (a high-level administrative office) in the Leipzig Council. See Jakob Christoff Beck and August Johann Buxtorf, *Supplement zu dem Baselischen allgemein historischen Lexico* (Basel: Johannes Christ sel. Wittib, 1744), 640.

148 Baruch, 'Das Hebammenwesen', 20.

149 Loytved, *Hebammen*, 96–97.

150 The only study to date devoted to this development in Germany is ibid. On the development of the maternity hospitals and man-midwifery within this particular context, see

the decision to create these offices was not always initiated by the municipal authority. The appointment of a Hebammenlehrer in Lübeck was the result of a five-year-long campaign of supplications, commencing in 1726, on the part of the *Ratschirurg* (council surgeon) Jacob Leonhard Vogel (1694–1781) to be compensated for performing obstetric operations.[151] Loytved concludes that the motivation driving Vogel's petitions related mostly to his personal financial situation; increasing competition between medical practitioners due to drastically sinking population numbers meant that Vogel had to seek new avenues of income to supplement his lagging private practice and the paltry retainer paid by the Lübeck Council.[152] Although the Council granted Vogel permission to receive payment from the city coffers for his operations, it ignored his requests to be appointed as a salaried 'Operateur' until Vogel offered to provide instruction to the city's midwives in 1728.[153] It took another three years and some four supplications for Vogel to finally convince the Lübeck Council of the necessity of employing him as a salaried Hebammenlehrer.[154]

Loytved is unable to find evidence that the Lübeck Council's appointment of a Hebammenlehrer was motivated by either depopulation anxieties or concerns that the city's midwives were not performing adequately, arguing instead that Vogel alone initiated the introduction of the Hebammenlehrer as a means of improving his income.[155] In Leipzig, however, both the prologue to Petermann's instruction and the entry of his appointment in the Council minutes suggest that the Leipzig Council was very much concerned about its population: 'many pregnant and parturient women, also foetuses and small children … have been left to their fate and cast into not little damage and danger to their health and life'.[156] Whereas Welsch had been concerned about holes in the city's midwifery provision principally in terms of a necessity to ensure the integrity of the common weal as fulfilment of God's divine intention, Petermann's appointment, which identified the plight of infants and mothers, had a more concrete target: reducing infant and maternal mortality. In the face of such grave concerns, the Council felt it could do 'no better than to obligate a

---

Schlumbohm, *Lebendige Phantome*, Loytved, ed., *Von der Wehemutter*, Metz-Becker, *Der verwaltete Körper*.

151 Loytved, *Hebammen*, 92–98.
152 Ibid., 92.
153 Ibid., 94.
154 Vogel was appointed in 1731 on a salary of 200 Mark Lübsch (=c. 66 Reichstaler) and Loytved suspects that the new burgomaster, who was the godfather of his fourth child, may well have played a significant role in swinging the opinion of the councillors in Vogel's favour. See ibid., 94–96.
155 Ibid., 98.
156 StadtAL, Tit. (F) XLIV.A.1a, 'Bestallungen zum Stadt Physicat ingl. Wegen derer kreisenden Weiber', 19r–21r, 'Amtsphysicus appointment (Dr. Benjamin Benedict Petermann)', 22 August 1715, 19r; Tit. (F) VIII Nr. 53, 'Protokoll zum Drey Rathen', 68–69.

certain Medicum' to attend poor women for free and wealthy women for a fee.[157]

It would be too easy to attribute Petermann's appointment to the project of human improvement that we call the Enlightenment; a number of studies on various aspects of urban social policy in late seventeenth and eighteenth-century German cities urge caution in this respect. Tanya Kervorkian finds that Leipzig's municipally run St Georg's Hospital, constructed in 1704 to house the indigent and orphans, was conceived and administered according to a 'religiously defined patriarchy' that perpetuated status and gender norms prevalent since the Reformation (at the latest) by deploying Scripture in word and image.[158] In his study of orphans and foster children in early modern Nuremberg, Joel F. Harrington suggests that changes in the circulation of children (in service, foster families, etc.) and the response of the urban authorities to issues of child abandonment did not spring forth from any ideological font, but instead from alternating cycles of supportive and punitive social policy which, with the exception of immediate reactions to crises, demonstrated little practical impact.[159] Similarly, historians have revised the much-touted theory that Enlightenment ideas and ideals were responsible for the abrupt end to the death penalty for child-murderesses in the eighteenth century, arguing instead that this was a matter of judicial efficacy: the decline in both the use of torture and the reliance on the confession as proof of guilt meant that courts had to find ways of punishing individuals for whom guilt could not be established firmly enough so as to warrant the death penalty.[160]

The Council's concern for Leipzig's mothers and infants was not motivated by humanitarian concerns, but rather constituted an extension of the Council's paternalist social policies that strove to uphold the 'common good' and appealed to 'God's assistance' in doing so.[161] To do this, the Council deployed an administrative practice that has been traditionally associated with territorial governments informed by the science of cameralism: the collection of information about its subjects. The gathering of statistical data about the resources of the state had been a trend followed by many territorial governments in the Germanies since the establishment of cameralism as an aca-

---

157 See the entry from 22 August 1715 in Tit. (F) VIII Nr. 53, 'Protokoll zum Drey Rathen', 68–69.

158 Kervorkian, 'The Rise of the Poor', 178.

159 Joel F. Harrington, *The Unwanted Child: The Fate of Foundlings, Orphans, and Juvenile Criminals in Early Modern Germany* (Chicago, IL and London: The University of Chicago Press, 2009), 292–93, 299.

160 Margaret Brannan Lewis, *Infanticide and Abortion in Early Modern Germany* (London: Routledge, 2016), 174–76. See also Richard van Dülmen, *Frauen vor Gericht. Kindsmord in der frühen Neuzeit* (Frankfurt am Main: Fischer Taschenbuch Verlag, 1991), 111–12. Jackson places the impact of a 'culture of sensibility' in England, for example, in the mid-to-late eighteenth century. See Mark Jackson, ed., *Infanticide: Historical Perspectives on Child Murder and Concealment, 1550–2000* (Ashgate: Aldershot, 2002), 88–90.

161 Tit. (F) XLIV.A.1a, 19r–21r, 'Amtsphysicus appointment (Petermann)', 22 August 1715, 19r.

demic discipline in the 1660s at Helmstedt University.[162] Traditional accounts of the frenzy of territorial states for statistics and facts about almost everything between their borders have tended to view the relationship between the state and its subject as a straightforward top-down hierarchy. However, as already discussed, the legislative, administrative and juridical efforts of the early modern states, which sought to regulate a vast number of areas of their subjects' lives, were part of a complex communicative process between the territorial government, government officials and the subjects themselves.[163] The sheer comprehensiveness of early modern Policey regulation necessitated the collation of local information about local circumstances; to carry this out, territorial governments relied heavily on the cooperation of low-level government officials on the ground, the subjects themselves and, as Karin Gottschalk has argued, officials employed by the communes.[164]

We can catch a glimpse of this communicative relationship in action on a local level in Leipzig. The Council decided when it appointed Petermann that it needed to get a handle on births in the city attended by Petermann because it was concerned about infant and maternal mortality in the city. Petermann was to provide regular reports to the Council on his attendance at deliveries, detailing the 'number, appearance, and quality' of each; he did so resolutely over the course of his appointment.[165] It is not evident that anything was done with the information supplied by Petermann and, given that most of the changes to the structure of municipal midwifery had taken place prior to Petermann's appointment, the details on difficult births do not appear to have informed any Council policy. Moreover, the visitation of medical office holders in the Ämter ordered by the Saxon government in 1723 did not affect the city's midwives. The Council was at this time concerned about the matter of illegitimacy and, in 1717, sought to control the problem, ordering registration of illegitimate pregnancies as well as baptised bastard children with the Leipzig Court and the interrogation of female offenders.[166] But Petermann was not employed to deal with such women; his services were destined for the broader community, for the honourable families both rich and poor (at least in theory) who would reap the benefits of his assistance and instruction of the midwives. Rather, the Council appears to have been applying the instruments of governance that, from the mid-eighteenth century onwards, would be a characteristic

162 'Statistik' had acquired an academic context in the 1660s and had since then been an important element in the education of territorial bureaucrats. See Johan van der Zande, 'Statistik and History in the German Enlightenment', *Journal of the History of Ideas* 71: 3 (2010): 411–32, 414.

163 An argument originally advanced by André Holenstein. See discussion in Karin Gottschalk, 'Wissen über Land und Leute. Administrative Praktiken und Staatsbildungsprozesse im 18. Jahrhundert', in Peter Collin and Thomas Horstmann, eds, *Das Wissen des Staates: Geschichte, Theorie und Praxis* (Baden-Baden: Nomos, 2004), 149–50.

164 Ibid., 167–69.

165 See Item 1 of Tit. (F) XLIV.A.1a, 19r–21r, 'Amtsphysicus appointment (Petermann)', 22 August 1715, 19v.

166 Schlenkrich, *Von Leuten*, 113.

practice of the German state: collecting information for information's sake in an effort to know the state of its subjects – in this case the number and type of difficult births in the city – through a form of proto-statistical information gathering.[167]

Although it was the Leipzig Council who ordered that this information be collected, as a medical official of the territorial government, Amtsphysicus Petermann's role demonstrates a reasonable level of interaction between local and state governments. Karin Gottschalk has suggested that the state 'involved the complexity and diversity of local circumstances into its political concept' because it had no other way of governing.[168] And yet in a city as large, as complex and as politically and economically independent as Leipzig, I argue that the relationship of the city to the territorial government was even more nuanced. The Leipzig Council clearly made recourse to emerging techniques of governance such as information gathering on a more regular and more de-tailed basis than could be afforded by intermittent visitations or the reports of the Amtsphysici in their sprawling districts. Leipzig's size and its extensive medical infrastructure made that possible. So as Leipzig drew upon adminis-trative practices gaining popularity amongst territorial government officials and in the burgeoning academic discipline of cameralism, it was in a far better administrative position, not only to put these knowledge-gathering techniques into practice but to do so from as early as 1715.

Petermann was to provide instruction to midwives and barber-surgeons and their apprentices 'according to need'.[169] The examination of the mid-wives, however, remained the responsibility of the Stadtphysicus Johannes Bohn.[170] By appointing Petermann, the Council was not issuing an outright negation of midwives' skills. Whilst the Council's letter of appointment blamed 'partly the negligence, partly the ignorance of the midwives and their so-called Bey=Weiber' – a claim peddled again and again in late eighteenth-century 'Enlightenment' discourses – Petermann's frequent praise of the midwives in his reports suggests that this negative attitude towards the midwives was not omnipresent.[171] It was not the general incompetence of midwives that so con-cerned him but rather the ability of midwives to master difficult births. Under-

---

167 Later conceptualisations of Statistik posited the practice as 'the proper study of the pres-ent state of civilized peoples with governments.' See Zande, 'Statistik', 424.

168 Gottschalk, 'Administrative Praktiken', 171.

169 Care of mothers and supervision of midwives made up the first four points of his ap-pointment letter. The other four points related to medico-legal work, epidemics, treat-ment of poor and rich, and fees. See Tit. (F) XLIV.A.1a, 19r–21r, 'Amtsphysicus appoint-ment (Petermann)', 22 August 1715.

170 Ibid., 19r–21r; Tit. (F) XLIV.D.1, 16–43, 'Appointment (Ehrlich)', 10 January–24 July 1713, 16–26; StadtAL, Tit. (F) XLIV.D.1, 'Kindermütter bey hiesiger Stadt betr. ingl. die angenommene Bey Weiber betr. 1673–1756', 44–45, 'Stadtphysicus Johannes Bohn re: Beifrau applicants', 6 April 1715, 45.

171 See, for example, Petermann's report from 23 January 1716 in Tit. (F) XLIV.D.3, 1–33, 'Hr. D. Benjamin Bendict Petermanns erstattete Berichte wegen schwerer Geburten de Ao. 1716', 23 January 1715–19 October 1723, 1v. Petermann wrote that 'the midwives present did not spare their part of the work'.

lying this focus on difficult births was a growing refusal to fatalistically accept that mothers and infants had to die. As the Council saw it, the solution to this problem lay in the better training of midwives and the employment of a dedicated physician who would be available to the poor for free.[172]

The office was attached to Petermann's person and he continued to occupy his position as 'certain medicum', supervising the midwives and providing the Council with regular reports on the difficult or fatal births he attended, from his appointment as Stadtphysicus in 1719 right up until his death in 1724.[173] It was certainly unusual for the Leipzig Council to permit someone employed by another jurisdiction to hold two offices simultaneously, which suggests further that the care of pregnant women and women in childbirth was considered important enough to warrant close cooperation between the Leipzig Council and the Leipzig Amt.[174] Whilst Petermann did not perceive his 'additional' responsibilities as the pinnacle of his career, it certainly helped him climb the greasy pole of medical offices.[175] He applied unsuccessfully for the office of Stadtphysicus in 1718 but was instead relocated as physician to the hospital of St Georg, 'where he could carry out his dissections and instruct the midwives'.[176] A renewed attempt in 1719 bore fruit. However, the Council was not prepared to allow Petermann to hold both offices simultaneously and insisted that he resign as Amtsphysicus.[177]

The circumstances surrounding Petermann's 1719 appointment are not evident from Council minutes but it is possible that like Vogel, Petermann was instrumental in persuading the Council of the necessity of his appointment. Certainly no one had held such a position in Leipzig prior to this point and this particular office appears to have been attached to Petermann's person[178]. When, in 1719, Petermann was accorded the office of Stadtphysicus by the Leipzig Council, he continued to occupy his position as 'certain medicum',

---

172 Tit. (F) XLIV.A.1a, 19r–21r, 'Amtsphysicus appointment (Petermann)', 22 August 1715, 19r–19v.

173 Tit. (F) XLIV.A.1a, 'Bestallungen zum Stadt Physicat ingl. wegen derer kreisenden Weiber', 29v, 'Stadtphysicus appointment (Benjamin Benedict Petermann)', 1719; Tit. (F) XLIV.D.3, 1–33, 'Petermanns erstattete Berichte', 23 January 1715–19 October 1723.

174 Petermann continued to carry out the broad range of medical tasks associated with the office of Amtsphysicus, such as medico-legal examinations, the examination of other medical practitioners and the management of epidemics.

175 It was not unusual for physicians to begin their career as Amts- or Landphysici (and sometimes military surgeons or physicians) before progressing to either an office of Stadtphysicus and, finally, moving into courtly circles as royal personal physicians. Such a hierarchical 'ladder' of offices is reminiscent of the way professorial chairs were obtained in university medical faculties, where a professor would rise through the rank of disciplines in a strict order.

176 Tit. (F) VIII Nr. 53, 'Protokoll zum Drey Rathen', 94–95.

177 Ibid., 96.

178 The entry in the minutes detailing Petermann's appointment has no occupational title, as was customary for general civic appointments, but was instead headed by Petermann's name. This suggests that, from the outset, the Council did not intend for the post to be a permanent fixture.

supervising the midwives and providing the Council with regular reports on the difficult or fatal births he attended, right up until his death in 1724.[179] Notably, on Petermann's death the Council did not deem it necessary to appoint a successor and responsibility for instructing the midwives and assisting in difficult births reverted to the Stadtphysicus.[180]

Enter the Stadtaccoucheur

When Stadtphysicus Petermann died in 1724, he was replaced by Johann Christoph Lischwitz (1693–1743), who later became ducal physician in Schleswig-Holstein and professor of anatomy and botany in Kiel. Like the Stadtphysici before him, Lischwitz was responsible for examining and instructing the midwives 'ex anatomia and whatever else is necessary for them to know'.[181] And like his predecessors before him, Lischwitz had been selected in part because the Council thought a physician's hand would be 'necessary' in 'difficult births' and 'because Dr Lischwitz is well versed in the theory and practice of anatomy'.[182] Lischwitz's appointment, however, was short-lived, and in June 1731 he was divested of office.[183] Responding in his defence, Lischwitz contended:

> According to the Stadtphysicus=Instruction I am obliged to assist them [the midwives] with counsel. That I have also done, but when I have myself operated *in partu foetus mortui* in the past years, used my [own] hands and spent nights and days in difficult *Casibus*, whereby [I] have carried out the office of a *Medici*, through several prescriptions of medicines with treatment by my own hands ... Thus in such *casibus* I have truly been able to have my troubles paid for by the right of law; considering that the *Operationes* do not belong to the Physicate [the remit of the Physician].[184]

Lischwitz's desire to be remunerated for the work he carried out with his hands reveals a deeper problem in the figure of this 'certain medicum': the social, intellectual and medical-corporate chasm between the work of the sur-

---

179 Tit. (F) XLIV.A.1a, 29v, 'Stadtphysicus appointment (Petermann)', 1719. See also Petermann's twice yearly reports in Tit. (F) XLIV.D.3, 1–33, 'Petermanns erstattete Berichte', 23 January 1715–19 October 1723.

180 Beck and Buxtorf, *Supplement*, 640.

181 UAL, Med. Fak. A01/52, Bd. 01–03, Medizinal Polizei, 327r–33r, 'Instruction for Stadtphysicus Dr Johann Christoph Lischwitz (sent by Leipzig Council to the Leipzig University Medical Faculty)', 1 May 1724, 330r. In his letter of appointment Lischwitz mentioned the appointment of a 'particular Medicus or Accoucheur', possibly a reference to Lischwitz's successor Hartrauff, however, there is no record of this appointment in the minutes of the Drey Rathen. See also StadtAL, Tit. (F) XLIV.A.1a, 'Bestallungen zum Stadtphysicat ingl. wegen derer kreisenden Weiber', 43–44, 'Letter from Johann Christoph Joseph Lischwitz to Leipzig Council', 1 June 1731, 44r.

182 See the entry from 30 April 1724 in Tit. (F) VIII Nr. 53, 'Protokoll zum Drey Rathen', 126–27.

183 See entry from 4 August 1731 in Tit. (F) VIII Nr. 61, 'Protokoll in die Enge', September 1730–12 May 1733, 32v.

184 Tit. (F) XLIV.A.1a, 43–44, 'Lischwitz to LC', 1 June 1731, 43–44.

geon and that of the physician.[185] Although physical assistance was part of his and his predecessors' remit, for Lischwitz getting his hands dirty with surgical obstetrics was not befitting of his station as a physicus. Physicians charged with the supervision of midwives were liminal figures in a medical world that, at least on paper, distinguished between the rights and obligation of medical practitioners in a very clear-cut, status–task-oriented manner. It was not so much the fact that man-midwifery was an unsavoury venture in itself due to the intimacy it necessitated with the female sex, but more so the mixing of the surgical with the art of physic – leaving the realm of advice and instruction and entering the theatre of surgery – that proved perturbing for these actors. At this stage at least, man-midwifery practice in early modern German cities did not afford the illustrious and wealthy career enjoyed by medical men across the channel, such as William Hunter.[186] Lischwitz, whose medical and academic career soared with professorial appointments in Leipzig and, finally, a position as personal physician to the Herzog of Holstein, was prepared to draw the line on the matter of surgical interventions. The Council did not agree that Lischwitz should be reimbursed for his extra troubles, yet it seemed to be aware of the tension between the surgical-obstetric and the 'medical' aspects of this hybrid role. Shortly thereafter, in 1732, it chose to put an end to the liminal existence of the Amtsphysicus/Stadtphysicus and had 'come to deliberate, whether one would like to provide the city with an Accoucheur'.[187]

According to Lischwitz's petition, the Leipzig midwives had ceased seeking his assistance in difficult births and had turned instead to 'the young Handkauff', who was presumably working as a surgeon in Leipzig at the time.[188] And it was this Johann Valentin Hartrauff who, after having 'registered himself for the position and completed several tests', was appointed by the Council as the city's inaugural Stadtaccoucheur on 24 August 1731 with an annual salary of 100 Taler (rising to 150 Taler in 1733).[189] The new post relieved the Stadtphysicus of all activity and responsibility in the area of child-

---

185 Stolberg has shown that physicians certainly learnt practical skills, however, these pertained largely to the realm of diagnosis, prognosis and therapy. Surgery was not the preserve of the physicus. See Michael Stolberg, 'Bedside Teaching and the Acquisition of Practical Skills in Mid-Sixteenth-Century Padua', *Journal for the History of Medicine and Allied Sciences* 69: 4 (2014): 633–61, 660.

186 Roy Porter, 'William Hunter: a surgeon and gentleman', in W. F. Bynum and Roy Porter, eds, *William Hunter and the Eighteenth-Century Medical World* (Cambridge & London: Cambridge University Press, 2002), 11–12.

187 See the entry from 24 August 1731 in Tit. (F) VIII Nr. 53, 'Protokoll zum Drey Rathen', 174.

188 Tit. (F) XLIV.A.1a, 43–44, 'Lischwitz to LC', 1 June 1731, 44r. No biographical information is available for Johann Valentin Hartrauff, presumably a surgeon as referred to initially as 'Herr' and later as 'Dr.' in Council minutes and reports.

189 See the entry from 24 August 1731 in Tit. (F) VIII Nr. 53, 'Protokoll zum Drey Rathen', 173–74. See Hartrauff's report to the Council from 8 July 1733 in StadtAL, Tit. (F) XLIV.D.1, 'Kindermütter bey hiesiger Stadt betr. ingl. die angenommene Bey Weiber betr. 1673–1737', 132–60, 'Stadtaccoucheur reports (Johann Valentin Hartrauff)', 29 November 1732–13 March 1737, 137.

birth and united the task of examining, supervising and instructing the mid-wives as well as carrying out necessary operative intervention in a single and permanent municipal medical office. Its first few incumbents, Hartrauff and his successor Johann Gottfried Breuer were surgeons, however, from 1759 on-wards, all of the city's Stadtaccoucheurs were academically trained physicians with a significant interest in anatomy and surgery.[190] Although it had agreed to create the office of Stadtaccoucheur, the Leipzig Council ensured that it would be in the position to get rid of Hartrauff as well as the office by putting him on probation.[191]

Conclusions

Over the course of the late seventeenth and early eighteenth centuries, the Leipzig Council and its medical officials embarked upon a relatively haphaz-ard and knee-jerk undertaking to improve midwifery provision in the city. Initial impetus for this action centred on concerns about depopulation that were to a great extent religiously motivated, for example, by fears over the proper way to baptise Lutheran infants, or inspired by the biblical maxim to go forth and multiply and the prevailing concept of charity. Not until the very early eighteenth century do we witness a statistical interest on the part of the Leipzig Council and its medical office holders in infant and maternal mortal-ity. However, the conceptual and practical link between depopulation and midwifery was forged in the latter seventeenth century.

The most enduring and 'radical' reform undertaken by the Council was to gradually intensify the supervisory and teaching role of the Stadtphysicus and, eventually, appoint a Stadtaccoucheur, a municipal official devoted ut-terly to the management and education of the city's midwives. All other meas-ures adopted during this period, however, aimed to repair and fine-tune rather than dismantle or radically alter the urban midwifery landscape: increasing the number of midwives under oath in the city, formalising existing practices such as the midwife–apprentice relationship or 'anatomical-obstetric' instruc-tion. With the exception of 'difficult' births, which through the introduction of the Stadtaccoucheur were formally integrated into the emerging field of (male) obstetrics, the radius of midwives' competence and their practice was left largely intact. Competition from male practitioners, so vivid across the Chan-nel in England, was negligible – that is to say that Leipzig's midwives appear not to have pursued complaints through the official channels; there is not one extant example of a midwife accusing a physician of encroachment (or vice

---

190 Subsequent Stadtaccoucheurs and their terms of office in Leipzig in chronological order: Johann Karl Gehler (1759–81/82), Johann Ehrenfried Pohl (1781–88), Christian Adolph Hartwig (1789–91/92), Carl Christian Friedrich Menz (1792–min. 1814).
191 See entry from 24 August 1731 in Tit. (F) VIII Nr. 53, 'Protokoll zum Drey Rathen', 174.

versa) in Leipzig prior to 1800.[192] The general consensus amongst the triage of Council, Stadtphysici and Stadtaccoucheurs was that, with a little bit of improvement here and there, the existing system of official midwifery would prove able to keep the kind of midwives commensurate with the status of the city. On a day-to-day basis it was thus to a great degree 'business as usual' for midwives in eighteenth-century Leipzig.

That the major changes to midwifery in Leipzig pre-date both the era of medical police and, more importantly, attempts to regulate midwifery on a territorial level ought to give pause for thought. This chapter has demonstrated that not only did these reforms occur on a local level, but the kinds of improvements undertaken by the Leipzig Council and its medical officials inscribed in the city's legal codex became a blueprint for later legislation relating to midwifery in all of Saxony. We might characterise the relationship between the state and the city thus: Despite its relative political autonomy, the Leipzig Council, with its various linkages through personnel to the territorial government, hewed closely to the administrative practices and ideas circulating in the late seventeenth and early eighteenth centuries, and put these into action. From around 1750 onwards, the state gathered up the discourses and practices generated in the city of Leipzig and cast them further afield, hoping to bring or reinstate order to the farthest 'backwater' and to educate the most 'ignorant' midwife. Where midwifery was concerned, territorial regulations did not germinate in the heads of a few state administrators, but instead were based upon the concrete example of urban midwifery regulation provided by the communal government in Leipzig. Measures to tackle the problem of depopulation by attempting to control infant and maternal mortality through improving midwife education and the structure of midwife apprenticeships in the city were realised by the first decades of the eighteenth century. It is this primacy of local governance and local solutions to local problems that we need to stress when analysing the relationship between communal authorities and territorial governments before 1800, not just within the context of midwifery but also in other aspects of social policy, as a recent study of school education policy in Saxony has demonstrated.[193]

This chronology and the particular relationship between Leipzig and the Saxon territorial government described here has an impact on how we think about medicalisation: Who medicalised? Who was medicalised? And how?

---

192 There is little evidence of disputes revolving around occupational propriety between these two groups. It is to be noted, however, that differences of opinion between a midwife and the Stadtaccoucheur rarely created a paper trail unless an unhappy client brought the issue of malpractice to the attention of the authorities. Such a case is analysed by Loytved, *Hebammen,* 104–9.

193 Töpfer finds that education policy was shaped largely by local authorities right through the eighteenth century. Even the major territorial ordinances of 1700 and 1773, which aimed to centralise and standardise schooling, were based largely on the exempla from local practice. See Thomas Töpfer, *Die "Freyheit" der Kinder. Territoriale Politik, Schule und Bildungsvermittlung in der vormodernen Stadtgesellschaft. Das Kurfürstentum und Königreich Sachsen 1600–1815* (Stuttgart: Franz Steiner Verlag, 2012), 293–309.

The now 'classical' interpretation of medicalisation as a product of the collusion of an ambitious medical fraternity en route to professionalisation with a state seeking to acquire a greater level of control over the bodies of its subjects presented by Ute Frevert and Claudia Huerkamp has been subject to significant critique.[194] Historians have instead come to think of medicalisation, in particular during the latter eighteenth century, as a process taking place both within and without the arena of governance and academia. One of the early critiques of the state/doctor medicalisation thesis was Franziska Loetz's study of Baden between 1750 and 1850, which stressed not only the gulf between Enlightenment discourse, on the one hand, and medical policy and practice on the ground, on the other. Loetz also argued that medicalisation was more than a mere political process conducted by elites, and entreated historians to consider the role of the 'medicalised' and to think about the process as a 'socialisation of medicine' rather than a 'medicalisation of society'.[195]

On a slightly different tack and taking his lead from Colin Jones' essay on the 'great chain of buying', Thomas Broman entreats historians to disassociate the process of medicalisation from the processes of medical professionalisation and enlightened absolutism. He argues instead that we ought to think about how medicalisation emerged as a product of a new culture of the press and literary criticism that made it possible for the eighteenth-century educated elite to declare its knowledge as a public good.[196] Other historians have caused us to revise our thoughts on the designs and footprint of the early modern 'state'. Mary Lindemann's study of health and healing in the Duchy of Braunschweig, as we have seen, argues that the public health apparatus that emerged during the eighteenth century as a product of a tumult of interests heeded no overriding general political strategy of medicalisation, modernisation or professionalisation. Eighteenth-century medical regulation instead dealt largely with issues of quackery and served largely to demarcate occupational propriety and censure occupational infringements.[197]

When considering 'medicalisation' prior to 1750, we ought to exercise similar caution against projecting an anachronistic concept onto a very peculiar culture of medical legislation, the main aim of which was the reinstate-

---

194 Although Frevert's study of Prussia mentions that the process of medicalisation took place largely on the level of 'explanatory paradigms' and 'norms' that structured the mentality of the various social classes, she argues that this process – the 'rationalisation of human behaviour, its orientation towards binding, designated standards sanctioned by the authorities [that] became part of the body economic' – was directed by doctors and health administrators. Huerkamp's study of Prussia focuses on the professionalisation of doctors as an occupational group, which she argues deployed strategies and resources to drive forward its professionalisation and was instrumentalised by the state. See Frevert, *Krankheit*, 15–16; Huerkamp, *Aufstieg*, 20–21.

195 Loetz, *Vom Kranken zum Patienten*, 317–18.

196 Colin Jones, 'The Great Chain of Buying. Medical Advertisement, the Bourgeois Public Sphere, and the Origins of the French Revolution', *The American Historical Review* 101: 1 (1996): 13–40; Broman, 'Zwischen Staat', 104–5.

197 Lindemann, *Health*, 139.

ment of a traditional social and medical order for the good of the community.
Keeping the equilibrium, not modernisation was the key motivation behind
the steps the Leipzig Council took to alter midwifery provision in the city. In
Leipzig the territorial government played a relatively small role in the changes
that took place to the structure of midwifery – at least in terms of its legislative
activity. And yet, as we have seen, the entanglement of medical officials within
both state and urban municipal structures was significant, allowing for the
flow of ideas and values from one level to the other. Changes to midwifery
provision in Leipzig were nevertheless largely local solutions to local problems. The next chapter will examine will now examine the local structure of
midwifery in early modern Leipzig.

Chapter Two
The Midwifery Landscape

Few women were complete novices when sworn into the municipal corps of midwives in Leipzig. In the seventeenth and eighteenth centuries childbirth was an event involving more individuals than just the mother and medical personnel. Women who gave birth in secret were suspected of attempting infanticide, hence it was important for witnesses to be present when a child was born.[1] On most occasions, however, birth was a festive occasion for the community of married women in the family and the neighbourhood, who would gather to tend the labouring woman.[2] When birth was imminent a midwife, possibly with an entourage of servant and apprentice in tow, would arrive to deliver the child. The number of women present at a birth could vary. Maria Schipgen, a 'persona pauper', gave birth in the presence of only one other woman and the midwife, whereas Mrs Thümler, the wife of a steward, was attended by four women as well as the midwife.[3] During the six weeks following the birth, this group of women would regularly tend the *Sechswöchnerin* (the new mother confined to her house during the six-week-long period of lying-in) and her infant by cooking, cleaning and generally celebrating the birth – festivities known as the *Kindbettzechen*. After lying-in the mother was churched and could resume normal household duties.[4]

The collective nature of childbirth meant that, in addition to the birth of their own children, women in early modern communities had ample opportunity to experience childbirth as an assistant. Thus most married women could claim direct experience of the techniques and the rituals employed by women known in the community as midwives. Maria Elisabeth Plau's letter of candidature from 1760 typifies the prevalent idea that this experience provided the valuable and necessary foundation for the office of midwife:

> I trust myself to carry the office of a midwife's apprentice and have a particular desire to do so, given that I have already borne four children myself, have lived in matrimony for nine years and have been frequently present during the labours of other women and have therefore accrued much experience of what one should do with labouring women during childbirth.[5]

1 Labouvie, *Andere Umstände*, 108–9.
2 As described by Labouvie in Labouvie, *Andere Umstände*, 104–5. On female relationships in early modern England, see Bernard Capp, *When Gossips Meet: Women, Family, and Neighbourhood in Early Modern England* (Oxford: Oxford University Press, 2003), 185–210.
3 StadtAL, II. Sekt. W (F) Nr. 319, 1–27, 'Hebammen. Verschiedene Beschwerden über Rosine Willendorf', 8 May–14 August 1717, 8–10, 18–19.
4 Labouvie, *Andere Umstände*, 198–279; Jacques Gélis, *Die Geburt: Volksglaube, Rituale und Praktiken von 1500–1900*, trans. Clemens Wilhelm (Munich: Diederichs, 1989), 281–93.
5 StadtAL, Tit. (F) XLIV.D.6b, Bd. I, 'Acta, Die Einrichtung der Kindermütter und Beÿweiber betr. de Anno 1757', 56–66, 'Beifrau appointment (Anna Held and Maria Plau)', 26 April–16 May 1760, 62.

Thus the basic criteria qualifying a woman to work as a midwife were: married status, participation in the ritual of female congregation at a birth, and experience of childbirth and motherhood.

Christina Rosina Hempel, the wife of a soldier in the Leipzig garrison, embodied these characteristics but, as we shall see, Hempel's experience of midwifery went further than mere neighbourly assistance.[6] In 1719 Hempel was appointed by the Leipzig Council to the office of sworn midwife. Strictly speaking, this appointment should have provided Hempel with the first opportunity to attend and deliver women independently. Yet both in terms of age and experience in midwifery, it marked an advanced stage in Hempel's working life. Her first foray into midwifery can be traced back to around 1703, when she was forty years old. Over the next ten years Hempel delivered some fifty children, a modest number which nonetheless laid the stepping stone between the duty of married women to provide assistance to neighbours and family members during childbirth and a desire to pursue midwifery in an official capacity. During the latter part of this decade, Hempel managed to 'apprentice' herself unofficially to two sworn midwives before eventually applying for a midwife office in 1713. Unsuccessful, she apprenticed herself unofficially once again to another well-established sworn midwife, Anna Sperling, before finally being appointed as midwife Sperling's sworn Beifrau (a midwife's official apprentice) in 1715, the year that the Council augmented the number of sworn Beifrauen.

Hempel's status as a Beifrau was somewhat illusory, for during this period she worked independently and delivered mothers without the supervision of a sworn midwife. On at least two occasions she attended women whose childbirth was so hopeless that the Stadtphysicus was fetched to extract the dead infant limb by limb from the womb, a procedure known to contemporaries as embryotomy.[7] When she finally obtained a sworn midwife office in 1719, Hempel was sixty years old and could boast some seventeen years of neighbourly and commercial experience in Leipzig. For a further six years she practised as a sworn midwife in the Vorstadt (extramural neighbourhoods) until she secured a much sought-after office in the the Stadt (intramural neighbourhoods), where she worked until her death three years later in 1728. When she died, Hempel had spent only around half of her midwifery 'career' in a sworn office.

Hempel's curriculum vitae exemplifies that possession of a midwife office was not the only way in which women might practise midwifery. In fact, the various informal routes into midwifery made up an integral part of the urban midwifery structure in early modern Leipzig. This chapter will sketch the breadth of that urban midwifery landscape, categorise its various 'official' and 'unofficial' actors and explore differences in status as well as variations in the tasks these women carried out. It will also examine midwife appointment

6   The following prosopographical information is derived from cross-reading a number of administrative documents.
7   Tit. (F) XLIV.D.3, 1–33, 'Petermanns erstattete Berichte', 23 January 1715–19 October 1723, 8r, 16r.

practices as a means of teasing out the kinds of formal and informal criteria involved in becoming a midwife. The final section will attempt to redraw the structure of the midwifery landscape to include all its various participants and reflect on the complicated relationships of dependency and authority that characterised urban midwifery up until the end of the eighteenth century.

Collating prosopographical information from various council administrative documents makes it possible to reconstruct the otherwise invisible careers of a number of Leipzig midwives prior to their official appointment. The trajectory that Hempel's working life followed – sporadic midwife activity followed by an apprenticeship or association with an established midwife and, finally, a sworn office – appears to have been quite common. There were, however, alternate routes into careers within the craft, for example, women could and did work as unsworn midwives and sworn Beifrauen could and did practise with greater degrees of autonomy than the structure of municipal sworn midwifery decreed. Many histories of midwifery have neglected these aspects of 'unsworn' (unofficial) midwifery, perhaps because their activities are not always readily visible in municipal records.[8] Others make only fleeting mention of the types of midwifery women pursued beyond the office. In Lübeck the authorities did occasionally appoint women who had not undergone the traditional apprenticeship, however, Christine Loytved argues that this was an aberrant practice as the succession from apprentice to sworn midwife was more or less automatic.[9] In contrast Claudia Hilpert classifies two groups of unsworn midwives in Mainz, those who worked without a licence for midwives and those who worked in competition to sworn midwives, suggesting that unsworn midwives were probably well-used within the community.[10] Mary Lindemann also finds that unsworn midwifery was widespread in eighteenth-century Braunschweig-Wolfenbüttel and, just as in Leipzig, made up most midwives' pre-office experience.[11]

There were a number of different avenues through which women could practise midwifery, but not all of these were to be found within the structure of official midwifery. The regulation in the cities that appears to give the urban midwife her status and her occupational identity is perhaps a *trompe d'oeil* obscuring a complex landscape of practice that skews our view of midwifery towards official duties and responsibilities, such as medico-legal testimony, serving the poor and indigent, and providing the Council with information on illegitimate or suspicious births. As Eva Labouvie has rightly critiqued in her studies of rural midwifery, it was not merely the local urban authority or the Church that shaped the activities and identity of the midwife, but more so the relationship between a midwife, her clients, their families and the community

---

8   For example, Hampe's and Schmitz's studies concentrate almost exclusively on sworn midwives. See Schmitz, *Hebammen in Münster*; Hampe, *Zwischen Tradition*.
9   Loytved denotes these women as 'Quereinsteigerinnen' (persons entering an occupation through informal channels). See Loytved, *Hebammen*, 75–76.
10   Hilpert, *Wehemütter*, 138–41.
11   Lindemann, 'Professionals?', 184–87.

more generally.[12] Conceptualising early modern midwifery as a landscape enables us to think both vertically and horizontally and to conceive of this urban structure as a complex form. In so doing, it serves to divert part of our attention away from the sworn midwife and towards unsworn midwifery, not as a lesser form of practice but as an integral and, in some instances, officially sanctioned part of late seventeenth- and eighteenth-century urban midwifery.

Sworn midwives

Organisation

Leipzig's sworn midwives made up by far the most numerous medical occupational group in the employ of the Council. By the early seventeenth century the corps of sworn midwives was headed up by an *Oberkindermutter* (senior midwife) and group of lay women, known as *geschworene Frauen* (sworn wives), who appear to have been appointed to collectively supervise the activities of the city's sworn midwives.[13] Such a multi-layered system of female supervision was commonplace in several large cities in the southwest of Germany during the fifteenth and sixteenth centuries. As Merry Wiesner has shown, in Nuremberg patrician women known as *ehrbare Frauen* (honourable wives) were enlisted to oversee the lower-estate midwives. Around the middle of the sixteenth century, however, the Nuremberg Council found it increasingly difficult to find willing volunteers and so replaced the honourable wives with women from the artisan estate and renamed them *geschworene Weiber* (sworn women).[14] A watered-down version of this structure may still have been in existence in Leipzig as late as 1725, where it appears to have been customary for a select group of women to be consulted on their preference for new midwife candidates.[15] Their actual involvement in midwifery, however, does not seem to have extended to consultation in deliveries or medico-legal duties. Nor are they present in the countless midwifery disputes, which suggests that their input was restricted to the selection of new midwives.

    Although not mentioned in the midwife instruction, it had long been customary for a sworn midwife to live and work within a designated part of the city and to draw many of her clients from the neighbourhood in which she

---

12   Labouvie, *Beistand*, 19.

13   There is only scant reference to these women in the extant sources. On the Oberkindermutter, see StadtAL, Straf. Nr. 236, 'Martin Scheiber and Martha Kist', 1613–20, 44r. In 1596 Mrs Cristoff Piemen, 'as in these matters a sworn wife', was called to examine an infant corpse in addition to the sworn midwives. See Straf. Nr. 67, 'Elisabeth Thier', 1596, 2v.

14   'Weib' denoted an honourable woman of lower social status. See Wiesner, 'Public/Private', 80–81.

15   StadtAL, Tit. (F) XLIV.D.1, 'Kindermütter bey hiesiger Stadt betr. ingl. die angenommene Bey Weiber betr. 1673–1756', 83–118, 'Beifrau appointments (Anna Greger and Johanna Veiß)', 22 November 1724–4 September 1725, 116.

lived. In 1728 four midwives operated within the city walls and three lived and worked in the suburban neighbourhoods sprawled in front of the city gates.[16] They were bound to serve the city and were required to first obtain permission from the Council when requested by women in the surrounding countryside.[17] Their number barely increased over the course of the century so that in 1757, the city's corps of sworn midwives numbered eight: five within the city walls and three without.[18]

Workload

Whereas in rural areas the midwife often belonged to the circle of women gathered around the pregnant woman in the weeks before birth to proffer advice on when the child would arrive, in Leipzig the midwife appears to have assumed a leading but less socially involved role.[19] In cities such as Leipzig, the demand on a midwife's services often outstripped her physical capacities, forcing her to economise on how much time she devoted to a mother's confinement.[20] Families, in turn, generally only sent for the midwife when the birth was thought to be imminent. A midwife's schedule of work was erratic, physically demanding and her shifts sometimes lasted days. Anna Stäps, for example, refused to attend one woman on the grounds that she had only just returned from a delivery and had a baptism scheduled the next day.[21] It was not unusual for a midwife already attending one mother to have to organise a 'replacement' to respond to the call for a midwife elsewhere.[22]

Because the skills of Leipzig's midwives (and Beifrauen) were in high demand, determining which deliveries were more urgent and which mother had priority over the other was a task that confronted most midwives (of all sorts) on a regular basis. By the mid-eighteenth century the Leipzig Council had acknowledged the problem of demand and specified the precise circumstances under which a midwife was permitted to leave a woman on her own during labour.[23] Those who acted contrarily received a fine or a reprimand.

16   Tit. (F) XLIV.D.5, 1–12, 'Kindermütter Attestata', 1727–28, 11.
17   See Item 15 of Tit. (F) X Nr. 23b, Bd. XIII, 58r–69v, 'Instruktion Kinder Mutter N.N.', 14 July 1758, 65r. The earliest midwife instruction I have found dates from 1758.
18   Tit. (F) XLIV.D.6b, Bd. I, 'Acta, Die Einrichtung der Kindermütter und Beÿweiber betr. de Anno 1782', 1–8, 37–8, 54–5, 'Stadtaccoucheur reports (Johann Gottfried Breuer)', 28 May 1757–14 July 1758, 1r.
19   Labouvie, *Andere Umstände*, 103–4.
20   This need to deal with a busy schedule and juggle simultaneous deliveries was reflected in the 1758 midwife instruction. See Items 4–7 of Tit. (F) X Nr. 23b, Bd. XIII, 58r–69v, 'Instruktion Kinder Mutter N.N.', 14 July 1758, 59r–61v.
21   StadtAL, II. Sekt. W (F) Nr. 332, 'Acta, Die inn: und vor der Stadt wohnende Wehmütter: und Beÿweiber, auch deren Amt und Verrichtung betr. 1717–1737', 13–16, 'Johann Jacob Gumbiß complains about Beifrau Anna Stäps', 14–19 November 1722.
22   For example, Stäps referred Gumbiß to the midwife Lorend. See ibid., 13–14.
23   Item 4 of the instruction reads: 'She should not leave any labouring person during the birth; however, if it occurs that another pregnant woman demands her assistance at the

The pressure on a midwife's services meant that despite the dictates of ritual and the ordinances, which bound a midwife to a particular mother for the duration of the delivery, her appearance at a birth was kept to a minimum. Midwife Johanna Sabina Raphel was called upon twice during one delivery in 1724. Unable to find a substitute in such a short time and sure that the child was already dead in utero, Raphel was forced to prioritise and decided to leave the woman she was attending in order to assist the other mother.[24] As an example from 1783 shows, if the midwife decided that it was still too early to attend, it was not unusual for her to leave her client in the care of her female attendees. Called to attend the wife of a printer, the Beifrau Dorothea Behnhold examined the woman a few times over the course of an hour. However, after seeing the birth was a while off and that the woman 'did not yet feel the pains of an imminent birth' she left, promising to return in just half an hour. After examining the second woman, who she found to be even further away from birth, Behnhold returned just in time for the onset of the real 'birth pains' of her first client.[25]

At the birth

Once the midwife arrived at a client's house, she set about examining the woman to see how far off the birth was.[26] According to her instruction, a midwife was to go about her work 'willing[ly]' and 'assiduously' demonstrating both 'modest and patient' behaviour towards everyone around her.[27] When the time came for the mother to push, the midwife became active. Erdmuth Dorothea Ulrich, for example, was described as 'insert[ing] her left hand into the birthing parts, the right [hand] onto the stomach of the labouring woman and impell[ing] the [woman] to push with all her power'.[28] Her duty towards the pregnant woman was not just obstetric; it was the midwife's duty to en-

---

same time, so she may, if there is time and no reason to fear danger at the first [birth], also if the permission of the pregnant woman and her kin [orig.] to whom she was first called is granted ... go to the other [woman], examine her exact circumstances, and remain by the woman who requires her assistance the most.' See Tit. (F) X Nr. 23b, Bd. XIII, 58r–69v, 'Instruktion Kinder Mutter N.N.', 14 July 1758., 59v

24 II. Sekt. W (F) Nr. 332, 'Acta, Die inn: und vor der Stadt wohnende Wehmütter: und Beÿweiber, auch deren Amt und Verrichtung betr. 1717–1737', 23–26, 'Heinrich Schütze complains about midwife Johanna Raphel', 1–7 September 1724, 17–18.

25 Tit. (F) XLIV.D.6b, Bd. II, 11–20, 'Midwife Christiana Behnhold is accused of negligence', 26 June–17 September 1783, 17–18.

26 The technical and ritual aspects of childbirth have been dealt with by Gélis, *History of Childbirth*. See also Labouvie, *Andere Umstände*.

27 See Item 1 of the midwife instruction in Tit. (F) X Nr. 23b, Bd. XIII, 58r–69v, 'Instruktion Kinder Mutter N.N.', 14 July 1758.

28 StadtAL, Tit. (F) XLIV.D.1a, 'Verschiedenes die Kindermütter oder Hebammen betr. 1680–1831', 2–7, 'Beifrau Eva Güntz complains about midwife Dorothea Ulrich', 21 February–2 October 1803, 18v–19r. For techniques employed by seventeenth-century midwives, see Schrader, *Memoirs Schrader* and Siegemund, *Court Midwife*.

courage a calm and 'sober' atmosphere in the birthing chamber. It was the midwife who would soothe the mother's fears and provide encouragement during the birth: she was to 'assist the women in labour in their need and pains according to her best knowledge and conscience', not with 'hard words' but by 'diligently speaking to the pregnant woman and explaining with modesty everything that she ... the woman giving birth, must do and necessarily must suffer'.[29] Once the child was born, the midwife cut the umbilical cord and delivered the placenta, which was to be shown to those present as proof that she had carried out her job properly.[30] If the child was strong, the midwife turned her attention to the mother, binding her belly and making her comfortable. Care of the baby was often left to the women present, yet frequently it was the midwife who bathed the child.[31] Swaddling the child was usually delegated to the midwife's assistant, either a Beifrau or her *Wickelweib* (swaddling woman), as was the changing of dressings in the first nine days after the birth.[32]

Baptism

Delivering babies was only one of the various tasks carried out by the midwife, some of which had no 'medical' functions whatsoever but were considered just as crucial by the both the Council and the community. Baptism was the most important of these. Midwives were responsible for both the physical and the spiritual well-being of the newborn infant and its mother. Since the Middle Ages midwives had been charged by the Church with the responsibility for carrying out emergency baptisms and this, more than any medical service, was a major reason why the Church and, following the Reformation, the urban magistrates licensed midwives. In the eighteenth century normal baptism generally occurred within three days of birth. This precluded the attendance of the mother, who was housebound and unable to set foot in a church until her ritual churching at the end of her six-week period of ly-

29 See Item 3 of Tit. (F) X Nr. 23b, Bd. XIII, 58r–69v, 'Instruktion Kinder Mutter N.N.', 14 July 1758.
30 Tit. (F) XLIV.D.6b, Bd. II, 11–20, 'Negligence (midwife Behnhold)', 26 June–17 September 1783, 12–14.
31 StadtAL, Tit. (F) XLIV.D.4, 1–21, 'Dorotheen Sophien Schröderin betr. Wegen Ausgebung Arzneÿ und Beschickung kreisender Weiber', 1722, 1–4.
32 Although the length of time was not specified in the midwife instruction, in the mid-eighteenth century postpartum care and swaddling through the midwife (or her Beifrau) ceased after nine days, as exemplified by a complaint from one midwife about her Beifrau, who refused to visit mothers on the ninth day. See letter from Regina Mend from 24 May 1754 in II. Sekt. M (F) Nr. 670, Bd. II, 'Hebammen. Verschiedenes 1748–59', 22–35, 'Beifrauen complain about Maria Teuhert and midwife Mend', 26 April–24 July 1754. Item 12 of the midwife instruction merely states that midwives should 'diligently visit women who had born their fruit and dutifully tend and care for them as well as the child ...'. See Tit. (F) X Nr. 23b, Bd. XIII, 58r–69v, 'Instruktion Kinder Mutter N.N.', 14 July 1758, 63v.

ing-in.[33] Indeed parents were often absent from the event. Instead, godparents were the main participants and it was the midwife's duty to carry the infant to church and hold it over the baptismal font to be christened.[34] Whereas the Leipzig Council generally tolerated unsworn women active in the obstetric side of midwifery, the task of registering a child for baptism was strictly reserved for the city's sworn midwives. Even Beifrauen, who frequently brought infants to church, were ordered to enter only the name of their allocated sworn midwife on the *Taufzettel* (baptismal certificate), which detailed the child's parents, godparents, and date of birth and which sworn midwives were required to submit to the church warden.[35]

As the numerous investigations into botched emergency baptisms and quarrels at the baptismal font suggest, the competence of midwives in conferring baptism correctly was just as critical in the eyes of both the Leipzig Council and the general populace as was their obstetric expertise. The extent of the Council's investigations suggests that it took complaints pertaining to baptisms very seriously. In 1728, for example, the midwives were reprimanded for not observing the 'relevant *Requisita*' (props and rituals) when carrying out emergency baptisms. This prompted the Council to reissue all instructions, with the new ones warning the midwives to baptise infants only with water and to say the 'Our Father' beforehand.[36] The death of an unbaptised newborn only a few years later in 1733 provoked a full-scale investigation by the Leipzig Council.[37] Moreover, in 1734 the Leipzig Schöppenstuhl (court of jurors) pronounced the failure to baptise a weak infant as 'negligence'.[38] A double baptism or the falsification of names entered in the Taufzettel likewise resulted in an investigation into the conduct of a midwife.[39] As discussed in Chapter One, baptism had been one of the battlegrounds of the era of confessionalisation and it continued to be a practice caught in the crossfire of doctrinal difference that pushed the stakes high for all involved in issuing the sacrament. In post-1648 Leipzig, the way one baptised or participated in a baptism had implications not only for the soul of the child, but also for the Protestant faith more generally. As we will see further on in this section, baptism was also an important financial factor for midwives.

33   For studies of the ritual and festivities of baptism as well as churching in a rural context, see Labouvie, *Andere Umstände*, 218–59. For the English context, see David Cressy, *Birth, Marriage and Death: Ritual, Religion, and the Life-Cycle in Tudor and Stuart England* (Oxford: Oxford University Press, 1997); 'Purification, Thanksgiving and the Churching of Women in Post-Reformation England', *Past and Present* 141 (1993): 106–46.
34   Tit. LX.B (F) Nr. 7, 250, 'Baptismal ordinance (proposal)', 1669; Labouvie, *Beistand*, 66–77.
35   StadtAL, Tit. (F) XLIV.6b, Bd. II, 'Die Einrichtung der Kindermütter und Beÿweiber betr. de Anno 1782', 41, 'Directive from Leipzig Council on baptism', c. 1785 (undated).
36   II. Sekt. W (F) Nr. 332, 70–73, 'LC vs midwives re: emergency baptisms', 28 June 1728.
37   II. Sekt. R (F) Nr. 442, 1–14, 'Hebamme Rein Nottaufe', 23 December 1733–08 January 1734.
38   See the Schöppenstuhl's pronouncement from 28 December 1734 in ibid., 12–13a.
39   II. Sekt. M (F) Nr. 760, Bd. I, 1–22, 'Wehmutter (Mend)', 15 March 1742–13 May 1743; II. Sekt. S (F) Nr. 2013, 'Acta (Stahlin)', 25 January–5 March 1774.

Policing illegitimacy

Sworn midwives were also supposed to act as a conduit of information on immoral or criminal female behaviour between clientele and the council authorities. Censuring aberrant female sexuality was an important task in the eyes of both the Church and the local authorities. In Saxony, as in most early modern societies, abortion and infanticide were capital crimes and sworn midwives were expected to report women they suspected of carrying out an abortion to the Leipzig Council without delay. Yet a sworn midwife's moral radar was supposed to pick up more than just individual criminal acts; the Council used her to police females in general. Although she was not required to register any 'untimely fruits' (foetuses less than four-and-a-half months old) with the *Leichenschreiberei* (municipal burial registry in Leipzig), her instruction stipulated that 'she should nevertheless inform Your City Court [of law] because of suspicious women'.[40] The sworn midwife was likewise to monitor the matter of paternity and maternity. Should she discover that 'persons have been wrongly stated as parents of the children ... or if something else suspicious should occur, [the midwife should] report this immediately to Your Honourable and Most Wise Council and its court of law.'[41] However, this policing role was not omnipresent and did not necessarily shape the relationship that midwives had to the married and honourable women in the community.

Historians have been quite ambivalent about the role of the midwife, with much of the debate revolving around whether or not the she was a figure of social-moral control or the leader of a subversive, female collective. Ulinka Rublack, for example, accounts for the increasing importance of midwives in the Germanies over the sixteenth and seventeenth centuries as the result of their role in policing female sexual deviance.[42] Studies using court records highlight the tension between the midwife as a figure of social and moral control, on the one hand, and assistance and collusion, on the other.[43] Ulrike Gleixner argues, for example, that the midwife was simultaneously 'good' and 'bad' because the various duties she carried out could be sorted into either one or the other category.[44] Laura Gowing also associates the midwife with this dual role, however, she sees a clear association between the role of the midwife and the social status of the woman she was dealing with; the everyday social relations (and tensions) between women were played out in the birth chamber, with only poor, itinerant mothers subject to punishment.[45]

---

40 The clause about registering 'untimely fruits' was repeated in 1770 after fears circulated about secret burials. See Tit. (F) X Nr. 23b, Bd. XIII, 58r–69v, 'Instruktion Kinder Mutter N.N.', 14 July 1758, 66v (Item 20).

41 See Item 22 of ibid., 67r.

42 Rublack, 'Public Body'.

43 Otto Ulbricht, *Kindsmord und Aufklärung in Deutschland* (Munich: R. Oldenbourg, 1990), 135–42, esp. 40.

44 Gleixner, 'Hebammen als Amtsfrauen', 96.

45 Laura Gowing, *Common Bodies: Women, Touch and Power in Seventeenth-Century England* (New Haven, CT: Yale University Press, 2003), esp. 149–76.

What was perhaps true for the seventeenth century, however, did not necessarily hold through the eighteenth. As Chapter Four will show, despite the continuing regulatory rhetoric of policing, the changing social and economic circumstances of the city meant that over the course of the eighteenth century, midwives and their apprentices became increasingly dependent on the fruits of deviant female sexuality as a source of income. Although illegitimacy was frowned upon in eighteenth-century Germany, it was not in itself a crime and could be dealt with in a variety of ways. At best, paternity could be established and the father coerced into marriage. However, many unwed pregnant women chose to give birth in one of the many lying-in houses run by women (and midwives) in the Vorstadt, sending the child to be raised by wet nurses in the country and either returning to service or taking up a wet nurse position themselves. What had emerged in the sixteenth and early seventeenth centuries as a problem of morals appears to have metamorphosed into a largely social problem that was solved, in turn, on a very local political level.

Hiding an illicit pregnancy remained a criminal action. The sworn midwife assumed a particular aura of authority when she was dealing with single women suspected of concealing a pregnancy or birth, most frequently domestic servants. When families discovered that their servant had already given birth but were unable to find an infant, most called for a sworn midwife.[46] Upon arrival the sworn midwife assumed the task of interrogating the woman suspected of killing her newborn child and looking for signs of a birth. Threatening to physically examine a woman was often the only means of duress a midwife had to apply in order to elicit a confession.[47] As in the case of Justine Stieler, once the midwife had taken care of the dead infant and its mother – in this case washing the dead infant and removing a piece of the placenta from the mother's womb – the midwife was expected to refer the matter without delay to the authorities, thereby setting an official investigation in motion.[48]

However, it is important to put these duties into perspective. Infanticide was a relatively rare phenomenon, even in a large city like Leipzig, with rarely even one charge per year.[49] Historians generally agree that there was a general increase in infanticide prosecutions from the 1570s into the first decades of the sixteenth century, and that the concern about the crime led to more detailed interrogations, longer trials and more convictions with the death penalty.[50] Certainly the legal framework introduced by the criminal codex govern-

46   See, for example, StadtAL, Straf. Nr. 654, 1–97, 'Maria Bohn, Johann Christoph Heÿden-
      reicher and Maria Schacher', 1711.
47   See Straf. Nr. 709, 1–112, 'Justina Elenora Stieler', 1741.
48   Ibid., 1r–v.
49   Data for Nuremberg bears this out, with a total of 58 cases of known infanticide between
      1520 and 1699. See Harrington, *The Unwanted Child*, 289.
50   Lewis, *Infanticide*, 51–56. A similar shift towards criminalising illegitimacy occurred in
      France, where, from the mid-sixteenth century onwards, illegitimacy cases came to be
      tried in criminal courts and concealment of an illegitimate pregnancy was automatically
      assumed as murder if the child died. See Cathy McClive, *Menstruation and Procreation in
      Early Modern France* (Farnham, Surrey and Burlington, VT: Ashgate, 2015), 24.

ing the Holy Roman Empire in the 1530s, the Constitutio Criminalis Carolina, had prompted this increased criminalisation of illegitimacy, yet the problem was largely one of perception: contemporaries felt that child murder was all around them and the rapidly developing culture of popular print, with its woodcuts and wild stories of monsters and witches devouring and harming children made the problem culturally larger than the metrics would have us believe.[51] Illegitimacy, not infanticide, was surely more of a numerical problem; the data for Nuremberg suggest that whilst illegitimacy rose substantially over the first half of the seventeenth century, it still only made out 4 per cent of total births in 1665.[52] And so we can safely assume that the policing function played by midwives was a relatively small aspect of a midwife's bread-and-butter work, although the psychological impact of these duties was perhaps disproportionately greater.

Medico-legal duties

The Leipzig Council also relied on its sworn midwives as medico-legal experts, as detailed in Section 21 of the 1758 instruction.[53] The practice of deploying midwives as medico-legal experts went back to the Constitutio Criminalis Carolina of 1532, which codified the use of torture in criminal trials throughout the Holy Roman Empire and enshrined the role of surgeons and midwives in reading the bodies of the dead and providing legal evidence of cause of death.[54] Although during the early eighteenth century many prominent legal scholars (some from Leipzig) began to attack the use of midwives as legal experts, midwives continued to be deployed by the Leipzig Council until the latter third of the eighteenth century.[55]

---

51 Lewis, *Infanticide*, 82–114. See also Chapter Three of Lyndal Roper, *Witch Craze. Terror and Fantasy in Baroque Germany* (New Haven and London: Yale University Press, 2004), 69–81.

52 Harrington finds no correlation between infanticide and illegitimacy rates. See Harrington, *The Unwanted Child*, 289. Drawing on various demographic studies, Wilson finds that at least 90% of births in seventeenth-century England were legitimate. See Adrian Wilson, *Ritual and Conflict: The Social Relations of Childbirth in Early Modern England* (Farnham: Ashgate, 2013), 7.

53 'When the Leipzig Council or the civic or territorial courts or the district office of Leipzig finds it necessary to examine female persons, she should go willingly and without delay to wherever said authorities demand, carry out the examination conscientiously, loyally according to her obligations, also without deference to the person, and report [her findings to the court]'. See Tit. (F) X Nr. 23b, Bd. XIII, 58r–69v, 'Instruktion Kinder Mutter N.N.', 14 July 1758, 66–67.

54 On the Carolina more generally, see John H. Langbein, *Prosecuting Crime in the Renaissance: England, Germany, France* (Cambridge, MA: Harvard University Press, 1974). On legal medicine more specifically, see Fischer-Homberger, *Medizin vor Gericht*, 53–57.

55 *Medizin vor Gericht*, 59–64. The last trial recorded in the Leipzig City Court's Strafakten during which a midwife was called upon to examine a female suspect is from 1769: Ristu Straf. Nr. 735 'Maria Elißabeth Peinick', 1769, 1r–v.

Once the Council heard of a suspected infanticide, it sent one or more sworn midwives to examine the woman and inspect the room.[56] If the suspect had already been incarcerated, the midwives were sent to the gaol to carry out the same procedure.[57] Difficulties encountered in adjudicating the 'evidence' called, even in 1749, for more midwives: a total of five midwives were sent to inspect the bedclothes of Regina Rademann on two occasions.[58] As previously ascertained, these types of situations were rare. As such, the type of interaction between midwife and mother in this context can hardly be representative of the type of relationship that a legitimate mother had with her midwife. Yet these extreme circumstances were the extension of a constant vigilance expected of the sworn midwife towards suspicious female persons, who were considered most at risk of aborting their pregnancies or murdering their newborn infants. And, if a midwife failed to provide the Council with all the information at her disposal, this constituted sufficient grounds for labelling her activities negligent. In 1769, for example, the Leipzig Schöppenstuhl lambasted the sworn midwife Mrs Zschach for not mentioning the whereabouts of a dead infant although this was known to her, and used this act of 'negligence' to denigrate her reputation and trustworthiness.[59] However, in the majority of cases surviving in the archives of the criminal court in Leipzig, the sworn midwives appear to have obliged, not hindered the cogs of justice, dutifully examining women and relaying their findings to the Leipzig Council.

Remuneration

Sworn midwives had been on the payroll of the Leipzig Council since the mid-sixteenth century at least.[60] Mid-eighteenth-century midwives received an annual allocation of 9½ Reichstaler, naturalia in the form of firewood and grain, and, for the midwives in the city, free accommodation in one of the Council's houses within the city walls (see Table 1).

---

56 In many instances, midwives were amongst the first to be called upon by the public and often notified the Council themselves. See also Erwin Ackerknecht, 'Midwives as Experts in Court', *Bulletin of the New York Academy of Medicine* 52: 10 (1976): 1224–28. For France, see Cathy McClive, 'Bleeding Flowers and Waning Moons: A History of Menstruation in France c. 1495–1761' (PhD thesis, Warwick University, 2004), 206–49; 'Blood and Expertise'. Although practices differed from place to place, the centrality of the midwife was a common theme. In the north of England, for example, women suspected of infanticide prior to 1750 were held by a 'jury of matrons' until the midwife arrived to conduct a physical examination. See Mark Jackson, 'Developing Medical Expertise: Medical Practitioners and the Suspected Murders of New-Born Children', in Roy Porter, ed., *Medicine in the Enlightenment* (Amsterdam: Rodopi, 1995), 147.

57 See, for example, StadtAL, Straf. Nr. 708, 'Johanna Margaretha Defer and Samuel Andreas Reinheckel', 1741.

58 Straf. Nr. 715, 'Regina Rademann', 1749.

59 Straf. Nr. 735, 'Maria Elisabeth Peinick', 1769, 46–47.

60 Thieme and Gerlach, eds, *Leipziger Eidbuch*, 153.

Table 1 Annual remuneration of sworn midwives and sworn Beifrauen (1758)

Annual remuneration from Leipzig Council (1758)	Sworn midwives	Sworn Beifrauen
Quarterly salary (*Quatembergeld*)	9½ Reichstaler* (2 Reichstaler, 12 Groschen per quarter)	2.63 Reichstaler (21 Groschen per quarter)
Grain (*Korn*)	1 *Scheffel* (bushel), 1 × ¼ Scheffel and 1 × ⅓ Scheffel (= c. 164 litres)	2 Scheffel, 1 × ¼ Scheffel and 1 × ⅓ Scheffel (= c. 267 litres)
Firewood (*Reißholz*)	1 *Schock* (= 7 ½ Reichstaler)	3 Schock (= 22 ½ Reichstaler)
Lodgings	Free apartment in the midwife house in Stadtpfeiffergäßgen (only for midwives stationed within the city walls). The eldest midwife has rights to largest and most comfortable apartment.	Beifrauen working within city walls receive accommodation in Stadtpfeiffergäßgen for which they pay rent of 12 Reichstaler per annum.

* Species Reichstaler (the minted coin in everyday use), not the virtual monetary unit ('Reichstaler') used in trade and banking throughout the German territories. Around 1700 one Species Reichstaler was equivalent of 32 'good' Groschen. For conversion rates used, see Anton Kirchhofer et al., Pierre Marteau webspace, entry on 'Holy Roman Empire: Money' (3 April 2008 (last page update)), available at <http://pierre-marteau.com/wiki/index.php?title=Money_(Holy_Roman_Empire)#Sachsen.2FMei.C3.9Fen_.28Saxonia.29>, accessed 20 October 2016.

Sources: StadtAL, Tit. (F) X.23b, vol. XIII, 'Instruktionen 1676–1800', 'Instruktion vor die Kinder Mutter N.N.', 14 July 1758, 67v–68r; Ibid, 'Instruktion für die Beÿfrau N.N.', 14 July 1758, 76r–76v; StadtAL, Tit. (F) XLIV.D.6b, vol. I, Acta, 'Die Einrichtung der Kindermütter und Beÿweiber', 307.

In comparison to other medical practitioners in communal employ, midwives were paid rather poorly; the barber-surgeon appointed to treat those reliant on poor relief earned 50 Reichstaler per annum and the Stadtaccoucheur some 200 Reichstaler.[61] To a certain extent this reflected the lower costs midwives incurred in treating their clients; surgeons and physicians were expected to pay for their equipment as well as the medicines, clysters, etc. they prescribed to their patients on alms out of their own salary.[62] Like the barber-surgeon, the salary sworn midwives received from the commune was intended as compensation for attending the city's alms recipients *pro bono*. However, this salarial discrepancy marked first and foremost the lower status of midwifery

61 StadtAL, Tit. (F) X Nr. 23a, 'Instruktionsbuch 1697–1732', 245–46, 'Instruktion des Chirurgi beÿ dem Allmosen=Ambte alhier', c. 1714; Tit. (F) X 23b, Bd. X, 'Instruktionen (1676–nach 1800)', 5–7, 'Instruktion für den Accoucheur', 1788–92. Such salary discrepancies were standard in most towns and cities. See, for example, Gabler, 'Hebammenwesen', 61.

62 The poor relief surgeon, for example, could only with some difficulty recoup expenses incurred over and above his salary.

and the women who inhabited the post: it was a highly tangible display of the social-economic logic of the Ständegesellschaft.

We therefore need to think about the salaries of medical officials in the seventeenth and eighteenth centuries as a social practice rather than mere reflections of the economic value of an individual or an occupational group. In Leipzig, as elsewhere in Germany, neither this salary nor allocations of naturalia had any bearing on real living costs; they were not regularly adjusted to match inflation. The sworn midwives' salaries, for example, remained stagnant between 1715 and 1779.[63] To give a rough idea of the real wage value, in 1724 a cow cost 9 Reichstaler, or roughly the amount a midwife received annually in cash. In 1762, 15 eggs would have cost around 3 Groschen and 3 Pfennig, and one (Saxon) bushel[64] of rye would have set a midwife back 21 Groschen and 6 Pfennig, or roughly two thirds of a Reichstaler.[65] A midwife's salary was certainly not sufficient to support a woman and her family, or even supplement familial income. Thus the cash element of a midwife's salary was a token amount which functioned as a symbol of the midwife's lowly place in the social structure of the city. Beifrauen, who were subordinate to the midwives, received only a fraction of the midwife salary, commensurate with their lower status in the midwifery hierarchy. Of far greater everyday value to many midwives were the rations of grain and firewood together with the free accommodation in the house in Stadtpfeiffergäßgen. These provided inflation-resistant basics that helped to alleviate everyday hardship.

A midwife's 'real' earnings came from the fees she charged her regular clients as well as the gifts offered by women and their families, in particular at baptism. Both the family and the godparents were expected to provide the midwife with a gift (either cash or material) at a baptism. Whereas the midwife's fee was fixed by the Leipzig Council, the value of the gift depended on the status and wealth of a midwife's client. In 1774 a midwife could demand one Reichstaler as her *Kindermutterlohn* (midwife's fee) and a further Reichstaler from unwed women she accommodated in her home during confinement: in that year the midwife Juliana Müller was accused of overcharging a woman, but by quoting these rates, managed to escape a fine for misconduct.[66] An electoral mandate on midwifery from 1818, designed to provide guidelines for fee schedules throughout the whole of Saxony, gives us a rough idea of what urban midwives could expect from families of modest means

63   Compare the following: StadtAL, Tit. (F) X.23a, Bd. III, 'Instruktionen (1676–nach 1800)', 257–59, 'Instruction für die geschwornen Beÿweiber', 16 April 1715; Tit. (F) X 23c, Bd. I, 'Eine Sammlung von Instruktionen [18th Century]', 74–79, 'Instruction E. E. Hochweisen Raths zu Leipzigk für die Beyfrau Rahel Reginen Pötschin', 1 April 1779.

64   A bushel in Saxony was not the same as a bushel elsewhere. Here equivalent to approximately 103 litres.

65   For conversions, see Kirchhofer et al., Pierre Marteau webspace, entry on 'Holy Roman Empire: Money'.

66   StadtAL, Tit. (F) XLIV.D.6b, Bd. I, 'Acta, die Einrichtung der Kindermütter und Beÿweiber', 158–285, 'Various complaints about the Beifrauen and midwives in Stadtpfeiffergäßgen', 14 July 1772–1810, 189–92.

which did not count as 'poor' (see Table 2). Women of social and economic means paid the midwife significantly more, and miserly clients ran the risk of angering the midwife if they did not pay a fee commensurate with their social status. In 1717, for example, Rosina Willendorf complained bitterly about receiving 'only four lousy Taler' from a merchant's wife. Accustomed to receiving 10 Taler from a lady of such wealth and standing, Willendorf was supposedly overheard spluttering spitefully to her fellow midwives: 'The slack cunt, her body looks like a smoked pig[!]'[67]

Table 2 Electoral fee schedule for midwives (1818)

Service *	Fee
Natural birth	1 Reichstaler
Swaddling	16 Groschen
Unnatural birth (presence of Accoucheur necessary)	1 Reichstaler and 8 Groschen
Resuscitation of an infant	1 Reichstaler
Setting a clyster (woman lying in)	2 Groschen
Setting a clyster (infant)	1 Groschen
Setting a clyster (other, non-pregnant women)	4 Groschen
Inserting a *Mutterkranz*** (uterine pessary)	8 Groschen

* The mandate advised that this fee schedule was to be used as a guideline only and that customary fees in each locality should remain as they were.
** A 'Mutterkranz' was a wooden, rubber or metal pessary that was inserted into the vagina either temporarily or permanently in the case of a uterine prolapse or incontinence. It had to be changed regularly, generally by a midwife. See entry for 'Mutterkranz' in Krünitz, *Oekonomische Encyklopädie*, vol. 99, 338–69.

Sources: StadtAL, Tit. (F) LX.A.18a, 'Churfürstliche Mandate 1768–1816', 'Mandat, die Erlernung und Ausübung der Geburtshülfe in hiesigen Landen betreffend. & Allgemeine Hebammenordnung', 2 April 1818, 106r.

The earnings of the sworn midwives working in the Vorstadt were much slimmer as these neighbourhoods were typically less affluent.[68] Urban centres throughout Saxony – in particular the Vorstadt communities – were not just affected by greater numbers of itinerant workers but also high levels of so-called *Hausarmut* (poverty experienced by settled residents) amongst artisans, whose level of production was often so low that it was nigh impossible for the

---

67   II. Sekt. W (F) Nr. 319, 1–27, 'Beschwerden (Willendorf)', 8 May–14 August 1717, 15.
68   In the sixteenth century, Feige found that around three-quarters of Leipzig's population with earnings below 200 Gulden per annum (roughly 14% of the taxable population) resided in the Vorstadt. See Wolfgang Feige, 'Die Sozialstruktur der spätmittelalterlichen deutschen Stadt im Spiegel der historischen Statistik – mit besonderer Berücksichtigung der niederen Schichten der Bevölkerung und mit einem Exkurs in das Leipzig des 16. Jahrhunderts' (Dissertation, Karl-Marx-Universität Leipzig, 1965), 219–44.

the household to accumulate wealth.[69] And working in the Vorstadt also brought with it additional costs. In order to pass through the city gates at night the gatemen often exacted a toll, which the midwives frequently had to pay out of their own pockets.[70] Hence, as we shall see here and in the following chapters, the city walls proved a major economic divide which midwives and Beifrauen alike were constantly trying to breach as well as defend; their livelihood depended upon both tactics.

Beifrauen (sworn apprentices)

As discussed in Chapter One, the Leipzig Council introduced sworn Beifrauen in the early eighteenth century to ensure a steady supply of skilled midwives. The institutionalisation of the apprentice midwife was a feature of the larger German cities. In Frankfurt am Main, for instance, one midwife-in-waiting and a further three apprentices, known as *Beyläuferinnen*, held office at the end of the seventeenth century, albeit without any regular remuneration.[71] In the much smaller and more provincial city of Braunschweig only one woman, known as a *Wärmefrau* (warming woman), occupied a comparable office.[72] As noted in the previous chapter, in Leipzig a fourth midwife known as the *Beÿ=Kindermutter* (an auxiliary midwife) had been appointed around 1673. However, the idea of having a widespread system of apprentices-in-waiting appears not to have been pursued with any vigour until four decades later.[73]

   Prior to 1715 the Leipzig Council generally appointed lay women directly to the office of sworn midwife, except when candidates had practised as sworn midwives in other localities, as was the case with Euphrosina Opitz of Wurzen and Catharina Ehrlich of Eilenburg.[74] Certainly none of the candidates who applied in July 1713 had previously held a Beifrau office, although almost all of them purported to have some level of experience in midwifery acquired through other, informal channels. Christina Hempel, for example, had as-

69   Simone Stannek, 'Armut und Überlebensstrategien von Frauen im sächsischen Zunft-handwerk des 16.–18. Jahrhunderts', in Katharina Simon-Muscheid, ed., *"Was nützt die Schusterin dem Schmied?". Frauen und Handwerk vor der Industrialisierung* (Frankfurt am Main: Campus, 1998), 100.

70   StadtAL, II. Sekt. M (F) Nr. 670, Bd. III, 'Hebammen. Verschiedenes über die Kinder-mütter, Wehemütter und Beifrauen (1756–69)', 96–98, 'Beifrauen complain about mid-wife Dorothea Westphal', 29–30 March 1769, 96.

71   Gabrielle Robilliard, 'Midwives in Early Modern Frankfurt am Main c. 1500–1700: Or-ganisation, Socio-Economic Status and Work Identity' (MPhil thesis, University of Cam-bridge, 2004), 37.

72   Lindemann, 'Professionals?', 183–84.

73   Tit. (F) XLIV.D.1, 1–6, 'Welsch to LC re: Beifrauen', 8–16 December 1673, 6.

74   StadtAL, Tit. (F) XLIV.D.1, 'Kindermütter bey hiesiger Stadt betr. ingl. die angenom-mene Bey Weiber betr. 1673–1756', 8–10, 'Midwife appointment (Euphrosina Opitz)', 9 September 1705–30 June 1706; Tit. (F) XLIV.D.1, 16–43, 'Appointment (Ehrlich)', 10 January–24 July 1713.

sisted the elderly midwives 'as a Beifrau' prior to 1713, but within an unofficial working relationship under two of the older midwives. Hempel was not appointed to the office of Beifrau until 1715.[75] After 1715 it became less usual for a sworn midwife to be recruited directly from the community of mothers. Although this did not preclude unofficial midwife activity, by the mid-eighteenth century it was rare for a sworn midwife *not* to have risen up through the ranks of the sworn Beifrauen first.

Like the sworn midwives, sworn Beifrauen were appointed under oath and were subject to their own Beifrau instruction. According to the instruction from 1715, Beifrauen were not permitted to practise independently, but were expected to take all their instructions from the sworn midwives.[76] During the birth the Beifrau was subordinate to the sworn midwife and the instruction ordered her to 'meekly assist the labouring women, speak to them in a friendly manner … to remind them of the urgency and to help [the mother] bring forth so much of her courage to assist the midwives to the best of her ability'.[77] In theory at least, there was a clear division of labour between the midwife, who carried out births and baptisms, and the Beifrau, who was supposed to carry out all the auxiliary tasks in the weeks following the birth: 'bathing, changing nappies, making the bed, washing, also when necessary tending the sick … giving mothers and their children their prescribed medicines'.[78] Although given permission to carry out emergency baptisms when the circumstances required, unlike sworn midwives, sworn Beifrauen had no duty to provide medico-legal evidence.[79] Nor were they, as already mentioned, permitted to carry the infants to baptism in their own name, but were instead required to do so on behalf of their allocated midwife.[80]

As with the sworn midwives, seniority determined the pecking order amongst the Beifrauen. It was not customary, as it was in Lübeck, for a Beifrau to automatically step into the shoes of her midwife-teacher.[81] Instead a complex ladder of entitlement based on seniority dominated promotions and reallocations. Upon the death of one of the midwives in the city, the protocol for promotion or reallocation followed a particular pattern:

Eldest midwife in Vorstadt	→	Deceased midwife's office (in Stadt)
Eldest Beifrau	→	Vacant midwife office in Vorstadt
New Beifrau	→	Vacant Beifrau office (anywhere)

---

75 Tit. (F) XLIV.D.1, 16–43, 'Appointment (Ehrlich)', 10 January–24 July 1713, 27–29.
76 See Items 3 and 5 of Tit. (F) X 23b, Bd. III, 'Instruktionen (1676–nach 1800)', 234–36, 'Instruction vor die geschworenen Beÿweiber', c. 1715 (undated).
77 See Item 3 of ibid.
78 See Item 6 of ibid.
79 See Item 14 of Tit. (F) X 23b, Bd. VIII, 'Instruktionen (1676–nach 1800)', 70–76, 'Instruktion für die Beÿfrau N.N.', 14 July 1758, 74v.
80 See Item 9 of Tit. (F) X 23b, Bd. III, 234–36, 'Instruction Beÿweiber', c. 1715 (undated).
81 Loytved, *Hebammen*, 75.

However, as we shall see below, both necessity and the will of the women themselves meant that this pecking order sometimes fell by the wayside.

Beifrauen also received a salary (see Table 1) consisting of cash and naturalia, however, the bulk of their income derived from the wage they received from their midwife-teachers. Unless attending a family receiving alms, a midwife was obliged to pass on a small portion of her fee to her Beifrau when the latter assisted or replaced her at a delivery. In 1803 this Beifrau wage came to 8 Groschen per delivery, or one-quarter of the minimum fee a midwife was entitled to charge.[82] Baptisms were generally more lucrative for Beifrauen, not least because they did not involve long hours and great physical exertion. Sworn midwives commonly sent out Beifrauen to carry infants to baptism on their behalf. Of the *Trinkgeld* (tip) offered by the godparents, Beifrauen were only required to pass on between 4 and 8 Groschen to their midwife.[83] For Beifrauen working within the city walls, the income derived from fees and gifts was – at least in theory – supposed to suffice for the rent these women paid to the Council (12 Reichstaler per annum). Perhaps the Council also assumed that the husbands of these younger women were still earning enough of a living to support the family. However, as will be explored in Chapter Four, Beifrauen working within the city walls were often forced to seek additional and sometimes 'illegal' avenues of income in order to pay their way, in particular towards the end of the eighteenth century.

Although midwives and Beifrauen drew upon a base salary from public coffers, the entire system of municipal midwifery in Leipzig was supposed to be more or less fiscally self-sufficient. The decisions made by the Leipzig Council thus sometimes reflected a desire for economy that might even override political or social considerations. As we have seen, the hierarchy of midwife and Beifrau underpinned the way individual incomes were both generated and allocated, making a Beifrau often dependent upon her midwife-teacher for income. It was this midwife-teacher (in some cases other midwives too) who would theoretically determine both how often the Beifrau would work and which of the midwife's clients she would attend. The case of Beifrau Maria Magdalena Thomäe demonstrates the importance of this relationship. In 1770 Thomäe's midwife Anna Hein had agreed to swap quarters with another midwife Dorothea Westphal. Although Thomäe had been instructed to accompany her midwife-teacher to the Rannstädter Tor, she pleaded with the Council to remain at the Grimmaisches Tor, arguing that because Hein permitted her to attend only the poorest clients, her earnings under Hein were meagre. The bulk of her income, Thomäe claimed, came instead through midwife Westphal. That Thomäe would want to remain with

---

82   Tit. (F) XLIV.D.1a, 2–7, 'Beifrau Güntz vs midwife Ulrich', 21 February–2 October 1803. The minimum fee was 1 Taler.

83   As the following dispute shows. See StadtAL, Tit. (F) XLIV.D.6b, 'Acta, Die Einrichtung der Kindermütter und Beÿweiber betr. de anno 1782', 29–37, 'Midwife Johanna Schulz complains about her Beifrau Christiana Behnhold', 23 February–18 March 1784, 36.

the midwife under whom she had the greatest earning potential carried weight with the Council and it promptly approved her request.[84]

This dependent relationship was a reciprocal one. Just as midwives were expected to provide Beifrauen with the opportunity to earn a living, so too were Beifrauen expected to financially support sworn midwives in old age and illness. The number of salaried midwife and Beifrau offices was strictly capped and most women held their office for life.[85] Because the Leipzig Council made no provision for incapacitated midwives unable to earn a living, problems arose when a midwife became too decrepit to carry out her office and had to be retired. When midwife Maria Grunert requested retirement in 1767, Stadtaccoucheur Johann Gehler recommended she continue receiving her salary and remain in her free midwife lodgings until her death. The Council initially agreed to appoint Beifrau Anna Hein to replace Grunert on one condition: Hein remain on her Beifrau salary and pay Grunert 9 Groschen for each child she carried to baptism. As recompense for moving to the city, the Council also offered Hein 12 Taler to cover her rental costs. Hein's promotion, however, was trumped by Juliana Maria Müller, a midwife in the Vorstadt. In return for taking over Grunert's lodgings, Müller offered to give Grunert half of her quarterly salary, her annual rations and 8 Groschen per child she delivered. The Council's decision to replace Grunert with Müller over Hein hinged largely on economic considerations. Whereas installing Hein would cost the municipal purse 12 Taler, promoting Müller to the city would cost nothing if the Council insisted Müller resided in the Vorstadt until Grunert's death. For Müller, who desired Grunert's more generously sized accommodation, this was a small price to pay and the Council appointed her as sworn midwife in the city.[86]

The situation became critical again in 1778 when the seventy-year-old midwife Maria Rosina Lorend took ill, leaving only two midwives working within the city walls. The Council initially wanted to appoint a 'good' Beifrau through whom Lorend could glean a living. Yet Stadtaccoucheur Johann Karl Gehler argued it would be more appropriate to appoint midwife Johanna Matthes, who had profited far more from Lorend's clientele and been promoted out of turn to midwife. For Gehler, Matthes was indebted to Lorend and should therefore shoulder the temporary burden of forgoing her own

84 Tit. (F) XLIV.D.6b, Bd. I, 'Acta, Die Einrichtung der Kindermütter und Beÿweiber', 120–48, 'Beifrau appointment (Johanna Schultz)', 1 December 1769–28 April 1770, 143–48.

85 Only two Beifrauen, Johanna Maria Werner and Christiana Elisabeth Jos, were divested of their office for misbehaviour (drunkenness) during the eighteenth century. See II. Sekt., M (F) Nr. 670, Bd. III, 'Hebammen. Verschiedenes über die Kindermütter, Wehemütter und Beifrauen (1756–69)', 50–87, 'Dismissal of Beifrau Johanna Werner', 19 April 1763–1 March 1764; Tit. (F) XLIV.D.6b, Bd. I, 'Acta, Die Einrichtung der Kindermütter und Beÿweiber de an. 1757', 226–32, 'Midwife Johanna Vogel complains about Beifrau Christiana Jos', 15 February–11 March 1782, 230–31.

86 Tit. (F) XLIV.D.6b, Bd. I, 'Acta, Die Einrichtung der Kindermütter und Beÿweiber betr.', 66–86, 'Beifrau appointment (Maria Thomäe)', 1 September 1767–20 November 1768, 82–86.

salary as Lorend's successor. The Council, more mindful of the costs involved with having two midwives at the same post, ignored Gehler's recommendation and appointed a Beifrau from the Vorstadt instead.[87] Lorend was able to keep her midwife salary and the newly appointed midwife remained on her Beifrau rations until Lorend's death. The resources for paying midwives were finite and such liminal situations necessitated that these resources be temporarily shared. Once again, the city's midwives and Beifrauen were expected to support each other financially in old age, and the Council ensured that the city fiscus did not have to venture additional funds for incapacitated midwives. The relationship between midwives and their Beifrauen was thus one of considerable financial dependence despite the infrastructure of municipal office. Neither the Leipzig Council nor any of its municipal medical officers questioned the basis of this dependent relationship, nor did they deem it necessary to alter the tradition of the eldest or the financial obligations between midwife and Beifrau. Thus, the social hierarchy expressed in the 'economic' practices within the profession discussed here was a vital aspect of ordering the day-to-day relations between a midwife and her apprentice in accordance with the structures and social mores of broader society.

Wickelweiber (swaddling women)

Wickelweiber was the name given to women engaged unofficially by sworn midwives as assistants-come-apprentices. As Wickelweiber were little more than apprentices without a sworn office, their identity emerged as the pendant to that of the sworn Beifrauen, with the term first appearing in administrative sources in the mid-1750s as a means of discriminating between the official and unofficial forms of midwife apprenticeship. As we have seen, before the Leipzig Council formalised midwifery apprenticeship in the early eighteenth century it was customary for a woman to 'hold to a midwife' for a number of years, during which time she assisted with deliveries, postnatal care and swaddling.[88]

Even after the Council established the office of Beifrau, midwives and women aspiring to a midwife office persisted in utilising the traditional pattern of unofficial apprenticeship. Christina Lorend's own protégé, Anna Rein, wrote in 1725 that she had 'already held myself to [midwife] Lorend for several years, and she has instructed me in everything that a Beifrau needs to

---

87   Tit. (F) XLIV.D.6b, Bd. I, 'Acta, Die Einrichtung der Kindermütter und Beÿweiber', 200–15, 'Beifrau appointment (Rahel Pötsch)', 12 June 1778–3 March 1779.
88   The midwife Christine Hempel, for instance, had assisted two elderly midwives for several years. See Tit. (F) XLIV.D.1, 16–43, 'Appointment (Ehrlich)', 10 January–24 July 1713, 27–29. Christina Lorend had likewise spent at least four years at the side of her mother, the sworn midwife Christina Hentschell, and even took over during her mother's long illness in 1713. See Ibid., 25.

know'.[89] Over a decade later in 1738, Anna Werner declared in her petition for an office that she had assisted midwife Lorend for nine years and Lorend now wanted Werner as her sworn Beifrau.[90] Reconstructing the careers of these women using biographical data gleaned from all known administrative sources related to midwifery in the city shows that between 1730 and 1800, at least eight sworn midwives and sworn Beifrauen began their working life by 'holding' to a sworn midwife.[91] If greater biographical detail were available for Leipzig midwives, this number would most likely be far higher.

This parallel system of apprenticeship flourished alongside the office of Beifrau and it proved difficult for both the Council and the Stadtaccoucheur to eradicate. Wickelweiber first emerged as an administrative problem when the city's seven sworn Beifrauen were compelled to defend their livelihood, clubbing together to oust a woman used by midwife Mend in 1754.[92] A further spate of angry petitions from the Beifrauen in 1756 prompted the Council to undertake an investigation into the use of Wickelweiber amongst the sworn midwives.[93] However, in 1758 the Stadtaccoucheur Johann Gottfried Breuer reported that the midwives continued to use their 'Mägde' (female servants), even after a spate of written complaints from the Beifrauen had led the Council to issue a warning that midwives continuing to do so would be divested of office. This had not deterred the midwives, who in Breuer's words 'begin again to use their women and in order to diminish their disobedience, claim that these arbitrarily appointed women would only tend the new mothers, not be in their [the midwives'] service ...', something Breuer claimed to be untrue.[94] In his next report, Breuer admitted the futility of the situation, suggesting the current Wickelweiber working in the city be appointed as Beifrauen in order to defray the problems between the midwives.[95] The Wickelweiber 'problem' appears to have resolved itself after this incident – at least subsequent Stadtaccoucheur reports are silent on the matter and there is no evidence of complaints against unsworn women from either Beifrauen or mid-

89   Tit. (F) XLIV.D.1, 83–118, 'Appointments (Greger and Veiß)', 22 November 1724–4 September 1725, 85.

90   Tit. (F) XLIV.D.1, 'Kindermütter bey hiesiger Stadt betr. ingl. die angenommene Bey Weiber betr. 1673–1756', 161–69, 'Midwife appointment (Maria Mößler) and Beifrau appointment (Anna Werner)', 29 May–9 July 1738, 165.

91   It was not possible to aggregate sufficient biographical data on all women involved in midwifery as they do not feature uniformly in the sources and the level of information provided on candidates varied greatly. Gaps in the coverage of the sources are also part of this problem. These eight sworn midwives were: Anna Maria Werner, Maria Rosina Lorend, Maria Rosina Tauhardt, Anna Maria Heinick, Magdalena Sophia Mäy, Dorothea Sophia Jäger, Christina Maria Bauer, Rahel Regina Pötsch.

92   See II. Sekt. M (F) Nr. 670, Bd. II, 22–35, 'Beifrauen vs Teuhert and Mend', 26 April–24 July 1754.

93   StadtAL, II. Sekt., M (F) Nr. 670, Bd. II, 'Hebammen. Verschiedenes 1748–59', 1–41, 'Leipzig Council investigates the use of swaddling women', 30 January–16 March 1756.

94   Tit. (F) XLIV.D.6b, Bd. I, 1–8, 37–8, 54–5, 'Stadtaccoucheur reports (Breuer)', 28 May 1757–14 July 1758, 1r–1v.

95   Ibid., 6r.

wives during the latter third of the eighteenth century. From an administrative
point of view, the role of the Beifrau and her position as apprentice appears to
have been consolidated after this time.[96] Until the latter eighteenth century,
however, 'holding' to a midwife constituted the earliest, pre-appointment experience of midwifery for most sworn midwives and Beifrauen.

Despite the name, a Wickelweib did not merely swaddle infants. Custom
dictated that a sworn midwife was to visit mothers lying in once or twice a day
for the first nine and sometimes the first fourteen days postpartum in order to
check on the mother, change any bandages or uterine pessaries, and swaddle
the infant. Midwives were well aware of the limits conferred by occupational
propriety and entitlement to office, and portrayed the work of their Wickelweiber accordingly. As Stadtaccoucheur Breuer mentioned in his report to the
Leipzig Council, although midwives seem to have used their Wickelweiber
just as they would a Beifrau, they were careful to create a discrete occupational area for the Wickelweib as a means of justifying her existence. In 1756,
for example, midwife Maria Lorend took her Wickelweib Sophia Mäy along
to deliveries but did not allow Mäy to 'touch or assist during labour'. She had
Mäy swaddle newborns if she had no time herself to do so, but did not permit
her to carry the children to baptism. Mäy confirmed Lorend's account, adding
that she only swaddled after the ninth or fourteenth day, after which time, she
claimed, midwives no longer looked after their clients personally.[97] Both
Lorend and Mäy were careful to situate the work of the Wickelweib in periph-
eral areas of midwifery so that it did not appear to clash with the tasks entrusted to the city's sworn midwives and sworn Beifrauen. Lorend, just like
other midwives, attempted to pass her Wickelweib off as a marginal figure.
Lorend even justified her use of a Wickelweib because she did not have her
own servant, who would otherwise carry out such menial tasks.[98]

Yet as the Council's 1756 investigation revealed, the tasks carried out by
Wickelweiber frequently differed little from those for which the sworn Beifrauen were appointed. Midwife Mend's Wickelweib, for example, was always
present at births and, according to Mend's outraged Beifrau Maria Zinck,
Mend even let her Wickelweib deliver children that came during the night.[99]
But why did midwives in some cases persist in using Wickelweiber instead of,
or sometimes in addition to, sworn Beifrauen? The relationship between a
sworn midwife and a Wickelweib was one of authority and subservience and,
as Chapters Four and Five will discuss in greater detail, the balance of authority between midwives and Beifrauen was delicate. Midwives expected their

96 Only one further case from 1759 provides 'hard' evidence that midwives continued to
    employ unsworn women. See the complaint by midwife Maria Reichardtin about the
    midwife Müller, who purportedly took her sister to help her in a birth. II. Sekt. M (F) Nr.
    670, Bd. II, 'Hebammen. Verschiedenes 1748–59', 72–76, 'Beifrau Maria Rosina Reichar-
    tin complains about midwife Müller', 31 March–1 April 1759.
97 II. Sekt., M (F) Nr. 670, Bd. II, 1–41, 'LC investigation swaddling women', 30 January–
    16 March 1756, 21–22.
98 Midwife Johann Krämpff also used her servant as a swaddling woman. See ibid.
99 Ibid., 2–3.

Beifrauen to act as servants, however, Beifrauen, with their instruction and office in hand, often overstepped the bounds of this relationship. Hence, at the heart of the problem was the realignment of authority and subservience that had to be (re)negotiated between a midwife and her Beifrau every time a new promotion altered the offices. Midwives like Mend often sought the service of a Wickelweib after the midwife–Beifrau relationship had broken down. For her own part, Mend was forced to take on her Wickelweib, claiming '[I] must admit that I can use her far better than any of the Beifrauen and if I have any clients left at all, that is purely the work of Mrs Teuhardt'.[100] As we shall see in Chapter Four, all parties involved in these disputes – the midwives, the Beifrauen, the Wickelweiber, the Council and the Stadtaccoucheurs – acknowledged that the disorder that the use of Wickelweiber provoked was of both a social and an economic nature; their attempts to steady the waters reflected this underlying understanding.

Until this point in time, unofficially appointed apprentice midwives were an integral feature of the midwifery landscape. The 'invention' of the Wickelweib as a field of 'illicit' activity discrete from the sworn Beifrau marks the point at which unofficial midwifery began to be pushed towards the margins of the midwifery landscape in Leipzig.[101] By firming up the structure of midwifery, the Council certainly did its bit to demarcate between official and unofficial midwifery, however, this structural divide, as will be discussed further in Chapter Four, was also formed by the women in all 'branches' of the profession.

Gassenmägde (female street servants)

In the latter seventeenth and early eighteenth centuries another 'way in' to midwifery existed in parallel to the triage of sworn midwife, sworn Beifrau and unsworn apprentice (later Wickelweib). Women working as *Gassenmägde* (female street servants) often side-stepped the traditional apprenticeship altogether on their way to becoming midwives. The Gassenmagd was part of a micro-system of neighbourhood governance and was a ubiquitous figure in seventeenth- and eighteenth-century communities. The Leipzig Council required each street in the extramural neighbourhoods to appoint a *Gassenmeister* (male street warden) and a Gassenmagd 'to serve the neighbourhood with the greatest conscientiousness' (Grimm's wording).[102] The Gassenmagd appears to have been subordinate to the Gassenmeister, whose principal task it was to

---

100 See Mend's letter from 24 May 1754 in II. Sekt. M (F) Nr. 670, Bd. II, 22–35, 'Beifrauen vs Teuhert and Mend', 26 April–24 July 1754.

101 As Hans-Christoph Seidel has noted for the first half of the nineteenth century in Berlin, there is no apparent evidence of male midwives using unsworn women (*Wickelfrauen*) to assist them. See Seidel, *Neue Kultur*, 391–93.

102 See the entry for 'Gassenmeister' in *Deutsches Wörterbuch von Jacob und Wilhelm Grimm*, (16 vols, S. Hirzel: 1854–1961), available at <http://dwb.uni-trier.de/de/>, accessed 21 October 2016, online version from 21.10.2016. This entry draws on the Leipzig Stadt-

be the Council's man-on-the-street for policing all aspects of urban Policey.[103] They were responsible for upholding civic order and keeping the peace in the neighbourhood; their palette of responsibilities embodied the early modern idea that social order rested on the two pillars of physical cleanliness and moral rectitude. Gassenmeister undertook regular property visitations to ferret out foreigners housed illegally as a measure to protect the community against criminality and disease.[104] They were also responsible for fire prevention, maintaining the wells, social disorder and policing unlawful sexual activity.[105]

The Gassenmagd performed a variety of tasks within her 'neighbourhood' which appear to have formed a 'natural' extension of the domestic and neighbourly duties expected of women. Midwifery, or at least neighbourly assistance in the birthing chamber, was one of these activities. Anna Drehseil, a sixty-four-year-old widow, had served as Gassenmagd in the extramural neighbourhood in the Gerbergasse (Hallisches Tor) for eighteen years when she applied to the Council for a midwife office in 1713. During that time she claimed to have tended the sick, washed the dead and assisted women during deliveries when no midwife was available.[106] The Gassenmagd in the Ulrichgasse at the Peterstor, sixty-four-year-old widow Anna Magdalena Kirchlöffel, not only had several 'emergency' deliveries under her belt but also maintained a side-line business by taking in unwed women for confinement.[107] A number of official complaints made by midwives and Beifrauen against the activities of the Gassenmägde between 1680 and 1717 suggests that assisting mothers at birth and tending women in confinement made up a reasonable share of a Gassenmagd's work. Certainly the practices of some Gassenmägde extended further than officially acceptable 'emergency' midwifery. Marie Schönwolff, a Gassenmagd in the Bettelgasse (Grimmaisches Tor), had a lively midwifery practice in 1696. All the women in her neighbourhood, together

---

ordnung from 1701. The Gassenmeister's counterpart within the city walls was the *Viertelmeister* (quarter warden).

103 See also Walther Rachel, *Verwaltungsorganisation und Ämterwesen der Stadt Leipzig bis 1627* (Leipzig: B. G. Teuber, 1902), 151–55.

104 Alexander Schunka, *Gäste, die bleiben: Zuwanderer in Kursachsen und der Oberlausitz im 17. und frühen 18. Jahrhundert* (Berlin: LIT-Verlag, 2006), 89. The Leipzig Council increased the responsibility of the Gassenmeister in the Vorstadt in the early 1700s. See Bräuer, *Der Leipziger Rat*, 69.

105 Gassenmeister in the Vorstadt had more far-reaching responsibilities than their counterparts within the city walls. See Rachel, *Verwaltungsorganisation*, 154–55. On Gassenmeister in the neighbouring town of Naumberg, see Siegfried Wagner and Ursula Dittrich-Wagner, *C-A-F-F-E-E, trink nicht soviel Caffe. Aus der Frühzeit der Naumburger Kaffee-Häuser* (Museumsverein Naumberg: undated), available at <http://mv-naumburg.de/kaffeegeschichte>, accessed 26 October 2016. On Berlin, see Rolf Kettler, *Eine kurze Geschichte des Abfalls* (Bundesamt für Umwelt, Wald und Landschaft, Abteilung Abfall, Switzerland: 2000), available at <www.booze.ch/cm_data/muell.pdf >, accessed 26 October 2016.

106 Tit. (F) XLIV.D.1, 16–43, 'Appointment (Ehrlich)', 10 January–24 July 1713, 22.

107 Ibid., 23.

with a number of women from other nearby streets, had appropriated Schön-wolff as their trusted 'midwife' in preference to the local sworn midwife, who had held office there for a number of years.[108]

Whereas unsworn apprentices and later the Wickelweiber were associated with a sworn midwife and generally made this association known, Gassen-mägde did not seem to have or make these associations public and usually portrayed themselves (when it is that we hear their voices) as occasional mid-wives.[109] Nonetheless, progression from Gassenmagd to sworn Beifrau or sworn midwife was a fairly normal, although by no means inevitable, occur-rence. Of the nine women known to have worked as Gassenmägde between 1680 and 1717, only three were appointed as sworn midwives. Many women made explicit reference to their role as Gassenmagd when they petitioned the Leipzig Council for a midwife office. Others, such as Euphrosina Opitz, who as a Gassenmagd had been accused in 1699 by sworn midwife Marie Plessing of encroachment and slander, did not.[110] Thus the number of women with this kind of experience entering the 'official' midwifery structure may indeed be higher than this figure suggests. Certainly, experience as a Gassenmagd was valued positively by both the Council and the community on two fronts. Firstly, it provided women with even more experience of assisting women in childbirth than customary neighbourly and familial assistance could offer. Secondly, the office of Gassenmagd could potentially raise the status of a woman's expertise in midwifery and the level of trust in which the community held her.

Although the roles of Gassenmagd and midwife were theoretically dis-crete, in reality there was significant overlap between the two, not just in terms of midwifery tasks but also in the standing both enjoyed in the local commu-nity. Both midwives and Gassenmägde assumed the role of a female in the service of the community. They both held the respect and trust (and some-times also fear) of the female neighbourhood and were both actively involved in a wide range of life events that took place within the domestic female sphere. They both shared the same socio-cultural space in the life of local communities and both trod a path between neighbourly assistance and the invigilation of social order. It is not clear why, but the Gassenmagd disap-peared as a direct rival to the sworn midwives around 1717, at about the same time that the Council began to seriously address the issue of training mid-

---

108 StadtAL, II. Sekt. K (F) Nr. 255, 1–6v, 'Kindermutter gegen Marie Schönwolff', 22–25 January 1696.

109 See, for example, the information gathered on the four Gassenmägde in II. Sekt. W (F) Nr. 332, 'Acta, Die inn: und vor der Stadt wohnende Wehmütter: und Beÿweiber, auch deren Amt und Verrichtung betr. (1717–37)', 1–9, 'Midwives complain about the Gassen-mägde', 30 January–10 March 1717, 4–7.

110 II. Sekt. P (F) Nr. 175b, 1–5, 'Hebammen. Marie Plessingen beschwert sich über die beiden Gassenmägde, welche den Frauen in Kindesnöten beistehen', 2 June 1699–17 July 1703; Tit. (F) XLIV.D.1, 8–10, 'Appointment (Opitz)', 9 September 1705–30 June 1706.

wives by introducing more sworn Beifrauen.[111] They did not withdraw from the midwifery landscape completely, however, and we have evidence of Gassenmägde taking in unwed mothers to lie in during the mid-eighteenth century, as will be discussed in greater detail in Chapter Four.[112]

Healers and nurses

Healers, nurses and women selling herbal remedies – women operating on the medical 'fringe' – were also active participants in the midwifery landscape in Leipzig. The proximity of midwifery to women's everyday tasks and to their role as mothers meant that it was relatively easy for women to branch out into healing and obstetrics. In particular during the first half of the eighteenth century, women might begin practising midwifery of their own accord without first entering into an unofficial apprenticeship or holding an office as Gassenmagd. This was most likely to be the case with women already operating in a healing or caring role, for example, Dorothea Sophia Schröder was reprimanded in 1722 for attending women during childbirth and dispensing labour-inducing medicines.[113] Another woman, Mrs Stöps, started practising as an unsworn midwife in 1707 after a long period of working as a *Leichenbitterin*, a woman who washed and laid out the dead for a living.[114]

The case of the wife of a garrison soldier Mrs Fritsch, who worked as a midwife without office between 1733 and 1736, suggests that these women held an ambiguous status and the Council showed some reluctance to sanction their activities. Stadtaccoucheur Johann Valentin Hartrauff reported in 1733 that Mrs Fritsch 'has been attending women giving birth as a midwife' and requested instruction from the Leipzig Council about what he should do. The woman, Hartrauff admitted, 'was not without skill' but 'had all the gifts of a gossipy woman ... and purports to know and do more than all other midwives are able.'[115] Hartrauff's concern lay not principally in the fact that Mrs Fritsch was practising as a midwife, but instead about whether or not this woman should be permitted to undertake 'difficult births' without another sworn midwife being present.[116] The Council, however, had little concern

---

111 The last complaint against a Gassenmagd dates from 1717, however, as records for the period between 1720 and 1748 are relatively patchy, it is difficult to ascertain whether this omission is meaningful.

112 For example, the daughter of a master carpenter in Rudolstadt spent her lying-in with the Gassenmagd in the Bettelgasse in 1742. See UAL, GA IV 205, 1–41, 'Schwängerungsacta', 1736–83, 36.

113 Tit. (F) XLIV.D.4, 1–21, 'Schröderin betr.', 1722.

114 StadtAL, Tit. (F) XLIV.D.1, 'Kindermütter bei hiesiger Stadt betr. ingl. die angenommene Bey Weiber betr, 1673–1756', 11–13, 'Midwives complain about Christina Hentschell and Mrs Stöps', 1707.

115 Tit. (F) XLIV.D.1, 132–60, 'Stadtaccoucheur reports (Hartrauff)', 29 November 1732–13 March 1737, 136–37.

116 Ibid.

about the activities of Mrs Fritsch and, to Hartrauff's exasperation, no recommendation was forthcoming.[117]

Activity on the medical 'fringe' was not a barrier to joining the ranks of
sworn midwifery. Mrs Stöps, the woman who washed and laid out the dead,
had been appointed as a sworn Beifrau by 1715. A healer from the nearby
town of Mockau, Dorothea Sophia Popp, was also appointed as a midwife in
1715.[118] Popp, who regularly travelled to Leipzig to heal, had petitioned several times for a midwife office in Leipzig prior to her appointment and had
also put herself forward for an office in the nearby town of Wurzen.[119] To
what extent she was involved in midwifery is uncertain; she was known to at
least one of the Leipzig sworn midwives who claimed in 1713, perhaps for
competitive reasons, 'that she had little knowledge of the office of midwife'.[120]
On the other hand, when Popp was finally appointed in 1715, Stadtphysicus
Johannes Bohn found her to have 'good knowledge' of midwifery, suggesting
that she had acquired at the very least some theoretical knowledge.[121] Experience in caring for the sick outside of one's own domestic sphere could actually
improve an aspirant Beifrau's or midwife's chances of selection, not least because of the good this could do a woman's public reputation. Johanna Matthes, for example, had worked as a sickbed and childbed nurse in her neighbourhood before she was appointed Beifrau in 1768 and used this experience
to bolster her application.[122] Indeed many of the women working unofficially
in this area paired midwifery with other types of healing. For example, Christina Hempel, who was later appointed to office, was said to 'apply internal
and external cures to the people'.[123] These women occupied an occupational
field that was poorly defined and in which midwifery and the care of new
mothers was only one aspect.

It is rare to hear from these women in person. In her supplication of
self-defence against the accusations of incursion from 1705, Christina
Hentschell was most careful to stress the usefulness of her work and the fact
that her activities were strictly in response to demand within her community:
she had 'been in this neighbourhood for some forty years, and in particular
during the evil time [presumably the plague epidemic of 1680] in places where
no midwife had wanted to go ...'.[124] It was important for these women to position themselves as vital to their local community without being seen to

117 Ibid., 140–41.
118 Tit. (F) XLIV.D.1, 44–45, 'Bohn re: Beifrau applicants', 6 April 1715.
119 Tit. (F) XLIV.D.1, 16–43, 'Appointment (Ehrlich)', 10 January–24 July 1713, 27.
120 Ibid.
121 Tit. (F) XLIV.D.1, 44–45, 'Bohn re: Beifrau applicants', 6 April 1715.
122 Tit. (F) XLIV.D.6b, Bd. I, 'Acta, Die Einrichtung der Kindermütter und Beÿweiber betr.',
    93–108, 'Beifrau appointment (Johanna Matthes)', 20 February–31 March 1768, 106–7.
123 Tit. (F) XLIV.D.1, 16–43, 'Appointment (Ehrlich)', 10 January–24 July 1713, 27–29.
124 See Hentschell's supplication, written in her own hand, to the Council from 2 September
    1705. Tit. (F) XLIV.D.2a, 'Varia, die Hebammen und das Hebammeninstitut betr. 1705–
    1812', 1–7, 'Midwives complain about Christina Hentschell', 14 August–2 September
    1705, 6r.

poach work from the sworn midwives. This was a relatively easy narrative to spin in terms of childbirth and the care of new mothers, and one that made use of the 'emergency'. These women derived their authority in childbirth largely from their position within the neighbourhood, at times, as was the case with Christina Hentschell, by assisting the sworn midwives here and there.[125]

As these women were not subject to licensing or occupational control mechanisms, our knowledge of them must be viewed through the narrow lens of conflict, largely between the sworn midwives and these 'outsiders'. Lay persons rarely initiated legal proceedings against these women. Indeed, it was overwhelmingly the sworn midwives and sworn Beifrauen themselves – not some higher authority – who fashioned and perpetuated the notion of illicit midwifery through accusations of encroachment. However, not all women who dabbled in midwifery were the objects of such conflicts. The activities of Popp, Kirchlöffel and Matthes, for example, were never called into question by the Council, the corps of sworn midwives or the community; at least, no such records have survived. These were women whose activities slotted peacefully into the midwifery landscape, did not pose a threat to the livelihood of the sworn midwives or cause an affront to their authority. We must keep in mind, therefore, that only a fraction of the women actually practising midwifery unsworn – be it independently such as Mrs Fritsch or looking after women in childbed such as Johanna Matthes – are captured in the municipal administrative sources.

Appointing midwives

When the Leipzig Council appointed the Stadtaccoucheur in 1731, it transferred the responsibility for the procedure of selecting candidates to this new office. The Stadtaccoucheur was now charged with the task of making enquiries into the 'Lebenswandel' (comportment and reputation) of women who petitioned for a Beifrau or midwife office, assessing their level of skill and knowledge, and compiling a list of candidates. The Council then made the final decision on who was to be appointed. Generally speaking, the Council followed the Stadtaccoucheur's recommendation.

This new way of determining which women became midwives replaced an older system of selection centred largely on the community of married women, similar to the midwife elections documented by Eva Labouvie for the rural Saar and Lotharingia regions.[126] Prior to the 1720s, consultation with the women of the individual neighbourhoods about which applicant they pre-

---

125 Hentschell claimed that the midwife at the Rannstädter Tor used her as an assistant-apprentice. See ibid.
126 Midwives there were appointed in official elections which were chaperoned by the local pastor and government functionary. However, the real selection process took place informally amongst the village women beforehand, so that usually only a single candidate stood for election. See Labouvie, *Beistand*, 99–116.

ferred appears to have been common practice. By 1725, however, the culture of the female collective was crumbling. Social stratification, in particular within the city walls, had rendered this practice redundant. Following the death of city midwife Dorothea Christina Seidel in July 1725, the Council shortlisted seven women, most of whom were already midwives or Beifrauen elsewhere in the Stadt or the Vorstadt. However, after consulting the women in the city as to which candidate should be appointed, the Council faced a major problem. The women 'did not want to reveal their thoughts, but had rather excused themselves that most of the women were unknown to them.'[127] With the breakdown of the traditional procedure of midwife selection, the Council instructed that the replacement midwife be appointed according to the recommendation of the Stadtphysicus Michael Ernst Etmüller. Christina Hempel, a sworn midwife of some seven years who, according to the Stadtphysicus, had 'the best knowledge and experience of how to treat women during confinement', was subsequently appointed.[128]

Many of the 1725 candidates that the women in the city claimed *not* to know lived and worked in the Vorstadt. They also largely belonged, as Chapter Three will discuss further, to the lower artisan estates:

> *Anna Martha Priebs:* Her first husband had been a horse dealer; her second husband was a country carriage driver. Priebs had worked as vice midwife to the midwife at the Grimmaisches Tor for four years.

> *Christina Hempel:* Wife (possibly widow) of a soldier in the city regiment. She served unofficially and officially as a Beifrau for seven years to one of the longest-serving midwives in the city. Following that she was appointed midwife in the Vorstadt, where she had worked for five years.

> *Johanna Regina Wagner:* Husband's occupation unknown. Wagner trained unofficially under her mother-in-law, the midwife at the Peterstor. Her sister-in-law was also a midwife in the city (1719–at least 1740). Midwife at the Peterstor for five years.

> *Anna Maria Rein:* Married to a brewery worker and unofficial apprentice to the city midwife Christina Lorend.

The fact that most held an office in the Vorstadt suggests that a rift between women of differing social status was a key issue in the breakdown of a traditional female collective surrounding birth that made it possible for low-estate midwives to be known to women of higher social status. As Chapter Five will demonstrate, women of the upper orders used sworn midwives just like the rest of the population throughout the eighteenth century.[129] We do not have the names of the women the Council actually consulted, however, this group of women would have almost certainly been restricted to the wives of burghers resident within the city walls, many of whom were comfortably off to

---

127 Tit. (F) XLIV.D.1, 83–118, 'Appointments (Greger and Veiß)', 22 November 1724–4 September 1725, 116.
128 Ibid., 117.
129 Midwives in London, who were often well-off and/or married to influential parishioners, typically counted gentry and well-ranked families amongst their core clients. See Evenden, 'Mothers and their midwives', 9, 16–19.

wealthy.[130] Their ignorance of the candidates suggests these were women who had little contact with women from either the Vorstadt or the lower artisan estates. But it is possibly also symptomatic of the fact that Leipzig was, demographically speaking, a city dependent greatly upon immigration.[131] The patriciate was porous; high levels of newcomers could increase levels of anonymity, even within the individual neighbourhoods. As reputation was the main criterion for determining skill and suitability, these women felt unqualified to pass judgement on candidates of whom they did not have first-hand knowledge. Thus, they abdicated their traditionally held right to determine who was appointed as their local midwife. But the ignorance of the women in the city may also have been due to occupational rivalry between the midwives and the Beifrauen. The complaints Beifrauen often made about their midwife-teachers (discussed at length in Chapter Four) suggest also that midwives were highly protective of their well-paying clients, often refusing to let their Beifrauen accompany them to deliveries or baptisms for fear their apprentices would reduce their earnings or even worse, poach their clients altogether.

The shift from the female collective to the Stadtphysicus in midwife appointments was therefore a structural solution to the problem of demographic and social change leading to the disintegration of a female collective that accommodated women from all social statuses. And yet this shift was neither sharp nor absolute. Although lay women may have no longer enjoyed much in the way of *formal* input into the appointment of midwives, their *informal* influence remained: not in opposition to, but rather as a structural aspect of midwife selection practices. Midwife selection was the point at which older traditional criteria and procedures intersected with the newer forms of selection born of social necessity. Early modern legislative culture was contingent on negotiation between governing bodies (i.e., local authorities and states) and ordinary men and women of all estates, who deployed 'an arsenal' of legal codes and customary law in order to implement, adapt or simply ignore legislation proclaimed by governing bodies on the level of everyday practice.[132] The shift to midwife selection at the recommendation of the Stadtphysicus (and later the Stadtaccoucheur) did not exclude women from the process of midwife selection, but the mix of the old and the new encouraged a culture of negotiation between lay women, midwives, municipal medical personnel and the Leipzig Council.

Thus, who worked as a midwife in late seventeenth- and eighteenth-century Leipzig was not determined exclusively by the Council or its Stadtphysicus and Stadtaccoucheur, but was still very much in the hands of the female community and midwives. This power to co-determine did not rest with these

---

130 Households with a taxable income of less than 200 Gulden per annum tended to reside in the Vorstadt during the sixteenth century. See Feige, 'Sozialstruktur', 219.

131 The city experienced extremely high levels of immigration, which balanced out the high mortality (amongst the highest of European cities). See Volkmar Weiss, *Bevölkerung und soziale Mobilität. Sachsen 1550–1880* (Berlin: Akademie-Verlag, 1993), 173.

132 Schlumbohm, 'Gesetze', 663.

groups' ability to legislate or decree. It rested instead on their right to contest
unfavourable and negotiate desirable situations with a largely responsive municipal authority. It also stemmed from their ability to use and apprentice
women from outside the corps of appointed sworn midwives. Although the
task of selecting midwives – the individual petitions, examination by the physician and, finally, appointment – appear more bureaucratic from 1725 onwards, the Council and the Stadtaccoucheur continued to use the traditional
criteria for selection and promotion.

The selection of midwives, as has been demonstrated by Mary Lindemann for other medical practitioners in eighteenth-century Germany, was
largely based upon non-medical criteria.[133] As Chapter Five will explore in
greater detail, for mothers and their families, being able to place their trust –
both a social and physical category – in the midwife 'qualified' a woman to
practice midwifery. Once the examination of midwives through the Stadtphysicus and the Stadtaccoucheur became common, obstetric and anatomical
knowledge was added to the social and physical criteria of selection. So, for
example, when the Stadtphysicus Johannes Bohn examined three candidates
in 1713 for their 'knowledge in obstetrics', he found only two suitably qualified.[134] Yet comportment, reputation in the community, familial links to midwifery, physical appearance, and family background were also crucial qualifiers. When recruiting a new midwife in 1713, the *Oberleichenschreiber* (senior
council officer responsible for recording deaths in the city) Georg Christoph
Winzer relied on both petition letters and personal interviews with candidates
and neighbours to make his assessment of each candidate, taking particular
care to note the nature of any illness, reliance on municipal alms, the number
of deliveries a woman claimed to have attended, and any idiosyncratic anec-
dotes or recommendations about her person. Anna Maria Kirchlöffel im-
pressed him with her personal and domestic cleanliness (which also carried
religious meaning as a sign of piety and godliness).[135] He likewise noted that
the neighbours of Johanna Sabina Netzold considered her 'knowledge of how
to attend women in labour learnt from books' to be so good that they gladly
employed her.[136]

These categories continued to determine the suitability of candidates
throughout the eighteenth century even though, as we will see in Chapter Three, chronological age was becoming more important in the eyes of the
Stadtaccoucheurs.[137] Stadtaccoucheur Johann Karl Gehler's descriptions be-
tray an intense interest in the character and demeanour of the aspiring mid-

133 Mary Lindemann, 'The Enlightenment Encountered: The German Physicus and His
    World', in Roy Porter, ed., *Medicine in the Enlightenment* (Amsterdam: Rodopi, 1995), 182–
    85.
134 Tit. (F) XLIV.D.1, 16–43, 'Appointment (Ehrlich)', 10 January–24 July 1713, 42.
135 Ibid., 23.
136 Ibid.
137 See, for example, the candidacy summaries provided by Gehler for Susanna Margaretha
    Hornung, Christiana Maria Bauer and Maria Christiana Stor in II. Sekt., M (F) Nr. 670,
    Bd. III, 50–87, 'Dismissal (Werner)', 19 April 1763–1 March 1764, 59–60.

wives, devoting far more space to these categories than to their level of knowledge or skill. Of Christiana Maria Bauer, for example, he wrote that 'she seems settled, modest, and polite. Her hands are quite good. Even though it appears to me that she were somewhat fearful and would not have the courage required in certain situations, I hope that she will gradually lose this natural stupidity the more experienced she becomes.'[138] So whilst medical personnel were becoming more involved in the selection of Beifrauen and midwives in mid-eighteenth-century Leipzig, this involvement did not consequently translate into a 'medicalisation' of candidacy criteria. Gehler and his successors merely assumed the defining characteristics of competence in midwifery – a good reputation, cleanliness, good hands, several children, and a friendly and calm manner – that had been the primary criteria for appointing a woman as a midwife and codified in oaths and instructions since the sixteenth century.[139] Moreover, sworn midwives and Beifrauen maintained a high level of control over any pre-appointment midwifery experience women might gain because this occurred unofficially.

As we have seen, promotion from a Beifrau office to a midwife office, or from a less lucrative office in the Vorstadt to one that assured a better-paying clientele in the walled city continued to be determined according to the traditional 'principle of the eldest' throughout the eighteenth century.[140] This meant that when a midwife or a Beifrau in the city died, she was replaced by one of the midwives in the Vorstadt, who was in turn replaced by the eldest Beifrau. A novice Beifrau was thus almost always allocated to one of the Vorstadt midwives. And when Beifrauen working under city midwives were promoted to the office of midwife, they invariably had to relocate to the Vorstadt, as the career trajectory of Anna Maria Hein demonstrates. Hein, a Wickelweib to one of the midwives in the city, was appointed Beifrau to that same midwife in 1758.[141] Two years later she was reallocated to another midwife in the city.[142] In 1767 Hein's midwife requested that Hein take over from her, however, one of the Vorstadt midwives was in line for that office. Hein was still promoted to the office of sworn midwife but moved out of the city into the Vorstadt at the Grimmaisches Tor, one of the larger Vorstadt suburbs.[143] After three years she moved to the Rannstädter Tor, a less attractive post because it involved attending women in the lazarette, but at the same time the district in

138 Ibid.
139 The oath dating from 1613, for example, specifies manner, skills, Christian belief and behaviour, tasks and the need to treat all women equally. See Ohne Sig., 51r–51v, 'Kindermuetter Aidt', 1613, 51r–51v.
140 A similar practice existed in many Dutch towns. See Marland, '"Stately and dignified"', 291–93.
141 Tit. (F) XLIV.D.6b, Bd. I, 1–8, 37–8, 54–5, 'Stadtaccoucheur reports (Breuer)', 28 May 1757–14 July 1758, 38r.
142 Tit. (F) XLIV.D.6b, Bd. I, 56–66, 'Appointment (Held and Plau)', 26 April–16 May 1760, 63r–65r.
143 Tit. (F) XLIV.D.6b, Bd. I, 66–86, 'Beifrau appointment (Thomäe)', 1 September 1767–20 November 1768, 85r–86r.

which most of Hein's clients lived.[144] Finally, in 1776, she was the eldest midwife in the Vorstadt and thus in line for promotion to the more lucrative city, where she remained until her death in 1799.[145] The principle of promoting the eldest endured throughout the eighteenth century. Even Stadtaccoucheur Gehler, who ardently believed in appointing youthful Beifrauen, felt no compulsion to overturn a system that rewarded maturity over merit or physical capacity.[146]

The voice of the local neighbourhood remained an important consideration for both Council and the Stadtaccoucheur into the latter eighteenth century. In 1763 the midwife Juliana Maria Müller accused her Beifrau Johanna Werner of being afflicted with the 'evil spirit' (spells of fainting or fitting).[147] After six weeks of investigations, the Leipzig Council dismissed Beifrau Werner because of her illness.[148] Just days later sixteen families petitioned the Council to testify that Werner had never once shown signs of the 'evil spirit' and had 'assisted the women according to duty and obligation'.[149] Stadtaccoucheur Johann Carl Gehler eventually recommended Werner be dismissed permanently, but his assessment of the situation was far from unequivocal. Not only had Werner's clients put in a good word for her, but most of her fellow Beifrauen had approached Gehler with a group petition supporting Werner's reinstatement on the grounds that they considered her a 'skilled, congenial and orderly midwife'.[150] Nor did Gehler think that Werner's illness was the 'evil spirit'. Although maintaining that Beifrau Werner should be kept on until a suitable candidate was found and he was able to learn more about her illness and its effect on her work as a midwife, he nonetheless recommended that her instruction be rescinded because the relationship between the midwife and her Beifrau had ceased to function.[151] Werner was dismissed, but evidently reinstated as she was working as a midwife the following year. Gehler's reticence in dismissing Werner was indicative of the weight accorded to the voices of the community and midwives in the matter of selecting (or in this case de-selecting) sworn midwives. And in the end, the will of the Beifrauen and the families at the Grimmaisches Tor was strong enough to effect Werner's reinstatement.

---

144 StadtAL, Tit. (F) XLIV.D.6b, Bd. I, 'Acta, Die Einrichtung der Kindermütter und Beÿweiber betr.', 120–48, 'Beifrau appointment (Johanna Sibylla Schultz)', 12 March–28 April 1770, 143–48.

145 Tit. (F) XLIV.D.6b, Bd. I, 'Acta, die Einrichtung der Kindermütter und Beÿweiber', 193–98, 'Beifrauen appointment (Rahel Leib and Christina Sophia Küchler)', 19 February–4 March 1776, 193.

146 Tit. (F) XLIV.D.6c, 'Acta, Die Einrichtung der Kindermütter und Beyweiber betr. de anno 1782', 54–74, 'Various appointments', 4 October 1782–22 January 1789, 57.

147 II. Sekt., M (F) Nr. 670, Bd. III, 50–87, 'Dismissal (Werner)', 19 April 1763–1 March 1764, 63.

148 Ibid., 68.

149 Ibid., 69.

150 Ibid., 61–62.

151 Ibid., 62.

Although there were all the outward signs of a tightly regulated and bureaucratic system of midwifery directed and sustained by the Leipzig Council
in the eighteenth century, lay women and midwives continued to exert a certain degree of control over the hiring and firing of the city's sworn midwives.
The newer structure of selection through the Stadtaccoucheur meshed with
older traditions, such as the principle of the eldest, relatively unproblemati-
cally. Moreover, Council provision of midwifery services through the city's
corps of midwives and Beifrauen made up only one part of the midwifery
landscape. The Leipzig Council had little intention of bringing the entire midwifery landscape under its supervisory eye. The micro-politics of who became
a midwife continued to hinge on largely social factors, which were controlled
and determined to a significant degree by midwives and the community in
conjunction with the Leipzig Council and its medical personnel.

The changing structure of the midwifery landscape

The array of practitioners operating within the midwifery landscape requires
us to reconceptualise the structure of midwifery in Leipzig depicted by the
regulations. What is clear is that a simple hierarchy with the Council at the
top and vagrant unsworn midwives at the bottom does not suffice; the relationships between the various actors were more complex than such a model
permits. As we have seen, the entry points into midwifery available to women
were numerous and their career paths as midwives varied (see Figure 2). Not
all women working as Gassenmägde or Wickelweiber became sworn midwives or Beifrauen; some were unsuccessful, others never even sought office.
Similarly many Beifrauen were left waiting in the wings for years on end, often dying before a vacant midwife office became available. It was not, for
many women, merely a case of working one's way up through the ranks.

How then can we conceptualise the structure of midwifery? Whether or
not a woman could practise as a midwife depended on one or more of the
following three factors. Firstly, sanctioning by the Council through office. Secondly, the acceptance of a woman's expertise by the community. And thirdly,
the support of an established midwife. So, for example, a sworn Beifrau's practice was underpinned by her office, the support of her midwife-teacher and
acceptance by the community. An unsworn midwife's claim to participate in
the midwifery landscape, on the other hand, rested only upon community
acceptance and – at most – the willingness of the sworn midwives and Beifrauen to tolerate her practice. Figure 3 visualises the complicated range of
associations between those involved in midwifery, the city authorities, and the
community that determined a woman's official and unofficial authority to
practise.

Although the Council, through its medical officials, certainly had its fingers in many parts of the midwifery landscape, its authority over midwifery
was weaker than one might expect. As the bottom-heavy diagram suggests, it

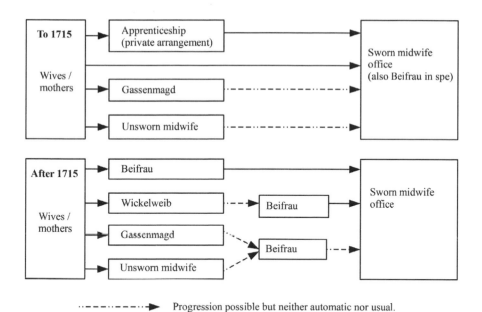

Figure 2 Potential career paths for women in the midwifery landscape, 1650–1810

Sources: StadtAL, Tit (F) XLIV.D, Hebammen, 1673–1852; Tit. (F) X, Ratsbeamte, 1590–1908; II: Sekt., 1568–1939.

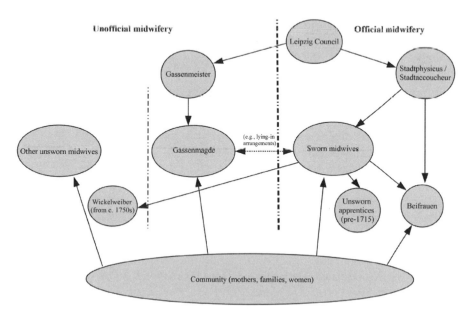

Figure 3 Relationships of authority within the midwifery landscape, 1650–1810

Sources: StadtAL, Tit (F) XLIV.D, Hebammen, 1673–1852; Tit. (F) X, Ratsbeamte, 1590–1908; II: Sekt., 1568–1939.

was the mothers and families, together with the midwives and Beifrauen themselves whose influence over whether or not a woman practised midwifery was
greater. For it was the pre-appointment milieu of the family and the neighbourhood in which a woman acquired her knowledge of childbirth, honed her
skills in midwifery, and began spinning the social networks that would enable
her to glean a living as a midwife. Unsworn midwives, and to a lesser extent
the Gassenmägde, were largely free from Council scrutiny. Their ability to
practice depended for the most part upon the willingness of mothers and
families to call upon their services. And whilst sworn midwives and Beifrauen
were directly subject to the control of the Council, the success of their practice
was equally dependent upon the preferences of women in the community
and – in the case of the Beifrauen – on the relationship to a sworn midwife.

Three parallel strands of midwifery emerge from this structure that may
be grouped roughly into a realm of 'unofficial' and a realm of 'official' midwifery, a distinction based primarily on legal entitlement to practise through
an office.[152] The first strand (in Figure 3 on the far right) was dominated by
midwives and Beifrauen with a sworn office but also encompassed the unsworn women they used as apprentices or assistants before the office of Beifrau was created. Wickelweiber, who stood in a direct relationship with the
sworn midwives, did not belong to this first strand of official midwifery, but
instead to the realm of unofficial midwifery. Although the sworn midwives
using them considered them to be their rightful apprentices, from the perspective of the Stadtaccoucheur and the Beifrauen these women had no legal entitlement to usurp the office of Beifrau. The Gassenmägde, who also held an
office but were not official midwives, made up the second strand. Women
working as unsworn midwives, some known as healers or nurses, and the
Wickelweiber made up the third and final strand. None of these strands of
midwifery were exclusive. Women could and did move relatively freely from
the second and third strands into the first. Movement in the opposite direction
from sworn to unsworn midwifery was, however, an infrequent occurrence as
sworn midwives and Beifrauen in Leipzig generally carried their offices to the
grave. Aside from death, there were only two ways to exit a midwife office:
grossly inappropriate behaviour or geographical relocation.[153]

Taking into account both official and unofficial midwifery, the structure of
the midwifery landscape throughout the seventeenth and eighteenth centuries
in Leipzig demonstrates a fairly flat hierarchy. For much of this period, midwifery had no explicit affinity to the incorporated medical groups in the city,
be it through familial ties (as the following chapter will demonstrate) or day-to-

---

152 There are parallels here to Mary Wessling's distinction between 'official' and 'customary'
     medicine. See Mary Nagle Wessling, 'Official Medicine and Customary Medicine in
     Early Modern Württemberg: The Career of Christoph Friedrich Pichler', *Medizin,
     Gesellschaft und Geschichte* 9 (1990): 21–44.
153 There is only one example of a Leipzig midwife moving to another town to take up a
     midwife office. See Tit. (F) XLIV.D.6c, 54–74, 'Various appointments', 4 October 1782–
     22 January 1789, 63–67.

day encounters with learned or artisan medicine. The only regular point of contact with the municipal medical apparatus and the Leipzig Council was appointment and swearing of the oath. This changed once the Council introduced formal lessons, however, more frequent contact with the Stadtaccoucheur and the emphasis placed upon training did not appear to substantially alter the relationship between official and unofficial midwifery. Nor did it change the necessity of accumulating experience as an unsworn apprentice or midwife – only few women were appointed without any experience whatsoever. And, with the exception of a new addition of age as a quasi-formal criterion, suitability for appointment continued to be assessed according to the older criteria of comportment, experience, knowledge and skill by the city's Stadtaccoucheurs.

Until the Leipzig Council, via its Stadtaccoucheur, began to stipulate what a midwife ought to know and which obstetric skills she was to master, it is important to remember that the sworn midwives, one of a number of officially sanctioned groups of 'medical' practitioners, were not tied to an official body of knowledge about the body. Although many displayed knowledge of – or at least acknowledged – 'book' medicine, their knowledge and skill was something to be judged by the mothers and honourable women of the neighbourhood. Epistemologically speaking, this put them on an even footing with the many forms of unofficial midwifery that existed in the city. The primacy of the community in this respect made it difficult and often undesirable, even towards the end of the eighteenth century, to prosecute unofficial midwifery. A further point to make here about unofficial midwifery is that it often occurred in a relationship of dependency with a sworn midwife. Wickelweiber, for example, were 'shadow' apprentices, performing all the tasks usually carried out by Beifrauen. And even some independently practising midwives had agreements with the sworn midwives to assist when needed or to field out the baptisms. Others accommodated single mothers during lying-in, calling upon midwives and Beifrauen to carry out deliveries and baptisms. Movement from unofficial to official midwifery was thus commonplace, even expected (from the community, midwives and the Council).

In many ways, the structure of midwifery was similar to a 'core' and a 'penumbra', terms that Laurence Brockliss and Colin Jones used to describe the structure of the medical world in early modern France.[154] Sworn midwives and sworn Beifrauen, whose official status rendered them quasi-tentacles of urban authority, made up the core group. This core of sworn midwives was neither incorporated nor hegemonic in itself, but the activities of those within it were defined by both ordinance and custom. The penumbra, a space with varying levels of proximity to the core, consisted of all those women practising midwifery unsworn (the other two strands of midwifery). Wickelweiber and Gassenmägde, who had no official business practising midwifery, and other

---

154 Laurence Brockliss and Colin Jones, *The Medical World of Early Modern France* (Oxford: Clarendon Press, 1997), 9–19. The level of medical incorporation in German cities was fairly similar. See Kinzelbach, 'Heilkundige', 120–26.

unsworn midwives inhabited the outer reaches of the penumbra. As we have seen, the physical border between the core and the penumbra was porous, particularly in the direction from the penumbra into the core. All these women were specialists to a greater or lesser degree in childbirth, baptism, infant health, maternal health – some even operated as general healers. And the fluidity with which they moved from the penumbra into the core attests to the symbiotic relationship between official and unofficial midwifery that persisted until well into the nineteenth century. The midwifery landscape was, as Robert Jütte has noted for medicine and healing more generally for the period before 1800, 'characterized by the lack of a monopoly and the openness of the system – at least from the point of view of the patient.'[155]

A recent contribution to an edited volume on medical pluralism has criticised Brockliss' and Jones' model of the medical penumbra on the basis of its assumption that there was a common set of concepts shared between popular and learned healers.[156] Matthew Ramsey calls instead for historians to think about difference as well as similarity between what he terms many concurrent 'epistemic communities' that were highly porous and did not preclude multiple membership.[157] From an epistemological perspective, however, there is little evidence of a distinction between women working as official and women working as unofficial midwives. As Chapter Four will explore, accusations of quackery and encroachment mostly revolved around claims about market entitlement, socio-occupational order and financial disadvantage, not questions of medical technique or knowledge. Furthermore, from the point of view of the community, the delineation between sworn and unsworn midwifery was far from absolute, and women and their families continued to use the services of unsworn midwives willingly. We should be more mindful of Ramsey's criticism, however, when contemplating the relationship between the midwifery landscape and the rest of the medical world. Was, for example, the readiness of midwives to acquire 'book' knowledge of midwifery evidence of a shared set of concepts with learned medicine, or, as Ramsey proposes, an instance of appropriation or translation?[158]

As Eva Labouvie has noted, during the early modern period the work surrounding childbirth and childbed in urban areas was no longer carried out by a single midwife but instead by a whole raft of different women. Confinement and lying-in were (at least in theory) the realm of the midwife and her apprentice, but other women might tend the woman, in particular during lying-in. Wealthier families might even take on an *Amme* (wet nurse) to look after the mother and child after the birth.[159] This process of specialisation was beginning to take place in eighteenth-century Leipzig but, as this chapter has

155 Robert Jütte, 'Medical Pluralism in Early Modern Germany', in Robert Jütte, ed., *Medical Pluralism – Past – Present – Future* (Stuttgart: Franz Steiner Verlag, 2013), 39.
156 Matthew Ramsey, 'Medical Pluralism in Early Modern France', ibid., 65–68.
157 Ibid., 77.
158 Ibid., 63.
159 Labouvie, 'Frauenberuf', 223–24.

shown, occupational differentiation was messy and contested: not one actor had been relegated a specific part in the production. Not even baptism, the one task legally entrusted to sworn midwives, was sacrosanct, with Beifrauen, Gassenmägde, Wickelweiber and unsworn midwives all making an appearance at the baptismal font at one time or another. Likewise, the taking-in of unmarried pregnant women was not alone the preserve of unsworn midwives; Beifrauen and some sworn midwives were also part of this semi black market in smothering the shame and dealing with the practicalities of illegitimacy. Midwifery in eighteenth-century Leipzig was an amalgam of old customs and new forms, of sworn and unsworn midwifery: there were still many means of practising midwifery open to women, and these all co-existed alongside one another for much of the century.

The structure of the midwifery landscape changed over the course of the eighteenth century, in particular during the latter half. As the number of Beifrauen grew in the early eighteenth century and their occupational role became better defined, the rivalries between sworn and unsworn midwives diminished. Encroachment was increasingly played out principally between sworn midwives and sworn Beifrauen. By the 1750s one strand of midwifery, that practised by the Gassenmägde, had disappeared from view completely – at least from the perspective of the midwives and the Stadtaccoucheur. We know, however, that these Gassemägde appeared to have carved a niche for themselves by 'specialising' in attending unwed women well into the latter eighteenth century. Unsworn midwives, in particular those attached to a midwife (such as the Wickelweiber), who had long been a feature of the midwifery landscape as unsworn apprentices, were now the primary target of complaint.

What this exploration of the midwifery landscape suggests is that the boundary between official and unofficial midwifery was blurred and continued to be so throughout the eighteenth century. Furthermore, despite increasing regulation, midwifery in all its forms was unable to emancipate itself as a profession from the traditional palette of female activities, in particular caring and healing. A well-established system of sworn apprentices may have reduced the visibility of unsworn midwifery and pushed it further towards the periphery of the midwifery landscape over the course of the eighteenth century. Yet unofficial apprenticeships, unsworn midwives and the use of Wickelweiber persisted. Sworn midwives almost always looked back upon several years of vital experience within the midwifery landscape. Until the late eighteenth century at least, this landscape in Leipzig was not the monopoly of women appointed by the Council to a sworn office but continued to incorporate, indeed rely upon, the midwifery and para-midwifery activities of a diverse array of unofficial midwives.

Chapter Three

Life-Cycle, the Household Oeconomy and the Meaning of Midwifery Work

The period from 1648 to the first decade of the nineteenth century proved to be an era of profound demographic change for Leipzig, as it did for urban centres all across Europe. Leipzig and its environs had sustained substantial population losses in the last ten years of the Thirty Years War.[1] Following the peace of 1648, mortality continued to outstrip fertility as epidemics and crop failures persisted as a regular feature of everyday life.[2] Yet the steady stream of economic migrants from the countryside ensured that the cities grew ever larger, sprawling beyond their walls into the surrounding villages and fields.[3] By 1750 the city's population, some 14,000 in 1650, had swelled to around 35,000, making Leipzig the second largest city in Electoral Saxony.[4] The population continued to grow modestly during the second half of the eighteenth century, reaching some 45,000 inhabitants in 1843.[5]

Leipzig's population growth went hand-in-hand with changes to the economic structure of the city. As the trade fairs picked up after 1648, so too did Leipzig's status as a merchant hub, and the trade fairs generated seasonal work. Manufacturing had also become a mainstay of the local economy and by the middle of the eighteenth century, some eighteen manufactories employing largely workers from the Vorstadt were producing luxury goods such as silk, velvet, gold and silver brocade just outside the city walls.[6] The pressure of a fast-growing population coupled with these new types of production and trade strained the traditional social and economic structures of the early modern city. Poverty became a huge problem, not just amongst those working in the manufactories, but also for families earning a living as artisans.[7] The task of dealing with poverty became an ever greater preoccupation of the paternalistic Leipzig Council.

---

1   Blaschke estimates losses of around two-thirds. See Blaschke, *Bevölkerungsgeschichte*, 94–95.
2   Harvest failures and speculation produced particularly bad 'hunger years' affecting Leipzig in the 1740s and the 1770s, effecting a dramatic rise in beggary. See Bräuer, *Der Leipziger Rat*, 67–68.
3   Weiss, *Bevölkerung und soziale Mobilität*, 56.
4   Blaschke, *Bevölkerungsgeschichte*, 140. Statistic for 1650 quoted in Beachy, *Soul of Commerce*, 22–23.
5   Blaschke, *Bevölkerungsgeschichte*, 140.
6   Czok, *Leipzig*, 28.
7   In 1739, for example, around 34% of the master linen weavers in central Saxony were forced to work as journeymen in the workshops of masters or to become beggars. See Helmut Bräuer, 'Arme Leute in Sachsen im 18. Jahrhundert', in Stadtarchiv Leipzig, ed., *Räume voll Leipzig 94. Arbeitsberichte des Stadtarchivs Leipzig* (Leipzig: Tangent Verlag, 1994), 74–76.

Historians have argued that the eighteenth century marked a watershed transformation in the definition of work. In the fifteenth and sixteenth centuries work was a moral force and one's occupation was tied inextricably to one's estate (*Stand*). During the eighteenth century, however, there emerged an economic concept of work as a productive force that realigned social distinctions along the line of 'useful' and 'not useful' work. Idleness and unemployment were marginalised as work became the focus of territorial governments and emerging nation states.[8] Since Max Weber's theory about the Protestant work ethic, there has been much debate as to whether Protestantism and Calvinism sowed the seed for the development of capitalism, however, work by Hans Medick seems to subdue enthusiasm for a Protestant teleology of work.[9]

Whichever way, the protoindustrial transformation had important implications for women's work. Historians working on England have argued that the demand for consumer goods increased dramatically over the period and, as much of protoindustrial production was carried out as piecework in the home, this appears to have created greater employment opportunities for women in particular.[10] Yet availability of work was one thing; social acceptability another. Paid female labour in the latter seventeenth and early eighteenth centuries was not spread evenly across society. In early eighteenth-century London, for example, Peter Earle finds working women ubiquitous amongst the poorer estates but rare to non-existent amongst the wives of gentlemen, professionals and skilled artisans.[11] For the Germanies there is a general consensus that there was a narrowing of opportunities for women to engage in commercial labour in many German regions from the Middle Ages.[12] However, in certain areas, women continued to be commercially active. Susanne Schötz notes that the participation rates of women in the Leipzig fairs peaked in the late eighteenth century, only to decline dramatically in the first half of the nineteenth as it became less culturally and socially viable for women to earn their own

8   Josef Ehmer and Peter Gutschner, 'Befreiung und Verkrümmung durch Arbeit', in Richard van Dülmen, ed., *Erfindung des Menschen. Schöpfungsträume und Körperbilder 1500–2000* (Vienna: Böhlau, 1998), 290. For a detailed overview of research on work from the Middle Ages into the early modern period, see Josef Ehmer and Catharina Lis, *The Idea of Work in Europe from Antiquity to Modern Times* (Farnham and Burlington: Ashgate, 2009).

9   Working on Pietists, Medick finds a Protestant ethic that lacked any 'spirit of capitalism'. See 'Introduction: Historical Studies in Perceptions of Work', in Josef Ehmer and Catharina Lis, eds, *The Idea of Work in Europe from Antiquity to Modern Times* (Farnham and Burlington: Ashgate, 2009), 16–17.

10 John Hatcher, 'Labour, Leisure and Economic Thought before the Nineteenth Century', *Past and Present* 160 (1988): 64–115, 75.

11 Peter Earle, 'The Female Labour Market in London in the Late Seventeenth and Early Eighteenth Centuries', *Economic History Review*, ser. 2, 42: 3 (1989): 328–53, 338. Earle, of course, focuses on remunerated work in his study.

12 See, for example, Ingrid Bártori, 'Frauen in Handel und Handwerk in der Reichsstadt Nördlingen im 15. und 16. Jahrhundert', in Barbara Vogel and Ulrike Weckel, eds, *Frauen in der Ständegesellschaft. Leben und Arbeiten in der Stadt vom späten Mittelalter bis zur Neuzeit* (Hamburg: Kramer, 1991).

living.[13] Women were also widely involved in medical activities throughout the early modern period.[14] This suggests, firstly, that an abundance of work open to women did not translate into higher social status and, secondly, that women's level of involvement in the world of work varied significantly from sector to sector. Moreover, focusing on commercial and remunerated work only provides part of the story – women worked but their activities are not so readily visible.[15]

The relationship between work and gender has been a focal point of historical research, with historians concentrating in particular on the gendered division of labour and on the question of how the emergence of capitalism caused this relationship to be redefined. Pat Hudson has argued that 'for the mass of the population the social position of women in medieval and early modern society was never simply one of inferiority and subjection because economic necessity made women indispensable partners in the work of household, farm and workshop as well as vital contributors to family incomes.'[16] For women work was not an 'occupation' in its own right, but understood instead as the social obligation of wives and daughters.[17] The family economy, Hudson thus claims, holds the key to understanding the decline of women's access to skilled work: as the family declined as a unit of production, so too did married women's work opportunities.[18] Sheilagh Ogilvie has criticised this transposition of the Anglosaxon experience onto Germany, arguing that during the eighteenth century in many parts of Europe (including Germany) it was not the market but institutional social capital deployed by guilds, the Church, etc. that prevented women and the poor from devoting more time to commercial work and, in so doing, stifling or delaying any 'industrious revolution'.[19] Lyndal Roper, in contrast, points to the shift from an ambiguous ideology of work to one focusing increasingly on remunerated work within the occupations that simultaneously tied women's 'domestic' activities into the central concept of *Nahrung* (early modern socio-moral concept of earning a living).[20] The neither-here-nor-there nature of women's work only resolved into a pattern of

13   Schötz, 'Von Kauffrauen und Kuchenweibern', 383–85.
14   Wiesner, *Working Women*. More recently for the English context, Deborah E. Harkness, 'A View from the Streets: Women and Medical work in Elizabethan London', *Bulletin of the History of Medicine* 82: 1 (2008): 52–85.
15   A point made by Harkness in her study of London. See 'A view'.
16   Pat Hudson and W.R. Lee, *Women's Work and the Family Economy in Historical Perspective* (Manchester: Manchester University Press, 1990), 3.
17   Ibid. Wiesner also notes this fusion of female identity with the work of the household in early modern Germany. See Merry Wiesner, 'Gender and the Worlds of Work', in Robert Scribner, ed., *Germany: A New Social and Economic History, 1450–1630* (2 vols, London: Edward Arnold, 1996), vol. 1.
18   Hudson and Lee, *Women's Work*, 5.
19   Sheilagh Ogilvie, 'Consumption, Social Capital, and the "Industrious Revolution" in Early Modern Germany', *The Journal of Economic History* 70: 2 (2010): 287–325, 320–21.
20   Lyndal Roper, *The Holy Household: Women and Morals in Reformation Augsburg* (Oxford: Oxford University Press, 1989), 27–31, 41–49.

male breadwinner / female housekeeper after 1800 once the differences between the sexes were construed as physiological and psychological disposi-
tions.[21]

As midwifery was per se a gendered occupation, it could blossom unfettered by guild restrictions. Between 1650 and 1800 we not only witness a
quantitative growth in the opportunities open to women working in the midwifery landscape in an official capacity – the number of offices more than
doubled. The growing city also provided greater opportunities for women to
work and support themselves as unsworn midwives and Wickelweiber by
looking after unmarried mothers during lying-in (see Chapter Four). Yet we
know relatively little about how the varieties of midwifery slotted into the economic existence of midwives and their households, an important consideration if we want to fully comprehend the specific relationship between economic activity and gender in the area of midwifery in the German cities.[22]
How did midwifery fit into the female life-cycle? Why did women become
midwives? How many women were financially reliant on midwifery? To what
extent did their households rely on the income from midwifery? And finally,
did this change over the course of the eighteenth century?

The data

Unlike the many illuminating studies of famous midwives, this chapter aggre-
gates biographical information on unknown and unpublished women.[23] The
patchiness of the records for the period between 1648 and the 1680s meant
that it was difficult to elicit substantial data on women working during these
decades. The demographic data in my main sample thus stems from material
collected on 43 women operating within the midwifery landscape in Leipzig
between 1695 and 1810. These 43 women were selected from the 118 midwives, Beifrauen, Wickelweiber and Gassenmägde known to be working in
Leipzig between 1695 and 1810. An effort was made to incorporate women
from all parts of the midwifery landscape: 17 of the 43 women in the sample
worked at some point in their lives as informal midwives, Gassenmägde or
Wickelweiber, although many eventually became sworn Beifrauen or mid-

21   Karin Hausen, 'Family and Role-Division: The Polarisation of Sexual Stereotypes in the
     Nineteenth Century – an Aspect of the Dissociation of Work and Family Life', in Rich-
     ard J. Evans and W. Robert Lee, eds, *The German Family: Essays on the Social History of the
     Family in Nineteenth- and Twentieth-Century Germany* (London and Totowa, NJ: Croom
     Helm; Barnes & Noble, 1981).
22   Evenden's study is one of the few to delve in detail into the relationship between mid-
     wifery and the household oeconomy. See Evenden, *Midwives*, 106–37.
23   For instance: Pulz, *"Nicht alles"*; Schrader, *Memoirs Schrader*; Thatcher-Ulrich, *Midwife's
     Tale*; Adrian Wilson, 'A Memorial of Eleanor Willughby, a Seventeenth-Century Mid-
     wife', in Lynette Hunter and Sarah Hutton, eds, *Women, Science and Medicine 1500–1700:
     Mothers and Sisters of the Royal Society* (Sutton: Stroud, 1997); Rattner Gelbart, *The King's
     Midwife*.

wives. Inclusion in the sample was based on the level of individual biographical information gleaned from council administrative records. Thus those women for whom I was able to amass a good deal of information from several different sources were more likely to be included in the sample. Yet the fact that during the eighteenth century most sworn midwives and Beifrauen appear in the administrative sources at least once (and frequently several) times over the course of a lifetime suggests that my sample is relatively representative.[24] Coverage of official and unofficial midwives was, of course, based on very different circumstances. Longevity in office, not status as a 'troublemaker', had the greatest influence on the level of coverage a sworn midwife enjoyed in the sources. Women working as unsworn midwives were seldom recorded in these administrative sources, other than when they came into conflict with clients (very rarely), with other midwives (more frequently) or came to the notice of the Council either directly or via the Stadtaccoucheur (quite rarely). Women who never made it as sworn Beifrauen or midwives but who worked inofficially are therefore probably (unavoidably) underrepresented in my sample.

For a small number of women, data from more than one source enabled me to pinpoint age and number of children reasonably accurately. These women were included in the sample without my having to pursue further genealogical research. In order to accumulate data on age, family size and socio-occupational milieu of additional subjects, I turned to the marriage and baptismal registers of the only churches in Leipzig to confer the sacraments: St Thomas and St Nikolai. As the marriage indexes in both churches are ordered alphabetically according to husband's surname, it was only possible to search for women for whom the husband's first name was known. In most cases the information elicited from the marriage register (midwife's maiden name, father's name and occupation, husband's occupation) was crucial for finding out when a midwife was baptised or how many children she had borne. Obviously, problems arose when a midwife had not married in Leipzig or the couple had not baptised its children in either St Thomas or St Nikolai, as was the case with recent immigrants or women raised in Leipzig who had married a 'foreigner' and left the city. Hence the sample may well underrepresent 'foreign' women working as midwives, which might, for example, artificially elevate the prominence of matrilineal ties amongst women in the midwifery landscape. Unable to collate data for each woman in the main sample on each category (children, marital status, husband's occupation, etc.), my statistical analysis for these demographic aspects is based upon smaller subgroups of women from the main sample of 43 women.

24 Using council administrative and legal records I was able to allocate a woman to each sworn midwife and Beifrau office for most of the eighteenth century, which indicates the high level of coverage (not just relating to appointment) most of these women enjoyed in the sources.

The following information was collected on as many individual midwives as possible:

1. Date(s) of marriage(s)
2. Names and occupation(s) of husband(s)
3. Date and place of baptism/birth
4. Names, occupations and place of origin of parents
5. Names and occupations of godparents
6. Baptismal dates of children
7. Names and occupations of children's godparents

Parallel to the quantitative analysis of the sample, I have utilised any further available prosopographical information concerning the 118 midwives known to be working during this period as supporting (anecdotal) evidence throughout this chapter.

Age: the demise of maturity

In early modern Germany 'age' was an abstract concept. Many Leipzig midwives, for example, were unaware of their precise date of birth and, when asked to provide their age in administrative or legal encounters, could often provide no more than a rough estimate in years. However, these figures were not simply plucked out of mid-air. As Pat Thane has recently concluded, the concepts of physical capacity and retirement from work have only been associated with a particular age since the twentieth century. In most premodern societies what both defined the ability to work and determined a person's stage of life was 'functional age', or 'the degree of capacity to carry out tasks'.[25] Eligibility for poor relief in early modern England, for example, depended on whether a person could feasibly continue working and control their affairs, not chronological age.[26] Other historians have emphasised the importance of visual significers on the body as markers for determining age – in particular old age.[27] Thane's suggestion that age 'is not fixed and ... has different meanings in different contexts' refers directly to old age, but her argument is just as applicable to conceptions of age more generally.[28] So, the age people gave corresponded to their functional capacity and the stages of the life-cycle. Chronological age was irrelevant inasmuch as there was no culture of tying capacity to a particular age in years. As this chapter will show, until the latter eigh-

---

25 Pat Thane, *Old Age in English History: Past Experiences, Present Issues* (Oxford: Oxford University Press, 2000), 4–5.
26 Ibid.
27 Lynn Botelho, 'Old Age and Menopause in Rural Women of Early Modern Suffolk', in Lynn Botelho and Pat Thane, eds, *Women and Ageing in British Society Since 1500* (Harlow: Longman, 2001), 60–61.
28 Thane, *Old Age*, 5.

teenth century, it was this functional understanding of age and her stage in the life-cycle that determined whether or not a woman was fit to practise as a midwife.

For statistical reasons this discussion abstains from calculating averages in order to produce a marker of general experience. The sample of women working as sworn midwives and sworn Beifrauen in Leipzig between 1695 and 1800 is comparatively small and the average ages derived are thus too susceptible to distortion. Depicting the scatter pattern of ages is far more meaningful and demonstrates two notable trends (see Figures 4 and 5).

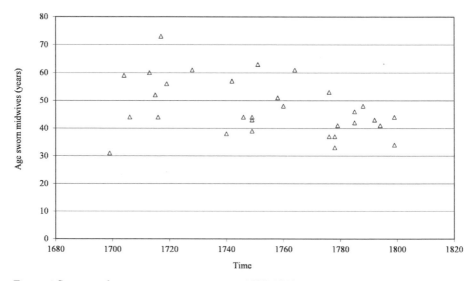

Figure 4 Sworn midwives: age at appointment, 1695–1810

Sources: KAL, Taufbücher; KAL Traubücher; StadtAL, Tit. (F) XLIV.D, Hebammen, 1673–1852; StadtAL, II. Sekt., 1568–1939; StadtAL, Straf. 1561–1856; StadtAL, Testamente, 1539–1847.

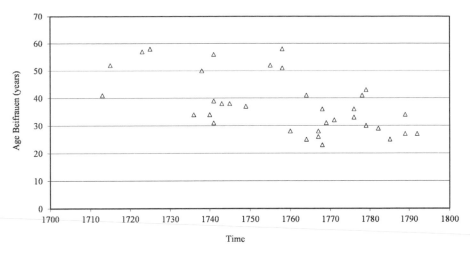

Figure 5 Beifrauen: age at appointment, 1695–1810

Sources: KAL, Taufbücher; KAL Traubücher; StadtAL, Tit. (F) XLIV.D, Hebammen,
1673–1852; StadtAL, II. Sekt., 1568–1939; StadtAL, Straf. 1561–1856; StadtAL, Testamente,
1539–1847.

Firstly, from around the 1780s both midwives and Beifrauen obtained office at
a younger age. Secondly, whereas the lowest chronological age of a sworn
midwife at appointment hovered at around thirty years throughout the century, Beifrauen became progressively younger as the century progressed (see
Figure 5). By the 1730s most Beifrauen were appointed in their thirties. After
1760 just under half of those appointed were in their twenties. From 1780
onwards no Beifrau older than forty years of age was appointed. As for the
sworn midwives, whereas roughly half those appointed prior to 1780 were
over the age of fifty at appointment, all women who gained office between
1780 and 1800 were younger than fifty.

Both sets of data indicate a similar trend over time towards a tighter range
of ages and the elimination of older recruits. Appointment ages prior to the
1780s demonstrate a mish-mash of the elderly, the middle-aged and the young,
reflecting the idiosyncratic individual life circumstances of novice midwives in
Leipzig. Whereas Dorothea Seidel, for example, was just 31 years old when
sworn in as a midwife in 1699, her fellow midwife Anna Sperling was appointed in 1704 at the ripe old age of 59. Seidel's youth was admittedly quite
exceptional, and only a few other women were appointed in their thirties.
Most offices went to women in their forties and fifties. In Leiden, where a
similar system of midwifery regulation was in place, the ages of women appointed as *stadsvroedvrouw* appear to demonstrate similar trends.[29] In seven-

29 Average age at appointment in Leiden was 39, by which stage candidates had already
    amassed a number of years of experience. See Marland, "'Stately and dignified'", 289.

teenth-century London, where ecclesiastical licensing was comparatively weak, women typically also began working as midwives in their thirties.[30]

This data suggests that functional rather than chronological age was the precondition for holding the office of sworn midwife until the latter decades of the eighteenth century. Prior to the 1780s, maturity was key in determining whether or not a woman was suitable for office. Most women were appointed as sworn midwives in their forties and fifties, towards the end of their reproductive prime. However, as the wide range of ages suggests, maturity was a slippery concept. Unlike in Leiden, where midwives had to be married with at least two children, the midwifery oaths and instructions produced by the Leipzig Council did not explicitly regulate the age or life-cycle of its midwives, leaving the matter instead to custom.[31] Maturity (post-childbearing state) was a desirable characteristic for sworn midwives from the perspective of the Council and the community, and many women were past their reproductive years when appointed and were aware this counted in their favour. Regina Meder, for example, stated in 1724 that 'my condition is such that because of my age nothing may count against [me], as I live in such a state in which desire ... has completely ceased'.[32] As Marland argues, municipal authorities all across Europe recognised maturity as a highly valuable attribute for municipally employed midwives. Maturity was tied to the contemporary medical notion that the post-menopausal woman was more neutral, stable and 'manly' than her pre-menopausal counterpart.[33] The cultural norm guiding the criteria for obtaining a midwife office, however, did not always apply to midwifery practice more generally and many sworn midwives gained years of midwifery experience either as apprentices or independent practitioners before reaching 'maturity'.

From the middle of the eighteenth century, we can see a trend associating the ideal midwife with younger women. Maturity, once a marker of experience and reliability, was gradually transformed into a state of fragility, lability and hostility. This transformation was the result of a new kind of encounter between midwives and male medical practitioners that subverted the rules of authority and maturity: formal midwifery lessons. This change corresponded more or less to the introduction of compulsory lessons for the midwives and Beifrauen taught by the newly appointed Stadtaccoucheur Johann Valentin Hartrauff (in office 1732–1740). In his report to the Leipzig Council in 1735, Hartrauff complained bitterly about the sworn midwives who regularly ex-

---

30   Evenden, *Midwives*, 112–13.
31   Marland, '"Stately and dignified"', 289.
32   StadtAL, Tit. (F) XLIV.D.1, Bd. I, 'Kindermütter bey hiesiger Stadt betr. ingl. die angenommene Bey Weiber betr. 1673–1756', 74–80, 'Beifrau application (Regina Meder)', 8 July 1724–25 January 1725, 74.
33   Marland, '"Stately and dignified"', 287–88. On the complex identity of mature women practising medicine in early modern England, see also Margaret Pelling, 'Thoroughly Resented? Older Women and the Medical Role in Early Modern London', in Lynette Hunter and Sarah Hutton, eds, *Women, Science and Medicine 1500–1700: Mothers and Sisters of the Royal Society* (Stroud: Sutton Publishing, 1997), 83–84.

cused themselves from his lessons: 'it does not please them that they should be tortured with so many questions and answers [and] that according to their opinion they do everything cleverly and God has not ever left their side'.[34] The Beifrauen, whose relationship with the sworn midwives was often rocky and for whom the lessons were often the best opportunity they had of learning their 'art' (see Chapter Four), were nevertheless generally present and willing to learn.[35] This level of absenteeism, Hartrauff warned the Council, would further the 'superstition, prejudice, oversight, unwilling behaviour and recalcitrance' that plagued the sworn midwives.[36] This was the moment in which the Stadtaccoucheur attempted – rather unsuccessfully – to turn the midwives into pupils; the moment in which the maturity and seniority of the city's sworn midwives was conflated with belligerence, stupidity and insubordination. By 1740 Hartrauff was convinced that the older Beifrauen were at appointment, the more likely they would be old, 'weak and grumpy' by the time they became sworn midwives.[37] From the perspective of the Stadtaccoucheur, maturity was no longer cast in entirely positive terms: old age had become an occupational liability and an impediment to learning.

Enshrining this new attitude towards maturity in practice proved itself, however, less straight forward. As Figure 5 shows, the number of novice Beifrauen in their reproductive prime (under forty years) during and after Hartrauff's term of office increased somewhat, but the ages of recruits continued to vary greatly. It was not until Johann Ehrenfried Pohl assumed the office of Stadtaccoucheur in 1782 that this preference for younger Beifrauen (and hence also younger midwives) translated into semi-coherent 'policy' and practice. Pohl's mentor and predecessor, Johann Karl Gehler, had also favoured youth in Beifrauen but had not implemented his ideas with any efficacy. Like Hartrauff, Gehler and Pohl's devaluation of maturity arose out of anxieties about the practical authority that it conferred which, when combined with belligerence, would hinder the learning relationship. Pohl's report to the city Council in 1785 sums up this newfound suspicion and frustration towards elderly midwives. Older women were:

> incapable of learning anything new, in part convinced too much of their own imagined knowledge that one could hope to educate them [to be] good midwives; if one such woman has tended mothers lying in, given *lavaments* or has been present at one or another confinements, she commonly believes that she already knows everything, although this does not give her any advantage over the others, nor does it make her more skilled

---

34   Tit. (F) XLIV.D.1, 132–60, 'Stadtaccoucheur reports (Hartrauff)', 29 November 1732–13 March 1737, 138.

35   See Hartrauff's report from 15 March 1736. Ibid., 140.

36   Ibid., 138.

37   StadtAL, Tit. (F) XLIV.D.1, 'Kindermütter bey hiesiger Stadt betr. ingl. die angenommene Bey Weiber betr. 1673–1756', 173–89, 'Midwife Maria M. Müller requests leave for Petersberg (Halle) and Beifrau appointment (Maria Lorend)', 17 May 1740–20 January 1741, 189.

in the work of a midwife, and [she] soon believes that she needs not learn anything further.[38]

What was now desirable in a midwife was the malleability and self-consciousness of younger years which meant that midwives, unfettered by 'old prejudices', could soak up 'the correct and truthful concepts of science'.[39] Experience acquired without the medical guidance of the Stadtaccoucheur was now treated with profound suspicion as 'unscientific'.

Pohl and Gehler were not just worried about insubordinate midwives. They were also greatly concerned about getting the best and the most out of the sworn midwives and Beifrauen. Both wanted to ensure the women appointed to the office of Beifrau and midwife would be active for a very long time, for the system of appointment was cumbersome and inflexible. As the number of midwife offices was capped, a Beifrau might have to wait ten or more years for a position. Moreover, the practice of inhabiting an office until death meant that at any given time, one or more of the most senior midwives were likely to be too frail or too ill to work, depleting the city both of experience and (wo)man-power. Pohl and Gehler were thinking consciously in terms of efficacy and productivity, attempting to engineer a corps of younger midwives. The youth of twenty-five-year-old Beifrau candidate Johanna Regina Gentsch, Gehler argued in 1785, was 'more a recommendation than an obstacle'. No Beifrau, he continued, should be appointed over the age of thirty so that when said Beifrau finally became a midwife twelve to fifteen years later, she would not be 'weary with the prospect of this onerous office before her, but may still be able and skilled in the service of the city'.[40]

From the beginning of his period in office in 1764 Stadtaccoucheur Gehler consistently favoured younger Beifrau candidates. He usually included women under the age of thirty in his shortlist of candidates, even when they had no or only little experience in midwifery.[41] Yet it was still quite rare for women that young to apply for an office and only one of the nine women who applied for a Beifrau office in 1771 was under the age of thirty.[42] Nevertheless, candidacy petitions suggest that the imperative amongst sworn midwives and Beifrauen to demonstrate maturity began to wane in the 1770s. It was not just a case of the Stadtaccoucheur cherry-picking young candidates; Gehler and

38   Tit. (F) XLIV.D.6b, Bd. II, 'Acta, die Kindermütter und Beiweiber betr. de Anno 1782', 53–62, 'Beifrau appointment (Johanna Regina Gentsch)', 12 November–9 December 1785, 59–61.

39   Ibid.

40   Ibid., 57–58.

41   See, for example, the candidatures of: Johanna Christiana Petsch (aged 26) in Tit. (F) XLIV.D.6b, Bd. I, 'Acta, Die Einrichtung der Kindermütter und Beÿweiber', 154–57, 'Midwife appointment (Dorothea Westphal)', 2–30 September 1771; Johanna Rosina Wegel (aged 27) in Tit. (F) XLIV.D.6b, Bd. I, 93–108, 'Appointment (Matthes)', 20 February–31 March 1768.

42   Ristu, Akten Teil 1, Nr. 185, Bd. I, 408–41, 'Ansuchungs-Schreiben um den, nach Absterben Juliänen Sharitas Zschachin ledig wordenen Kinder-Mutter und beÿfrau Dienst (1775)', 1775.

his successor Pohl had no lack of fresh, young candidates from whom to choose. In 1776, for example, all of the shortlisted applicants were aged between 30 and 36.[43] As the century drew to its close, ever fewer Beifrau candidates were over the age of forty, and many were in their early thirties as a younger generation of women clambered to become sworn Beifrauen.[44]

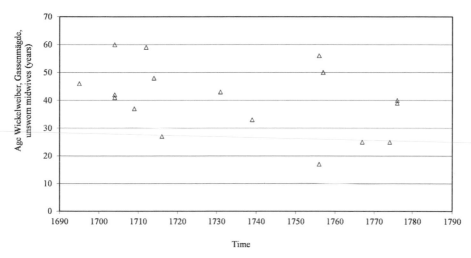

Figure 6 Wickelweiber, Gassenmägde and unsworn midwives: age when commenced working as midwives, 1695–1810

Sources: KAL, Taufbücher; KAL Traubücher; StadtAL, Tit. (F) XLIV.D, Hebammen, 1673–1852; StadtAL, II. Sekt., 1568–1939; StadtAL, Straf. 1561–1856; StadtAL, Testamente, 1539–1847.

Although the age spread of women practising midwifery without an office – the Wickelweiber, Gassenmägde and other unsworn midwives – was erratic and broad, it also demonstrates a similar downward trend towards the end of the eighteenth century (see Figure 6). If we take into account that for many of these women, there is insufficient information on the length of time they were involved in midwifery before they became visible in the sources, these groups of unsworn midwives were probably far younger when they began in midwifery than depicted in Figure 6. This suggests that even before the Stadtaccoucheurs began to consciously lower the age of new Beifrau recruits, youth was not a barrier to becoming involved in the various varieties of unofficial midwifery. Thus, until the late eighteenth century, maturity was largely associated with the *office* of sworn midwife, not the act of assisting women during

43 Tit. (F) XLIV.D.6b, Bd. I, 193–98, 'Appointment (Leib and Küchler)', 19 February–4 March 1776, 193.

44 None of the Beifrau candidates in 1775 was over 40. See Ristu, Akten Teil 1, Nr. 185, Bd. I, 408–41, 'Ansuchungs-Schreiben (Zschachin)', 1775. This trend also occurred in Mainz, where the average age of midwives at oath fell from 50 in the 1770s to between 30 and 40 at the end of the century. See Hilpert, *Wehemütter*, 53–55.

delivery and childbed per se. Younger women *learning* midwifery – irrespective of setting – was culturally and socially conceivable before the trend towards young midwives and Beifrauen gained momentum. Maturity in a midwife only assumed a negative connotation once sworn midwives were turned
into pupils in the lessons of the Stadtaccoucheur. Thus two trends coalesced to
produce this new situation: Firstly, maturity ceased to be a marker of ability
and suitability for the office of sworn midwife as the focus shifted towards
teachability and the acquisition of a particular type of knowledge gleaned in
formal lessons. Secondly, socio-economic conditions towards the end of the
eighteenth century appear to have made it increasingly necessary for young
women to exploit the opportunities for paid work that this shift opened up to
them.

Marriage and motherhood: from matron to working mother

Motherhood and wifehood were key elements in the identity of early modern
midwives all across Europe. Unmarried and childless midwives such as Justine Siegemund and Angélique le Boursier du Coudray, whose practice extended beyond the bounds of the local community, were exceptions to the
norm in the same way that their midwifery careers were also extraordinary.
Indeed, even at the height of her success and fame as the court midwife in
Brandenburg in 1690, Siegemund felt compelled to defend her childlessness
in the introduction to her midwifery manual.[45] And the childless and unmarried du Coudray simply adopted herself a family in lieu of a husband and
children.[46]

In Leipzig the women appointed to the office of sworn midwife were most
likely to be married, not widowed. This demographic pattern, which appears
to have been common since the late sixteenth century at least, continued into
the first half of the seventeenth century.[47] The eighteenth century demonstrates a similar proportion of women married with only one-quarter of newly
appointed midwives widowed at appointment.[48] Beifrauen, who tended to be
younger than midwives when appointed, demonstrate an even lower rate of
widowhood in the eighteenth century – a mere 3 per cent.[49] Of course, many

---

45   Lynne Tatlock, 'Volume Editor's Introduction', in Justine Siegemund, *The Court Midwife.
      Justina Siegemund,* trans. Lynne Tatlock (Chicago, IL: The University of Chicago Press,
      2005), 1.
46   Rattner Gelbart, *The King's Midwife,* 58.
47   Five of the seven midwives listed in the 1590 oath were married, two widowed. See Ohne
      Sig., 28, 'Kindermuetter Aidt', 1590, 28. Marital status could be obtained for 40% of
      midwives known to be working between 1583 and 1650 (21 out of 52 women). 71%
      (15 no.) of these women were married.
48   Marital status could be identified for 61% of midwives in the sample. Of these, only 26%
      were widowed at appointment.
49   91% of the sample was used to derive the rates of marriage and widowhood for Bei-
      frauen.

of these women would end up as widows during the course of their career; a few would remarry, many would not. Midwifery was not, however, a last resort for widowed women. Whilst it was culturally conceivable for a midwife to be widowed, midwifery continued to be a task for women who could draw upon both their experience of childbirth and their honourable status of wife and mother within the community.

The fact that most midwives in Leipzig were wives and, as we shall see, mothers when they began to practise has something to do with the age at which they began working: most women were married by the age of thirty and, when widowed, many remarried if they could. However, it is also related to the meaning of marriage as a social institution during this period. The adoption of Lutheran doctrine in the wake of the sixteenth-century Reformation fundamentally changed the status of marriage and family. Whereas in the Middle Ages legal and guild restrictions on establishing a household meant that only a small proportion of the population could actually marry, the decline of feudalism and the abolition of clerical celibacy following the Reformation meant that that marriage came to prevail as the main form of social organisation and the cornerstone of society in general.[50] Lutheran reformers recast marriage as a secular institution, but simultaneously counted the conjugal state as the first Godly ordinance. Marriage (and the begetting of many children) thus became an integral mechanism of social and political order. The Lutheran legacy of conjugality as the 'natural order' endured until well into the eighteenth century.[51]

The married state was, in this respect, an honourable state. Wives were responsible not just for the running of the household but also for the behaviour of female members within it. Thus a wife's role as Hausmutter (mistress of the house) was to safeguard the integrity of the household. In turn this provided her husband, the Hausvater (master of the house), with the honour required to participate in burgher society.[52] The honour that women derived from the married state was an important aspect of a midwife's identity. In the eighteenth century a sworn midwife or Beifrau was expected to diligently pursue a 'Christian honourable peaceful life' which, in Lutheran Leipzig, entailed wifehood and motherhood.[53] Indeed reputation, which formed one of the

50   Large sections of medieval society were destined to spend life unmarried and there were several institutional barriers to forming an independent household: Men and women from the upper echelons of society frequently became monks, nuns and priests. Serfs were not permitted to establish their own households until they held land. And merchant and artisan journeymen were likewise forbidden from entering conjugality until they had established their own businesses or acquired the status of master tradesman. See Wunder, *"Er ist die Sonn"*, 59.

51   Richard van Dülmen, *Kultur und Alltag in der Frühen Neuzeit. Erster Band. Das Haus und seine Menschen 16.–18. Jahrhundert* (2nd edn, 3 vols, Munich: Verlag C.H. Beck, 1995), vol. 1, 157–64; Wunder, *"Er ist die Sonn"*, 66–69; Roper, *The Holy Household*, 133–64.

52   Wunder, *"Er ist die Sonn"*, 250; Dülmen, *Das Haus*, vol. 1, 164.

53   See Item 1 of Tit. (F) X 23b, Bd. III, 234–36, 'Instruction Beÿweiber', c. 1715 (undated), 234–36.

criteria of appointment, was also based on the honour of the household and
marital life. Those whose marriages were not peaceable, such as sworn midwife Catharina Ehrlich, were treated with suspicion and required to prove
their honour through the medium of attests from families in their neighbourhood of residence.[54]

The married state was the unwritten rule for most women working in the
midwifery landscape – for sworn midwives, Beifrauen, Wickelweiber, Gassenmägde and unsworn midwives alike. The group of 'unsworn' midwives in the
sample demonstrates similarly high levels of marriage (83 per cent were married). Unmarried women might only operate within the midwifery landscape
if they partook in some kind of informal apprenticeship or servant role under
female relatives who were midwives themselves. Maria Magdalena Thomäe,
for example, was just seventeen years old when she claimed to have begun
learning the art of midwifery from her grandmother. And Regina Pötsch had
already been working alongside her mother, a sworn midwife, for some time
when she married at the age of twenty-five in 1775.

As the age of midwives and Beifrauen decreased over the course of the
eighteenth century, combining midwifery with rearing a family became increasingly common. Midwives with one or more young children to care for
were not unheard of prior to 1700. In 1605, for example, the sworn midwife
Magdalena Ackermann's three youngest children (should they have survived
infancy) would have been aged five, eight, and twelve – all 'dependent' according to contemporary understandings of childhood.[55] Yet others, such as
Dorothea Adler, were appointed when their children were all grown up.[56]
What both Ackermann and Adler had in common was that they were no
longer in their childbearing years when they obtained office.

A century later it was quite common for women with young families to
begin learning or practising midwifery. Five of Christina Lorend's six children
were under the age of thirteen when she began assisting her mother, a sworn
midwife, in 1709.[57] On appointment to the office of sworn midwife in 1716,
her three youngest children were aged between nine and thirteen. Anna Doro-

54   Tit. (F) XLIV.D.1, 16–43, 'Appointment (Ehrlich)', 10 January–24 July 1713, 29–41. At-
      tests were standard fare in an appointment, however, Ehrlich had to produce additional
      documents in this case.
55   The spacing of her births (2+ years) suggests that many of her children survived at least
      part of the first year of life. See KAL, Tauf. Thom., 1584, 94b; 1587, 117a; 1589, 135b;
      1593, 172b; 1597, 199b; 1600, 275a. The age of adulthood varied according to the situa-
      tion (involvement in business matters, participation in legal matters or ability to carry
      arms) as well as between the sexes. In legal terms, however, a child was able to be prose-
      cuted as an adult from the age of fourteen. See Wunder, *"Er ist die Sonn'*, 35–36.
56   Ackermann's youngest would have been fourteen years old when she was appointed. See
      KAL, Tauf. Thom. 1584, 96b (Erhard); 1585, 104b (Anna); 1588, 125a (Maria); 1591,
      150a (Magdalena); 1592, 159a (Magdalena); 1593, 172b (Thomas); 1596, 189b (Wil-
      helm). Evenden notes that most midwives in seventeenth-century London had completed
      their childbearing years by the time they were licensed. See Evenden, *Midwives*, 113–14.
      On Quaker midwives, see also Hess, 'Midwifery Practice', 67.
57   Aged 18, 13, 9, 8, 6 and 4 years.

thea Braun began helping her mother, a Beifrau, in 1715 when at least one child from her first marriage was just four years old. In 1725, when she petitioned the Leipzig Council to replace her deceased mother as Beifrau, Braun was thirty-six years of age and had borne nine children, the youngest of whom would have been under ten (if still alive). Johanna Sophia Stranz became a Beifrau in 1743 and was also the mother of five children under the age of fourteen at the time. When she was appointed as a sworn midwife five years later, her three youngest ranged between eight and thirteen years of age.[58]

Stranz, Braun and Lorend's experiences were not exceptional. As the century progressed, the number of Beifrauen with children aged thirteen years or younger rose from 67 per cent in the period before the introduction of the Stadtaccoucheur (1695–1731) to 100 per cent in the period following Gehler's appointment (1763–1800). Some, such as Beifrau Maria Margaretha Hornung, were still in the midst of childbearing when appointed: Hornung became a Beifrau in 1764, but died in childbirth just three years later, leaving one young daughter behind.[59]

Sworn midwives, who likewise tended to be younger in the late 1700s, were also more likely to have young children than in the century before. Around 64 per cent of Leipzig sworn midwives working in the eighteenth century appear to have had young, dependent families.[60] Indeed, the trend towards sworn midwives with young families followed that of the Beifrauen. Whilst only half of the sworn midwives had dependent children prior to 1763, this figure jumped to 89 per cent for the period 1763–1800. Evidence from Lübeck suggests a very similar pattern. Most of the sworn midwives working in 1791 there were raising dependent children under the age of ten, and a few were still in their childbearing years when sworn into office.[61] Those who were already practising as unsworn midwives, Wickelweiber or Gassenmägde prior to obtaining an office were almost certainly combining raising a young family and/or childbearing with midwifery. Thus the majority of women working within the midwifery landscape were not elderly; for much of the period under scrutiny they were mothers of young children. Although working as a midwife with a young family had never been unusual, over the course of and, in particular, towards the end of the eighteenth century, it slowly became the norm for both women learning midwifery and women in *sworn* office.

58 Tit. (F) XLIV.D.1, 83–118, 'Appointments (Greger and Veiß)', 22 November 1724–4 September 1725, 104.
59 StadtAL, Leichenbücher, 7 August 1767 (Susanna Margaretha Hornung). See also her mother's will in StadtAL, Ristu, Testamente, Rep. V, Paket 216, Nr. 3, 'Testament: Maria Dorothea Westphal', 1768.
60 Of the 22 sworn midwives who were known to have children, 14 had children under the age of 14.
61 In Lübeck 8 of the 11 midwives in office in 1791 (appointed between 1770 and 1786) had at least one child under the age of 10 (73%). Four women had two or more. However, most women in this cohort (8 of 11 women) had ceased childbearing by the time they assumed office. See Loytved, *Hebammen*, 169–71.

Socio-economic milieus: the artisan midwife

Most midwives, Johann Georg Krünitz reasoned in his *Enclyclopaedie* (1781–
89), 'are from the lowest rabble, of coarse reason and peasant morality'. This,
he continued, was all because 'excepting the large cities, no midwife can live
from her services, not even badly. Why then should a sensible woman … de-
vote herself to this onerous business, if she is able to make a living in another
way?'[62] Krünitz's harsh words were in the spirit of his time. For many amongst
the burgeoning chattering elite, rural Germany was the badlands of eighteenth-century society and for decades the countryside had been the primary
target of cameralist-driven, 'enlightened' absolutist directives. But if the midwives in the large and bustling city of Leipzig were not considered by critical
contemporaries to belong to the social 'rabble', who were they? So far, we
have established that they were predominantly married, often no longer in
childbearing years, in their thirties, forties or fifties, and often had young children. But in what kinds of social and economic milieus did they operate? And
how did this change over the course of the eighteenth century?

Social and geographic origins were formative aspects of social status and
social identity throughout the early modern period. For the day labourer, just
as for the council elder, social standing depended upon where one came from
and whom one could count as family and kin. In the Germanies, society was
organised into *Stände*, a complex hierarchy of social estates that had developed during the Middle Ages and remained the guiding principle of social
organisation until the late eighteenth and early nineteenth centuries. The social hierarchy of the Stände affected social and political status within society
at large, for example, between the status of the king, the noble and the peasant or burgher. From the sixteenth century onwards, the concept of the Stände
began to include a specific space defined by work, reflecting the growing interests of those incumbent of an Amt (government office) and, in particular, of
the artisans.[63] Yet the structure of the Stände also applied to the microcosm of
the household to differentiate between household members according to gender, age and social status. Thus married persons belonged to the *Ehestand*,
journeymen to the *Gesellenstand*, and the elderly to the *Stand der Alten*. This
ideal Ständegesellschaft (society of estates) was inherently and demonstrably
based on the principle of a divinely ordained, vertical hierarchy of inequality.
Every person in that hierarchy, whether at the bottom or the top, was bound
to uphold the order of the Stände.[64] Membership of a particular Stand was
absolute and based on birth, occupation and social status; the Stand defined

---

62   See entry for 'Heb=Amme' in Krünitz, *Oekonomische Encyklopädie*, vol. 22(ii), 542.
63   The most famous expression of this new concept of the Stände is Hans Sachs' 'Stände-
       buch' in which he describes in prose and picture the entire gamut of society, including
       the so-called 'unehrlichen' (dishonourable persons). In particular, Sachs accorded each
       artisan trade its own place in society. Sworn midwives, however, were not included. See
       Hans Sachs, *Eygentliche Beschreibung Aller Stände auff Erden* (Frankfurt am Main, 1568).
64   Richard van Dülmen, *Kultur und Alltag in der Frühen Neuzeit. Zweiter Band. Dorf und Stadt
       16.–18. Jahrhundert* (3 vols, Munich: Verlag C.H. Beck, 1992), vol. 2, 176–78.

the social, political and economic space in which each person operated. His or her ability to move about within the Stand was circumscribed by the opportunities and possibilities that family and household provided. Social and political rights were, at least in theory, conferred upon individual persons by the Stand, as were social worth and status – not the other way around.[65]

This began to change in the eighteenth century as work emerged as a key determinant of social status. However, the social identity of women in the seventeenth and eighteenth centuries was still bound up in the individual social milieu of the household and family and, therefore, the Stand to which the household belonged. At the head of each household stood the Hausvater, the male head of the family to whom all members of the household – wife, children, servants and apprentices – were subordinate. In his role as patriarch, the Hausvater was responsible for both the material well-being and the moral rectitude of his household. Although the wife, the Hausfrau or Hausmutter, enjoyed a certain level of authority over the organisation of the household and housework, it was the Hausvater who represented the household to the outside world and participated in the almost exclusively male world of civic politics and guild life.[66] The patriarchal organisation of society into the Stände on a macro-level and into households governed by the Hausvater on a microlevel meant that the social status of menfolk – fathers, husbands, brothers and, to a lesser extent, sons – was a major determinant of a woman's social identity throughout all phases of the female life-cycle.[67]

Thus there are four occupational markers that enable us to gauge the social environment in which Leipzig midwives operated over most of their life-cycle:

1. Father's occupation
2. Occupations of midwife's godparents
3. Midwife's husband's occupation
4. Occupations of the godparents of a midwife's children

Much of this information could be gleaned from the baptism and marriage records of the churches of St Thomas and St Nikolai. Church scribes generally recorded the names, occupations and residential status of men and, in the case of godparents, also of women. The use of occupation to define social environment is, however, not without its problems. It is not so much the potential unreliability of these sources that is the greatest cause for concern, but rather the problem of pinning down occupational identity itself in the early modern period. Historians have come to the conclusion that in the seventeenth and eighteenth centuries, very few people pursued a single occupation, either at any one time or over the course of a lifetime. Work in early modern

---

65 Ibid., 181.
66 *Das Haus*, vol. 1, 38–55.
67 On the 'thin' type of occupational identity accorded to women's work during this period, see Hudson and Lee, *Women's Work*, 3.

times was characterised by two phenomena, namely 'irregular work rhythms and the flexibility with which people combined various occupations and sources of income'.[68] Furthermore, the kind and variety of work people actually carried out did not always tally with the occupational labels recorded in official documents.[69] Recording of multiple occupational data for the husbands of midwives is not unusual.[70] Even more common was the interruption of work by war, which meant many artisans and day labourers endured lengthy periods as soldiers before returning to Leipzig and resuming their occupations. But how may we categorise the artisan-turned-soldier-turned-artisan-again, or the artisan journeyman who periodically worked in a shop during the fairs? Which form of work was the most important mark of social identity?

I suggest getting around this by focusing on socio-occupational milieus. By looking at the range of occupations that feature in a midwife's broader social environment, that is the occupations of parents and godparents, it is possible to discern certain trends towards discrete occupational milieus or clusters of related occupations.[71] Individual occupations have been grouped into thirteen categories which reflect the basic conceptual boundaries contemporaries made between different types of work and how they distinguished status within an occupational category: military (above the rank of officer), military (below the rank of officer), master artisan, artisan journeyman, domestic servant, minor official, academic (notary, schoolteacher, etc.), merchant/vendor, medical crafts/professions, clerical, day labourer, musician, other.[72]

68 Josef Ehmer and Peter Gutschner, 'Probleme und Deutungsmuster der "Arbeits-gesellschaft" in der Gegenwart und in der frühen Neuzeit', in Gerhard Ammerer et al., eds, *Tradition und Wandel. Beiträge zur Kirchen-, Gesellschafts- und Kulturgeschichte. Festschrift für Heinz Dopsch* (Vienna: Verlag für Geschichte und Politik, 2001), 315.

69 For example, state-employed Physici commonly carried out several simultaneous roles and tasks unrelated to their medical practice in late eighteenth-century Germany. See Lindemann, 'Enlightenment Encountered', 182–84.

70 Maria Sophia Mößler's husband, for example, was registered in three separate documents: firstly as a notary, then a student, and finally the admissions scribe at the hospital. The husbands of two other midwives Maria Plau and Josephina Popp were both recorded as artisans (probably journeymen) and so-called *Markthelfer* (fair assistants), the men hired by foreign merchants during the trade fairs to oversee shops.

71 Godparents, often relatives, were usually selected from within the social and occupational circles within which a household operated. In Leipzig it was common to name three godparents, two of whom belonged to the same sex as the child. Parents often selected godparents from a slightly higher social sphere than the parents. See Dülmen, *Das Haus*, vol. 1, 85–87; Martina Wermes, 'Die Analyse von Patenschaften und ihr Wert für sozialgeschichtliche Untersuchungen – dargestellt am Beispiel Leipziger Familien', *Genealogie. Deutsche Zeitschrift für Familienkunde* 24: 5–6 (1999): 592–601, 598.

72 These categories attempt to reflect the socio-occupational divisions that existed between types of work, rather than differences in economic status in Leipzig.

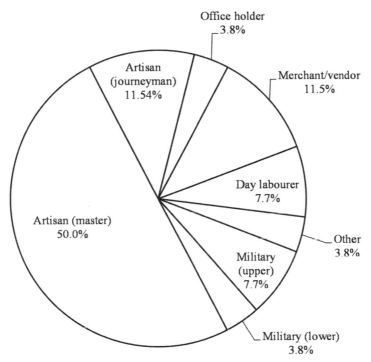

Figure 7 Midwives: occupation of father, 1695–1810 (sample size: 26 no.)

Sources: KAL, Taufbücher; KAL Traubücher; StadtAL, Tit. (F) XLIV.D, Hebammen, 1673–1852; StadtAL, II. Sekt., 1568–1939; StadtAL, Straf. 1561–1856; StadtAL, Testamente, 1539–1847.

For just over half of these women in the main sample (26 no.), information exists on the father's occupation (see Figure 7). The data reveals an unambiguous trend. An overwhelming 50 per cent of midwives' fathers were master artisans and a further 11.5 per cent were journeymen, making the artisan class the best represented occupational grouping.[73] The variation in individual occupations within this grouping, however, was vast and included bakers, butchers, bookbinders, tanners, shoemakers, bag-makers, hosiers, bottle- and basket-makers. The next largest groupings were merchants/vendors (of which 2 of the 3 were horse dealers) and military personnel, each of which made up 11.5 per cent of the sample. Day labourers made up 7.7 per cent of the group and minor officials a mere 3.8 per cent. Not one midwife from this sub-sample came from a family where the father was involved in a medical craft or profession, indicating that midwifery did not belong to the various social milieus of physicians, surgeons or apothecaries. It is worth remembering that most of this data is derived from midwives' church marriage records and represents occupational information for established family heads in middle or old age.

---

73   This is hardly surprising, given that artisans made up the largest Stand (estate) in society.

Indeed many midwives' fathers were in fact deceased by the time their daughters married.

The weighting towards the ranks of the artisan continues in the next sub-sample of 39 first husbands and 8 second husbands for whom occupation is known (see Figure 8). Of all first and second husbands combined, 38.3 per cent were master artisans and a further 31.9 per cent artisan journeymen.[74] The next largest group was made up of merchant/vendors (6.4 per cent) consisting of a horse dealer, a starch dealer and a fair assistant, followed by the group of domestic servants (also 6.4 per cent). Only one husband, a journeyman barber-surgeon, pursued a medical occupation.[75]

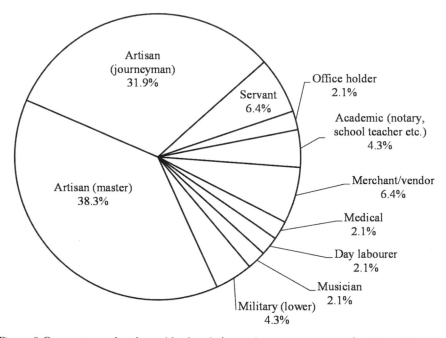

Figure 8 Occupations of midwives' husbands (second marriages included), 1695–1810, (sample size: 39 no. first husbands, 8 no. second husbands)

Sources: KAL, Taufbücher; KAL Traubücher; StadtAL, Tit. (F) XLIV.D, Hebammen, 1673–1852; StadtAL, II. Sekt., 1568–1939; StadtAL, Straf. 1561–1856; StadtAL, Testamente, 1539–1847.

Occupations requiring university study are noticeably underrepresented, with only one husband recorded firstly as a student, then as a notary and, finally, as

---

74 Journeymen in any trade were generally quite poor as they drew a wage and had no proper guild affiliation.
75 To compare: almost half of the Lübeck midwives working in 1791 were married to journeymen and just under one-third to military officers. See Loytved, *Hebammen*, 168. In late eighteenth-century Göttingen some 72 of midwives were married to artisans. See Hampe, *Zwischen Tradition*, 34.

an admissions scribe in the hospital. One further husband was noted as a 'literati' (probably academically trained) and schoolmaster. Of the artisan and merchant groupings, many would have been literate and numerate. Maria Erdmuth Medel's husband, a book printer, possibly also had a university background.[76] Each of the remaining categories (military, minor official, day labourer and musician) comprised less than 4 per cent. The very low numbers of day labourers – the non-specific, unincorporated mass of often itinerant workers known as *Handwerker* in the cities and *Tagelöhner* in the countryside – are particularly worth noting as this occupational grouping formed the backbone of the 'resident poor' in Leipzig.[77] This suggests that midwifery was the preserve of women whose households were well integrated into local communities. Women working in midwifery unofficially in various capacities do not appear to vary in terms of socio-economic background from sworn midwives and Beifrauen – hardly surprising considering that most midwives started practising midwifery in these unofficial roles.

How stable were these occupational milieus across generations amongst Leipzig midwives? By looking for occupational consistencies between fathers and husbands and incorporating data on godparents (both midwives' own godparents and the godparents they chose for their children), we can get an idea of how common it was for midwives to remain within a particular socio-occupational and economic milieu. The pool of women for whom both data on both the father's and the husband's occupation is available is small, but for eight women a clear correlation between the two criteria is apparent. Three of them demonstrate highly closed occupational affiliation:

1. *Beifrau Maria Alsdorff,* whose father was a burgher and master furrier in Leipzig, was baptised in 1666 with godparents from furrier and comb-making families.[78] When she married in 1686 Alsdorff reinforced her ties (as well as those of her paternal household) to the fur trade by marrying another burgher and master furrier.[79]

---

76 Those involved in the printing trade were largely educated and many even sported a university education. See Hazel Rosenstrauch, 'Leipzig als "Centralplatz" des deutschen Buchhandels', in Wolfgang Martens, ed., *Zentren der Aufklärung III: Leipzig. Aufklärung und Bürgerlichkeit* (Heidelberg: Verlag Lambert Schneider, 1990), 108–9; Axel Frey, 'Der "Leipziger Platz". Buch- und Verlagswesen', in Axel Frey and Bernd Weinkauf, eds, *Leipzig als ein Pleißathen. Eine geistesgeschichtliche Ortsbestimmung* (Leipzig: Reclam Verlag, 1995), 129–30.

77 Also belonging to this group were retired (and often incapacitated) soldiers, servants, manufacturing workers and much of the mass artisanal estate (e. g., low-level shoemakers, tailors, etc.). See Helmut Bräuer, 'Leipzigs Messen und die armen Leute während der frühen Neuzeit', in Günter Bentele et al., eds, *Leipzigs Messen 1497–1997. Gestaltwandel – Umbrüche – Neubeginn, Teilband 1: 1497–1914* (2 vols, Cologne: Böhlau, 1999), vol. 1, 324–25.

78 KAL, Tauf. Nik. 1666, 331 (Maria Magdalena Höpfner).

79 KAL, Trau. Nik. 1686, 143 (Johann/Hans Georg Altorff).

2. *Juliana Charitas Zschach* also remained affiliated to the very same guild to which her father Tobias Zeüner, a burgher and hosier, belonged by marrying the hosier Abraham Zschach in 1730.[80]

3. *Sworn midwife Maria Grunert,* the daughter of a burgher and horse dealer in Leipzig, could likewise prove an occupationally homogeneous lineage in the horse trade. Grunert's godparents were a country carriage driver's wife and the wife of a horse dealer (all burghers in Leipzig).[81] Maria married Christian Grunert, a horse dealer and *Einwohner* (non-burgher resident of Leipzig) from the city of Gera in Thuringia, in 1723.[82] It is difficult to be certain whether Grunert's marriage to a non-burgher entailed a step down the social ladder or rather constituted a strategic move to strengthen business ties with horse dealers, breeders and carriage drivers outside of Leipzig.[83] What we do know is that by 1741, Christian Grunert was working as a country carriage driver and the couple rearticulated their ties to the horse business when they baptised their first child in 1724: all three of the godparents they secured for their daughter were horse dealers.[84]

For a number of other midwives it is possible to identify a cluster of related occupations over the generations that sometimes extended beyond the boundaries of a particular guild. Maria Magdalena Thomäe's familial connections reveal an occupational cluster around leather clothing: her father was a master bag-maker and Thomäe married a master shoemaker.[85] Dorothea Ulrich's father was a master baker and burgher in Pegau, a town close to Leipzig. Dorothea married a keeper of a beer inn in 1773 who, by 1789, was working as a starch merchant (starch being an important commodity in the baking trade).[86] Sometimes, however, an occupational connection could hide upward mobility over a generation, as in the case of Johanna Sybilla Schulz, whose father earned a living combing wool. Wool-combing, like spinning, was a cottage industry and was carried out as piecework by urban day labourers (*Handwerker*) or by the inmates of the municipal workhouses (*Zuchthäuser*) erected in many

---

80 Trau. Nik. 1730, 476 (Juliana Charitas Zeüner).
81 Ibid. 1702, 455 (Maria Magdalena Biltz).
82 Ibid. Nik. 1723, 215 (Christian Grunert).
83 Horse-dealing and carriage driving were less reputable but often lucrative trades. Dealers were often suspected of selling sick horses and drivers of stealing the contents of barrels (esp. grains). Carriage drivers were, therefore, particularly dependent on building up trusting relationships with horse dealers and inn-keepers abroad. See entry for 'Landkutsche' in Krünitz, *Oekonomische Encyklopädie,* vol. 60, 315–16. See entry for 'Fuhrmann', ibid., vol. 15(i), 433–35.
84 Tauf. Nik. 1724, 208 (Maria Regina Grunert).
85 KAL, Trau. Thom. 1759, 151 (Johann Heinrich Thomä).
86 The starch trade was particularly important in the eighteenth century for a variety of reasons. It was the basis for face powder (fashionable) and a vital resource for a variety of other trades, e.g., book-binding, cooking, pastry-making, cotton-printing, linen and cotton manufacturing and laundering. The largest starch-producing regions in Germany were close to Leipzig in Halle, Weißenfels and the region around Dresden. See entry for 'Stärke' in Krünitz, *Oekonomische Encyklopädie,* vol. 169, 732–33.

European towns during the late seventeenth and eighteenth centuries.[87] Schulz's father, however, managed to find work as a fair assistant (*Markthelfer*) for a foreign merchant during the Leipzig trade fairs, which appears to have paid off for the family, for when Sybilla was baptised, three merchants served as her godparents.[88] Years later Sybilla married 'up', taking a journeyman in the silk-makers' guild as her husband in 1760.[89] Thus Sybilla's occupational milieu remained within the cloth-making crafts but she was now associated with the artisan Stand through her husband.

Whilst this socio-occupational data demonstrates that midwifery was a type of work most open to women from artisan households, it does not offer any information on the social and economic status of various trades and occupations. Although most artisans could refer to the honour and virtue of their guild, there was substantial variation in the level of social status accorded to each artisan craft and this was often city-specific. In general, the status of a craft depended upon the vintage of the craft or the guild, how full its coffers were, the material worth of the end product, and the 'cleanliness' of the work.[90] So whereas goldsmiths usually crowned the hierarchy of craftsmen, those who worked with cheaper materials and whose craft processes were rougher and dirtier – tailors and shoemakers, for example – found themselves at the lower end of the occupational status spectrum. Many crafts in the German territories such as tanning, weaving, pottery-making and barbering (i. e., work that entailed contact with blood, mud and body parts) were considered too filthy and dishonourable to warrant a guild at all.[91] There could also be significant variation in wealth between masters within the same guild. In Leipzig the textile industry (including cloth, linen, fur and leather) assumed particular economic importance during the fifteenth and sixteenth centuries, although this did not always correlate with wealth and power. Whereas the fur-makers' guild was quite wealthy, the linen-makers' guild was the least respectable and economically weakest of all the textile guilds, with linen weavers typically earning less than a day labourer.[92] Leipzig's position as an international hub of commerce and trade meant that horse-dealing and long-dis-

---

87   See entry for 'Wollkämmer' in ibid., vol. 240, 107.

88   Tauf. Nik. 1738, 566 (Johanna Sybilla Behnhold). Markthelfer were both numerate and literate. They were invested with a great deal of responsibility in the general running of shops and stalls. Hence, foreign merchants commonly employed the same Markthelfer at each fair. See Krünitz, *Oekonomische Encyklopädie*, vol. 84, 588.

89   Trau. Nik. 1760, 192 (Johann Gottlob Schulz). Silk was a luxury good and was produced in manufactories in Leipzig, where silk-workers also had their own guild. See Krünitz, *Oekonomische Encyklopädie*, vol. 152, 457–59.

90   Dülmen, *Dorf und Stadt*, vol. 2, 94.

91   Ibid. The tanners in Leipzig were organised in a guild that was reasonably respectable. However, as Kathy Stuart argues, the social *reality* of honour and dishonour was less straightforward, in particular within non-artisanal milieus. See Kathy Stuart, *Defiled Trades and Social Outcasts: Honor and Ritual Pollution in Early Modern Germany* (Cambridge: Cambridge University Press, 1999), 48–49.

92   Feige, 'Sozialstruktur', 173–80.

tance transport were significant, although unincorporated, occupations in the eighteenth-century.[93] That so many daughters and wives of artisans and journeymen became midwives suggests, moreover, that midwifery was indeed a respectable and honourable occupation for a woman and her household.[94]

It is worth noting which occupational groups do not feature amongst the husbands, fathers and godparents of midwives. The wives of lawyers and merchants, the two occupational groups that made up the ruling elite throughout the period, did not become midwives.[95] Nor, it seems, did the wives of clergymen or higher-status council employees. Most interestingly, no midwives were married to physicians, surgeons or pharmacists. Not even the lower status medical occupations – that is, barber-surgeons, barbers, veterinary surgeons, tooth-pullers and bath-house surgeons – are represented amongst the husbands of Leipzig midwives, so it appears that these women entertained no familial connections to learned or incorporated medical practitioners.[96] This does not take into account marital relationships with non-guild and non-academic healers (herbalists, soothsayers, etc.) that made up a large proportion of the medical 'marketplace' in Leipzig. However, the fluidity of the boundaries between sworn and unsworn midwives means that the wives and daughters of

93   See entry for 'Kutscher' in Krünitz, *Oekonomische Encyklopädie*, vol. 57, 450. Transport was one of the burgeoning branches of commerce throughout the early modern period, according to Dülmen, *Dorf und Stadt*, vol. 2, 103–4. As an indicator of the importance of the transport trade in 1700, the ratio of horses to humans was 4.5 times higher in Leipzig than in Dresden. See Katrin Keller, 'Kursachsen am Ende des 17. Jahrhunderts – Beobachtungen zur regionalen und wirtschaftlichen Struktur der sächsischen Städtelandschaft', in Uwe Schirmer, ed., *Sachsen im 17. Jahrhundert. Krise, Krieg und Neubeginn* (Beucha: Sax-Verlag, 1998), 153.

94   Disputes over honourability increased during the eighteenth century, as the guilds became increasingly more exclusionist and pedantic about upholding guild honour. See Stuart, *Defiled Trades*, 222.

95   Artisans ceased to be represented on the Leipzig Council in 1548, after which lawyers and merchants came to dominate. See Beachy, *Soul of Commerce*, 45–47. The Leipzig fairs and international trade – and with that the merchant class – were by far the most important and economically influential trades in the city and aspiration to that class was high. See Keller, 'Kursachsen am Ende des 17. Jahrhunderts', 146; '"Gemeinschaft des hantwergs weiber und kinder". Zunft und Familie im Leipziger Handwerk des 16. Jahrhunderts', *Sächsische Heimatblätter* 36: 2 (1990): 74–79, 77.

96   Connections between medical practitioners and midwives appear to be more pronounced in other areas of Europe. There are several examples of midwives in early modern English communities claiming a connection to barber-surgeons and even physicians, for example, the Quaker midwife Sarah Harris, whose father was a 'practiser of physick'. See Hess, 'Midwifery Practice', 57–58. London midwife Eleanor Willughby worked closely with her father, a man-midwife. See Wilson, 'A Memorial of Eleanor Willughby'. And on the Continent the Frisian midwife Catharina Schrader was married to a barber-surgeon. See M.J. van Lieburg, 'Catharina Schrader (1656–1746) and Her Notebook', in Hilary Marland, ed., *"Mother and Child were Saved". The Memoirs (1693–1740) of the Frisian Midwife Catharina Schrader* (Amsterdam: Rodopi, 1987), 6–7. However, Germany's most famous early modern midwife had no such familial connections to the 'medical' world; Justine Siegemund was the daughter of a pastor and the wife of a steward and secretary. See Siegemund, *Court Midwife*, 4–5.

medical practitioners and healers may well have been practising midwifery for family and neighbours, but did not need to acquire the financial and social benefits that a midwife office would bestow upon them.[97] Certainly recent work on domestic medicine has highlighted the difficulties in separating out 'home-made' medicines and medical care from commercial medical activities.[98] Indeed the only woman in our sample with explicit connections to medical occupations was the unsworn midwife Johanna Christiana Winter, wife of a journeyman barber-surgeon. Winter had sought an appointment as a midwife primarily because her husband had been unable to find work in Leipzig.[99] This example suggests that service-for-fee midwifery (sworn and unsworn) amongst families within the medical milieus was restricted to those in the lower ranks of medical practice (e.g., barber-surgeons and journeymen) and to those in financial need. Familial connections to any kind of medical practitioners appear to have been largely irrelevant for both midwives and the community.

The socio-occupational data on Leipzig midwives suggests that by the seventeenth century, midwifery (and perhaps this is indicative of women's work more generally) had become a phenomenon of the lower estates; most midwives working in this period came from and remained within the middle and lower artisan or lower military milieus.[100] Over the course of the eighteenth century, so Wiesner, the status of midwifery slipped further, as fewer wives of master artisans became midwives. This lends credence to the argument put forward by a number of historians of women's work that the world of work underwent a process of classing and gendering as early as the late Middle Ages, be this due to economic crisis or institutional barriers and professionalisation.[101] For Leipzig, Keller argues that the economic distress of the sixteenth

97 Lynette Hunter notes that late sixteenth- and seventeenth-century aristocratic women who carried out health-care work within their local communities (in particular in rural communities) thought of their work as a devotional or social-charitable act. By the seventeenth century the recording and discussion of medical receipts and remedies by aristocratic women had become 'a social medium for exchange, a leisure activity' within the context of court life in London. See Lynette Hunter, 'Women and Domestic Medicine: Lady Experimenters, 1570–1620', in Lynette Hunter and Sarah Hutton, eds, *Women, Science and Medicine 1500–1700: Mothers and Sisters of the Royal Society* (Stroud: Sutton Publishing, 1997), 101–3; 'Sisters of the Royal Society: The Circle of Katherine Jones, Lady Ranelagh', in Lynette Hunter and Sarah Hutton, eds, *Women, Science and Medicine 1500–1700: Mothers and Sisters of the Royal Society* (Stroud: Sutton Publishing, 1997).

98 See Elaine Leong, 'Making Medicines in the Early Modern Household', *Bulletin of the History of Medicine* 82: 1 (2008): 145–68.

99 Ristu, Akten Teil 1, Nr. 185, Bd. I, 408–41, 'Ansuchungs-Schreiben (Zschachin)', 1775, 410v.

100 Wiesner finds that the exodus of midwives from the urban elite in Nuremberg actually took place in the fifteenth and sixteenth centuries, when women of the upper estates assumed a supervisory role over lower-status midwives and the wives of craftsmen and minor officials. See Wiesner, 'Early Modern Midwifery', 96.

101 See variously Bártori, 'Frauen in Handel und Handwerk'; Keller, 'Zunft und Familie'; Sheilagh C. Ogilvie, *A Bitter Living: Women, Markets and Social Capital in Early Modern Germany* (Oxford: Oxford University Press, 2003); Susanne Schötz, 'Zur Mitgliedschaft

century lowered the number of master craftsman households able to sustain themselves from 61.3 per cent to 45.8 per cent, forcing women in the lower artisan estate to seek an additional income, largely outside of the home in washing, sewing, hawking or midwifery.[102] Yet the pressure to find new sources of income in sixteenth-century Leipzig was not just felt by women. Less wealthy artisan masters also sought to inhabit lower-level offices, such as the Gassenmeister, well master or gatekeeper, as a means of augmenting the family finances and potentially also the status of the household within the community. Others invested in property, brewed beer or branched out into the business of trading goods.[103]

During the eighteenth century the household model reliant on more than one source of income was the norm rather than the exception. With the economic squeeze brought about by an increasing population and an archaic and anachronistic culture of guild corporatism and enclosure, this dependency on more than one source of income increased. Fewer journeymen were able to set up a workshop of their own and ever more were relegated to a lifetime of wage work in another man's business. The profile of these journeymen families demonstrated greater similarity to those of other 'wage' earners: the urban day labourers, career domestic servants and minor officials whose numbers had swelled considerably during the seventeenth century amidst high levels of urbanisation and the expansion of princely administrations.[104] The 'double burden' of reproductive *and* productive work remained the norm for most women throughout the ensuing centuries. The Leipzig data suggests that in the eighteenth century, the more wealth and status a family had, the more likely it was that wives' and daughters' work would be restricted to reproduction and domestic labour.[105] This process was not a disassociation from the artisan world per se, but rather a gradual dissolution of paid female work from the more 'respectable', middling milieus.

Yet in addition to these socio-economic factors, the occupation of midwife was coming to mean something quite different to women in the latter eighteenth century. The need for a varied household income, the introduction of Beifrauen and the concerted effort on the part of the Stadtaccoucheurs Gehler and Pohl to appoint younger women converged together to transform the office of midwife from an occupation tied largely to a woman's mature life-cycle phase to one a woman would pursue from her youth to her grave. Because of

von Frauen in der Leipziger Kramerinnung im Spätmittelalter bzw. zu Beginn der frühen Neuzeit', in Henning Steinführer et al., eds, *Leipzig, Mitteldeutschland und Europa. Festgabe für Manfred Straube und Manfred Unger zum 70. Geburtstag* (Beucha: Sax-Verlag, 2000); Wiesner, 'Gender'.

102 Keller, 'Zunft und Familie', 74–75.

103 'Handwerkeralltag im 16. Jahrhundert', in Karl Czok and Helmut Bräuer, eds, *Studien zur älteren Sächsischen Handwerksgeschichte* (Berlin: Akademie-Verlag, 1990), 39–40.

104 Michael Mitterauer, *Grundtypen alteuropäischer Sozialformen: Haus und Gemeinde in vorindustriellen Gesellschaften* (Stuttgart: Frommann-Holzboog, 1979), 58–63.

105 As Keller finds. See Keller, 'Zunft und Familie', 75.

changing economic circumstances, young households were becoming dependent on the kind of long-term security, however paltry, that a Beifrau and a sworn midwife office could guarantee.[106]

Midwifery, family and household

Having examined the demographic and socio-occupational profile of midwives, it is now time to explore the material basis of midwifery work and how this particular type of early modern women's work fit into family life and the household oeconomy.[107] In the traditional guild-oriented model of work that dominated in most early modern urban communities, women's work was located within the household and the workshop without any clear demarcation between a woman's labours within the home for the family and her work in the family business. As the wife of a master craftsman, a woman's work incorporated both domestic and commercial tasks. Early modern women were primarily identified through their husbands or fathers and assumed the social, economic and occupational status of their menfolk.[108] The transfer of identity was not merely an expression of patriarchal authority or a vacuous shift of status from husband to wife or from father to daughter. During this period the labels 'wife of' and 'daughter of' were primarily economic categories, in particular amongst artisans. Although largely barred from the guilds in their own right, women were more than just 'helpers' on the side-lines; they were active and productive actors in their husbands' and fathers' businesses.[109] Hence the wife of a shoemaker was known as 'Mrs Shoemaker' because she was directly

106 This demonstrates parallels with Mitterauer's findings that domestic service, another field of work open to women, was also transformed during this period from a near universal rite of passage (that is, something most people belonging to the lower and middle estates did between childhood and marriage) to a life-long occupation. See Mitterauer, *Grundtypen*, 62–63.

107 I use 'oeconomy' here to stress the focus on the household as simultaneously a 'domestic' and 'commercial' unit. See the use of this term in Elaine Leong and Sara Pennell, 'Recipe Collections and the Currency of Medical Knowledge in the Early Modern "Medical Marketplace"', in Mark S. R. Jenner and Patrick Wallis, eds, *Medicine and the Market in England and Its Colonies, c.1450–c.1850* (Basingstoke: Palgrave Macmillan, 2007), 136–37.

108 Van Dülmen differentiates between five factors that determined social status in the early modern period: 1) property and wealth, 2) occupation, 3) degree of political influence, 4) family and kin, 5) comportment. See Dülmen, *Dorf und Stadt*, vol. 2, 181–84.

109 Darlene Abreu-Ferreira, 'Work and Identity in Early Modern Portugal: What Did Gender Have to Do with It?', *Journal of Social History* 35: 4 (2002): 859–87, 859–60; Merry Wiesner, 'Spinning Out Capital: Women's Work in Preindustrial Europe 1350–1750', in Renate Bridenthal et al., eds, *Becoming Visible: Women in European History* (3rd edn, Boston, MA, 1998), 6; Katharina Simon-Muscheid, ed., *"Was nützt die Schusterin dem Schmied?". Frauen und Handwerk vor der Industrialisierung* (Frankfurt am Main: Campus, 1998), 24–30.

involved in the business of crafting and selling the shoes produced in her husband's workshop.[110]

Working women (that is most women) in early modern cities were not only involved in the running of the family business. Many women married to artisans, and in particular to men who out-sourced their labour as day labourers, domestic servants or minor public officials, would frequently draw on additional income from a great variety of activities.[111] Washing, sewing, spinning and hawking were common types of work pursued by women, but they might also assume minor municipal offices, which often required literacy and numeracy. In Nuremberg, for example, women also worked as licensed employment agents for domestic servants (*Zubringerinnen*) and appraisers who inventoried the movable estate of deceased persons for the communal inventory register (*Unterkeuflinnen*).[112] Midwifery was one such type of work that women often pursued in addition to their commercial and domestic household work. Yet, even when a woman sought additional avenues of income carrying out tasks entirely unrelated to her husband's occupation, she was still known as the wife of the shoemaker. How then did these additional occupations and additional sources of income contribute to the identity of a woman?

Supplications submitted for sworn midwife and Beifrau positions in Leipzig demonstrate that the occupation and the residential status of the husband, not the various additional occupations of the wife, functioned as the key identifier. Women who washed, sewed or worked as nurses were identified through the occupation of their husbands. After appointment, however, a midwife or Beifrau was usually identified as the sworn midwife of a district rather than through her husband. A paucity of sources involving midwives in non-midwifery related matters makes it difficult to gauge what sorts of labels midwives were conferred in everyday matters. However, not one of the five wills found for midwives or midwives' husbands refers to a woman's work as a midwife. Christiana Dorothea Behnhold's husband, for example, even omitted the fact that his wife had been working as a sworn Beifrau for over ten years, although he instructed that his wife be permitted to continue with her hat-making business.[113]

---

110 Merry Wiesner Wood, 'Paltry Peddlers or Essential Merchants? Women in the Distributive Trades in Early Modern Nuremberg', *Sixteenth Century Journal* 12: 2 (1981): 3–13, 6–7.

111 Keller, 'Handwerkeralltag', 16–17; Ogilvie, *A Bitter Living*, 351. For a summary of the broad range of wholesaling and selling activities carried out by women in Leipzig's markets, see Susanne Schötz, *Handelsfrauen in Leipzig. Zur Geschichte von Arbeit und Geschlecht in der Neuzeit* (Cologne: Böhlau, 2004), 426–23.

112 These women were mostly the wives of artisans and minor officials. See Wiesner Wood, 'Paltry Peddlers', 7.

113 StadtAL, Testamente Rep. V, Paket 236, Nr. 3, 'Testament: Paul Ludwig Lehnhold', 1782. Inexplicably, Paul Ludwig Behnhold was recorded as 'Lehnhold', however, a comparison of his family members leaves no doubt that he was the husband of the midwife Christina Dorothea Behnhold.

What this suggests is that although urban sworn midwives were acknowledged as belonging to a particular occupational group, on a public and official level the occupational label of 'midwife' was not a formative aspect of *household* identity. However, on a local, everyday level midwives and other women working in midwifery within a neighbourhood were prominent figures within the community. As this chapter will later discuss, as the eighteenth century progressed, midwifery increasingly became the oeconomic mainstay of households plagued by unemployment or underemployment. Yet despite greater reliance on female labour, the occupational identity of 'midwife' was not strong enough to trump the social environment of the household and the socio-occupational status of the husband. Women worked as midwives, but their occupation did not emancipate them from the identity of their husbands.[114] Despite increased training opportunities and the transformation of midwifery to an occupation pursued by women across most of their adult life rather than in just one particular phase of the life-cycle, working midwives continued to retain the identity of their menfolk. Eighteenth-century midwives remained anchored within the larger social environment into which they were born and into which they married. However, what *concrete* role did midwifery play in the family oeconomy? And what kinds of households did midwives have?

House-ownership amongst midwives was minimal and largely restricted to the less affluent neighbourhoods outside the city walls. In 1713 one of the women shortlisted for office, the widow of a day labourer, owned the house in the Vorstadt in which she lived.[115] Another sworn midwife working around this time, the wife of a basket weaver, also owned a house in one of the Vorstadt neighbourhoods.[116] Most midwives rented, in particular those stationed within the city walls. In order to ensure the presence of sworn midwives in the city, the Leipzig Council provided the women stationed there with free accommodation in one of its properties in Stadtpfeiffergäßgen. Almost all sworn midwives stationed in the city appear to have been reliant on this accommodation. By the middle of the eighteenth century, finding affordable rental accommodation was also becoming a problem for midwives and Beifrauen working in the traditionally cheaper Vorstadt. According to a midwife who petitioned the Council in 1738, there was growing reluctance amongst the Vorstadt burghers to allow midwives to hang their signs out the front of their

114 There are parallels here to what is known about the famous 'King's Midwife', Mme du Coudray. Du Coudray engineered the careers of her niece and her niece's husband, both of whom were trained by her and worked alongside her during her teaching missions. Although she intended her niece alone to be her successor and obtained a royal *brevet* for this very purpose, she was well aware that a married woman with an independent occupational identity was socially unacceptable. Thus she devoted considerable effort to the securing of a permanent position as a teacher of childbirth in Bordeaux for her niece's husband Coutanceau, throwing in the outstanding midwifery skills of her niece as 'part of the package deal'. See Rattner Gelbart, *The King's Midwife*, 238–40.

115 Tit. (F) XLIV.D.1, 16–43, 'Appointment (Ehrlich)', 10 January–24 July 1713, 22–25.

116 Ibid.

houses and, as a result, midwives were being forced to pay exorbitant rents.[117] Without drawing any causal link between the two, this midwife was at pains to also mention the increasing demand placed on her services by 'unmarried women', the care of whom made up a sub-business for many Vorstadt midwives and Beifrauen. The two were, however, undoubtedly linked. Despite the financial benefits these neighbourhoods derived from such women (to be discussed at length in Chapter Four), midwives who provided this service to unmarried women devalued a neighbourhood's respectability.

Reallocations and promotions ensured that Leipzig midwives were relatively mobile within the city. These moves often entailed physically moving the household to another neighbourhood, particularly when the new post took a woman from the Vorstadt into the walled city or vice versa. Whilst this might have been relatively unproblematic for women in rented accommodation, it caused difficulties for those whose husbands had a stable and geographically fixed business, in particular artisans with expensive workshops or trades requiring the space and resources of the Vorstadt. Some families appear to have circumvented the nuisance of moving house by maintaining two abodes. Anna Martha Priebs, the wife of a carriage driver, rented a flat at the Grimmaisches Tor in addition to her family house (probably at the Rannstädter Tor) in order to comply with her instruction.[118] Others petitioned the Leipzig Council to remain in their neighbourhood, a plea that was rarely ignored. In 1769, for example, Maria Sabina Herrmann requested a midwife office in her own neighbourhood at the Peterstor on the grounds that she and her husband, a cotton smoother, had recently installed a new workshop at great expense and the cost of renting a second set of lodgings for the sake of Maria's office would prove beyond their means.[119] Hermann's request was granted by the Council but six years later, when promoted to an office within the city walls, she was instructed to reside (at least overnight) in one of the free Council-owned apartments in Stadtpfeiffergäßgen.[120]

Both Hermann and Priebs lived (at least some of the time) physically separated from their families and households, which suggests that midwifery could draw a physical and spatial boundary between domestic life and work life more than many other types of women's work. And this may have altered the social and oeconomic dynamic between husband and wife. Husbands and families had not only to get used to the erratic and long hours a midwife worked out of the home, but also become accustomed to the semi-permanent

---

117 Tit. (F) XLIV.D.1, 161–69, 'Appointment (Mößler and Werner)', 29 May–9 July 1738, 170–71.

118 Tit. (F) XLIV.D.1, 83–118, 'Appointments (Greger and Veiß)', 22 November 1724–4 September 1725, 108–9. The fact that Priebs' second husband was well off enough to acquire burgher status just after they married in 1717 suggests that the family was relatively comfortably off.

119 StadtAL, Tit. XLIV.D.6b, Bd. I, 'Acta, Die Einrichtung der Kindermütter und Beÿweiber betr.', 112–19, 'Beifrau appointment (Medel)', 2–4 December 1769, 116–17.

120 Tit. (F) XLIV.D.6b, Bd. I, 193–98, 'Appointment (Leib and Küchler)', 19 February–4 March 1776, 193.

absence of the person traditionally so integral to the family business and the running of the household. Perhaps through the economy of makeshift, these women had ceased to have high levels of involvement in either their husbands' or their domestic work.[121]

Whilst the work of a midwife took her out of the home, most midwives resided in their own households. Midwives may have been lone practitioners, but many could only carry out their task when they drew on the assistance provided by their households. Indeed family members were often directly involved in a midwife's practice. Daughters were frequently inveigled into their mothers' practices, as we shall see later on this chapter, and both midwives and Beifrauen used their female servants to carry the birthing stool, act as a messenger and sometimes even to assist them during deliveries. Information on whether or not midwives typically kept servants is scarce. However, in 1784 both the sworn midwife Johanna Sybilla Schulz, the wife of a silk maker in one of the manufactories, and her Beifrau Christiane Behnhold, the wife of an instrument maker, each kept a servant and used them to communicate with one other.[122] Neither of these women appears to have been particularly well off, yet the servant seems to have been integral to their midwifery practice.

Husbands were also involved in their wives' work. Because midwifery was both a nocturnal and 'out-of-house' occupation, husbands sometimes figure as safeguards of the household and its occupants. Beifrau Maria Zinck's husband, for example, regularly accompanied his wife whenever she was called out at night to an unfamiliar woman or house.[123] Husbands also shared the burden of nocturnal disturbances, getting out of bed to answer anxious knocks at the door in the middle of the night. In 1719 it was Dorothea Seidel's husband who rose to tell a messenger that his wife had only just returned from a delivery and was too exhausted to attend another.[124] Husbands also assumed a vital organisational role in their wives' work, particularly at night. Whilst in the middle of a delivery, midwife Johanna Sabina Raphel received news that one of her clients required urgent attention. Unable to leave the labouring woman in front of her, midwife Raphel sent a message to her husband asking him to arrange for another midwife to attend the woman.[125]

Husbands could also be held responsible for acts of negligence ('Verwahrlosung'). In 1764, for example, the Beifrau Johanna Maria Werner delivered the child of an indigent single woman. For some unknown reason (the records

121 The entwinement of domestic work and midwifery visible through the rural Maine midwife Martha Ballard's diary around 1800 may not have been characteristic of Leipzig's busy midwives. See Thatcher-Ulrich, *Midwife's Tale*.

122 Tit. (F) XLIV.D.6b, 29–37, 'Midwife Schulz vs Beifrau Behnhold', 23 February–18 March 1784, 32–36.

123 Tit. (F) XLIV.D.6b, Bd. I, 56–66, 'Appointment (Held and Plau)', 26 April–16 May 1760, 58r–58v.

124 StadtAL, II. Sekt. S (F) Nr. 1023, 'Hebammen. Eine Beschwerde über Dorothea Seidel', 26 October–15 November 1719, 1–5.

125 II. Sekt. W (F) Nr. 332, 23–26, 'Schütze/Raphel', 1–7 September 1724, 23–26.

could not be found) the matter ended up being investigated and, interestingly, the accusations of negligence were levelled at both Beifrau Werner and her husband.[126] Yet a midwife's reputation and honour did not hinge entirely on the behaviour of her husband. Candidates for a midwife office were subject to investigations by the Council into their comportment ('Lebenswandel') and their standing within the community. Badly behaved husbands could cast a shadow on the suitability of applicants, but did not disqualify them altogether. Catharina Ehrlich, for example, who was known for her tempestuous relationship with her husband, was required in 1713 to produce additional evidence of her good comportment to the Leipzig Council.[127] And of another applicant, Christina Lorend, the Council scribe was careful to note that her husband, after getting himself into debt, had fled Leipzig leaving his wife and six children to fend for themselves.[128] Yet whilst Ehrlich's marital disharmony and the debts of Lorend's husband were considered noteworthy, neither actually hindered either woman from obtaining an office. Lorend's absentee husband may indeed have been a recommendation, inasmuch that a midwife office would ensure her a livelihood. Family life was a crucial aspect of a candidate's reputation, but as far as the Stadtaccoucheur was concerned, the most explicit criticisms targeted the behaviour of midwives, their penchant for drink or their roughness of hand, rather than the unseemly character of their spouses.[129]

Research on women's economic involvement in the artisan workshop has provided us with insight into the essential but poorly visible role women played within husband-led households.[130] A midwife's practice, however, was not an auxiliary function in the same way as the work carried out by the wife of an artisan was. As we have seen, midwifery practice relied upon both paid and unpaid labour supplied by family and household dependents. This reflected the entanglement of commercial and social relations and transactions women maintained more generally within the local community that differentiated the world of women's work from that of men. Midwifery really was a 'family' affair, even in the city where it was practised commercially: a midwife was dependent upon the labour of her daughters, daughters-in-law, sisters and female servants. Like the wife in the artisan workshop, the midwife's husband was an integral part of a midwife's practice, even when his level of involvement stopped short of the birthing chamber. As we will now see, in financial

---

126 II. Sekt., M (F) Nr. 670, Bd. III, 50–87, 'Dismissal (Werner)', 19 April 1763–1 March 1764, 51.
127 Tit. (F) XLIV.D.1, 16–43, 'Appointment (Ehrlich)', 10 January–24 July 1713, 27–29.
128 Ibid., 22–25.
129 See, for example, Breuer's shortlisting of five candidates in 1758. See Tit. (F) XLIV.D.6b, Bd. I, 1–8, 37–8, 54–5, 'Stadtaccoucheur reports (Breuer)', 28 May 1757–14 July 1758, 6.
130 Cavallo's study of women's economic activity and value within the artisan workshop/ household shows that the entwinement of female household members in production was significant and that women were economically active across the life-cycle. See Sandra Cavallo, *Artisans of the Body in Early Modern Italy*, trans. Liz Heron and Sandra Cavallo (Manchester: Manchester University Press, 2007), 160–80, esp. 76–77.

terms midwifery became an increasingly important part of the household oeconomy over the course of the eighteenth century as many households became increasingly dependent upon women's paid work.

Midwifery and the household oeconomy: the forces of poverty

Surveying the large collection of supplication letters of aspirant midwives and Beifrauen, it becomes clear that poverty and desperation were significant factors motivating women to take up commercial midwifery. The stories of financial need recounted by women are tales about incapacitated husbands, woefully inadequate household income and perilously large families. In a world without a culture of occupational health and safety, earning one's 'daily bread' could prove itself an unhealthy, even fatal pastime. Johanna Christina Bähr's husband, for instance, was plagued with chronic ill health caused by his work which required him to sit all day long. In 1775 Bähr decided to ease the burden on her poor husband by looking for work and submitted an impassioned but unsuccessful plea for a Beifrau office.[131] Juliana Charitas Zschach, who eventually gained an appointment as Beifrau in 1741, petitioned the Council in 1740 with the sole argument that she, her husband and their three children were experiencing extreme economic hardship.[132] For Beifrau candidate Rahel Sophia Lehmann, poverty and the Christian ideal of the large family had conspired to become a financial liability. Not one of her offspring was able to contribute to the household oeconomy, plagued as they were with 'weakness and miserable bodies'.[133]

Pressures on the artisan employment market and the particularly protectionist behaviour of the guilds in the eighteenth century was a further incentive for women to seek work as midwives. Johanna Dorothea Findeis, the wife of an ailing tailor, petitioned the Council for a midwife office after the tailors' guild prohibited her from continuing to run the business on behalf of her husband.[134] The wife of a barber-surgeon journeyman, Johanna Christina Winter, likewise turned to midwifery after her husband was barred from practising within Leipzig and it became necessary that she 'be able to honestly earn my bite of bread for myself and my husband through this office'.[135]

An even greater problem appears to have been pressure on the number of master artisan positions available, which meant that more and more craftsmen were doomed to a lifetime as journeymen. The finite number of master

---

131 Ristu, Akten Teil 1, Nr. 185, Bd. I, 408–41, 'Ansuchungs-Schreiben (Zschachin)', 1775, 417.

132 Tit. (F) XLIV.D.1, 173–89, 'Müller (leave) and Beifrau appointment (Lorend)', 17 May 1740–20 January 1741, 183.

133 Tit. (F) XLIV.D.6b, Bd. I, 66–86, 'Beifrau appointment (Thomäe)', 1 September 1767–20 November 1768, 71r–72r.

134 Findeis' supplication was unsuccessful. See ibid., 70r–71v.

135 Ristu, Akten Teil 1, Nr. 185, Bd. I, 408–41, 'Ansuchungs-Schreiben (Zschachin)', 1775, 410.

titles permitted by each guild ensured that the most common way of acquiring a title and workshop was to marry the widow of a former master craftsman.[136] As this pressure continued over the course of the eighteenth century, it became increasingly normal for masters to employ more journeymen than apprentices.[137] Dorothea Christina Seidel's husband Andreas, for example, was still a journeyman carpenter when Dorothea died at the age of fifty-seven in 1725. A journeyman's existence was both socially and economically precarious, which directly affected the household. Journeymen were generally not covered by the guild-based system of welfare provision and were dependent on either public alms or private bequests and loans in times of hardship.[138] Maria Erdmuth Medel's husband, a printing apprentice, was already ailing and, without recourse to guild assistance, was unable to support the family when she was appointed Beifrau in 1768. In these rather bleak economic circumstances it became necessary for wives to seek a reliable source of income as the economic mainstay of the household. The office of sworn midwife was attractive; not only did it provide a source of monetary income, but also wood, grain and, at some later stage, a free roof over the family's head. And it was for life.

The case of the midwife Maria Catharina Vogel, who moved to Naumberg (a small city near Leipzig) to take up a sworn midwife office in 1787, provides us with a rare and wonderfully explicit example of the relationship between midwifery and the household oeconomy, and how midwifery could overturn the notion of female work as complementary to the household oeconomy. For the Vogels, Maria's work as a midwife was the financial rock upon which their existence was built. Her husband's wig-making and hairdressing business was sporadic, mostly during the trade fairs, and hardly produced enough for the family to live on.[139] After Maria had applied for permission to resign her office, the Council summoned her husband Johann Vogel to explain how he planned to pay the taxes he owed the city. They also asked him how he planned to support his wife should she fail to find her feet in Naumberg. He replied (with a hint of tongue-in-cheek) that he would 'win back his clientele again which he had lost because he had to follow his wife, a midwife in the Vorstadt, out of the city.'[140]

Not only was Johann rather nonchalant about leaving Leipzig, he was also content to let his wife assume the role of main breadwinner and follow her wherever necessary. His wife, Johann told the Council, was to travel alone to

136 This was the case in eighteenth-century Salzburg and Vienna. See Mitterauer, *Grundtypen*, 106–16.

137 Between 1647 and 1794 the proportion of journeymen to total workshop workforce in Salzburg and Vienna employed in artisan master workshops rose from 42% to 60%. Ibid., 63.

138 Stannek, 'Armut', 103–8. Also noted by Loytved, *Hebammen*, 168.

139 See Vogel's petition to the Leipzig Council dated 7 November 1782 in Tit. (F) XLIV.D.6b, Bd. I, 158–285, 'Various complaints', 14 July 1772–1810, 236.

140 Tit. (F) XLIV.D.6c, 54–74, 'Various appointments', 4 October 1782–22 January 1789, 66.

Naumberg. He would only follow her, he continued, once she had 'acquired a sufficient clientele'.[141] The opportunity, he proffered, might even provide both of them with a new chance of improving their livelihood: if Maria was successful, Johann intended to ply his trade in Naumberg but continue to work in Leipzig during the fairs. If not, he planned to return with her to Leipzig.[142] Johann added that he certainly hoped his wife would be able to make something of herself in Naumberg. Responsibility for the couple's livelihood was placed squarely with Maria, but Johann was confident that she was up to the challenge. After all, he explained to the councillors, 'his wife is not at all dim and will know how to feed herself.'[143]

Poverty is a recurrent theme in the biographies of women working within the midwifery landscape in Leipzig, yet the letters of supplication for midwife and Beifrau offices suggest that this was not the main reason offered by women. Women who argued their cases through a rhetoric of need were not given preference over women who did not (irrespective of whether the latter were, in fact, poor). At the same time, women pleading poverty were not considered unserious contenders. Although poverty alone rarely landed a woman a midwife office, the plea of poverty voiced by many women resonated with the general idea that the allocation of lower public offices, such as that of sworn midwife and Beifrau, could constitute an act of paternal provision and compassion for those who might otherwise be forced to join the ranks of the 'deserving poor' and become dependent upon public alms.[144]

An analysis of four cohorts of supplications (1713–25; 1738–40; 1760–69; 1770–75 (see Figure 9) shows that the number of women citing an incapacitated or un(der)employed husband during the eighteenth century ranged from 20 per cent of supplicants in the 1738–40 cohort and peaked at 36 per cent in the 1760–69 cohort, which coincided with the final, economically devastating years of the Seven Years War. Women who only mentioned unspecific poverty were even fewer in number in each cohort. Therefore, we can conclude that acute financial stress constituted the basis of at most 40 per cent of all supplications across the eighteenth century. In other words, the majority (around two-thirds) of all known aspirant Beifrauen and sworn midwives cited motivating factors unrelated to poverty or financial need when making a case for appointment.

---

141 Ibid., 65.
142 Ibid.
143 Ibid., 66.
144 This contrasts with Lindemann's findings for Braunschweig that the discourse of poverty was a strategy to prove deservedness and that the category of deservedness alone was a reason for the authorities to employ a midwife. See Lindemann, 'Professionals?', 181–82.

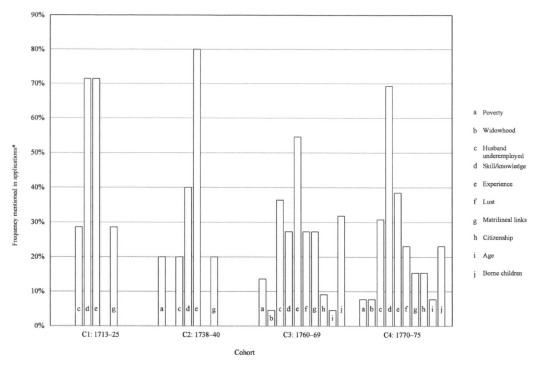

Figure 9 Motivations for applying for a midwife or Beifrau office, 1713–75

* Multiple motivations per application petition.

Sources: StadtAL, Tit. (F) XLIV.D.1, 'Kindermütter bey hiesiger Stadt betr. ingl. Die angenommene Bey Weiber betr.', 1673–1756, 16–118, 161–89; StadtAL, Tit. (F) XLIV.D.6b, 'Die Einrichtung der Kindermütter und Beÿweiber betr. de Anno 1757', 1760, vol. I, 58–66, 120–57; StadtAL, Ristu. Akten Teil I, Nr. 185, Ansuchungs-Schreiben um den, nach Absterben Juliänen Sharitas Zschachin ledig wordenen Kinder-Mutter und beÿfrau Dienst, 1775, vol. I, 408–41.

This suggests that in economic terms, midwifery meant different things for different women. Women from families with middling means probably saw in midwifery an extra source of income, less important (but probably desirable) for the financial health of the household. We know, for example, that Beifrau Maria Sabina Herrmann's husband had the wherewithal to install a very expensive workshop in their house at the Peterstor.[145] Similarly, the husband of Beifrau Christiana Dorothea Behnhold, an instrument maker, left a total of 300 Taler in cash to his five children when he died (just over the annual salary of the Stadtaccoucheur). He also bade his wife Christiana keep the profit from her business in making hats. This suggests that the couple drew upon at least three different sources of income: instrument making, midwifery and hat-making.[146]

145 Tit. XLIV.D.6b, Bd. I, 112–19, 'Beifrau appointment (Medel)', 2–4 December 1769, 116–17.
146 Testamente Rep. V, Paket 236, Nr. 3, 'Behnhold', 1782.

Even as a Beifrau, Behnhold appears to have been well established in the Vorstadt neighbourhoods around the Rannstädter Tor.[147] But she was also a rather shrewd businesswoman and, by owning her own set of baptism robes, she was able to keep the borrowing fee (between 2 and 4 Groschen) per christening that would have otherwise been due to her midwife-teacher.[148]

All in all, neither the Behnhold nor the Herrmann household could have been solely dependent on an income from midwifery. For those households in which husbands were plagued by underemployment, unemployment or illness, midwifery was a lifeline that steered the family away from dependence on alms. For others – in particular those from established artisan households – midwifery was an additional regular source of familial income that could shore up, sometimes even enhance, moderate living standards. These women cited other grounds for seeking an office, as the following sections will discuss.

Midwifery as a family tradition

For many Leipzig midwives, midwifery was 'in the blood'. Some inherited their occupation from female relatives, others married into the family of a midwife. Whereas it is quite easy to identify occupational transfer from a midwife to her daughter-in-law, the true extent of matrilineal occupational inheritance remains a largely hidden phenomenon. A woman always assumed her husband's surname on marriage, obscuring matrilineal links. It is possible to link mothers to daughters by tracing maiden names in the Leipzig marriage registers. However, the frequency of second marriages coupled with multiple 'sets' of children renders this task difficult. Mobility poses a further obstacle. A number of women migrated to the city at an advanced age and are therefore not traceable in either the marriage or baptismal registers. Nonetheless, the majority of Leipzig midwives – even those of foreign birth – had resided in the city long enough to be captured at some vital event in the church records. Although a number of relationships between midwives and Beifrauen reveal themselves in the council administrative sources, tracing a small sample of women in the marriage and baptism registers uncovered a much higher rate of congenital and conjugal relationships. Some twenty women could be identified as being related to another midwife or Beifrau.[149] This figure is most likely underestimated.

The two most common relationships within this small group of midwives were those between 1) mother and daughter, and 2) mother-in-law and daughter-in-law. In almost all of these cases the daughters-in-law were also appren-

---

147 Tit. (F) XLIV.D.6b, 29–37, 'Midwife Schulz vs Beifrau Behnhold', 23 February–18 March 1784, 36–37.
148 It appears to have been unusual for a Beifrau to own her own christening robes. Ibid., 32–36.
149 This figure (20 no.) is based both on women in the original database of midwives (177 no.) as well as on those women in the main sample used to elicit age spans who were found to be related during the course of research in the church registers.

ticed, either officially or unofficially, to their mothers for some period of time. Beifrau Maria Dorothea Westphal's youngest daughter, Maria Magdalena Hornung, for instance, had already acquired considerable experience in midwifery at her mother's side when she was appointed as a Beifrau in 1764.[150] Mother and daughter appear to have continued working together from time to time thereafter, despite the fact that Hornung was officially allocated to another sworn midwife.[151] Rahel Regina Pötsch was also probably trained in midwifery by her mother, midwife Christina Maria Bauer. When appointed Beifrau in 1779 she was allocated to Bauer, and mother and daughter continued to work together until at least 1792.[152]

It is possible that the practice of training a daughter-in-law occurred only if no daughter was available. The well-established sworn midwife Christina Hentschell, for example, taught her daughter Christina Lorend the art of midwifery after Lorend, abandoned by her husband in Dresden, returned to Leipzig to live with her mother in 1709. In 1713 Lorend was appointed Beifrau, but it was only in 1716 that her mother took on her own daughter-in-law (Lorend's sister-in-law) Johanna Regina Wagner as her informal apprentice. Lorend, who was also made a sworn midwife in 1716, had probably continued to assist her mother unofficially until her promotion. Bereft of her 'apprentice', Hentschell appears to have turned to the next closest female relative.

Occupational transfer of midwifery could span more than two generations of women, which suggests strong parallels to traditional artisan patterns of occupational transmission. Another midwife, Maria Magdalena Thomäe (née Bracht), who applied for a Beifrau office in 1767, could count her familial connections to midwifery through her grandmother *and* her mother-in-law.[153] With such a pedigree, it was probably no coincidence that Maria Magdalena subsequently married into the family of one of the city's most well-respected midwives, Susanna Magdalena Thomäe.[154]

Matrilineal or conjugal links to midwifery are by no means only found amongst sworn Beifrauen and midwives. Women working as unsworn midwives, even those who never acquired a sworn office, also demonstrate familial connections with midwifery. The daughter of Beifrau Maria Magdalena

150 II. Sekt., M (F) Nr. 670, Bd. III, 50–87, 'Dismissal (Werner)', 19 April 1763–1 March 1764, 59–60 and 75–76.
151 Westphal had a tempestuous relationship with her Beifrau, which no doubt encouraged her to use her daughter instead. See StadtAL, II. Sekt. M (F) Nr. 670, Bd. III, 'Hebammen. Verschiedenes über die Kindermütter, Wehemütter und Beifrauen (1756–69)', 88–95, 'Maria Westphal complains about her Beifrau Maria Groß', 25 July–28 November 1765, 88–89.
152 Tit. (F) XLIV.D.6b, Bd. I, 200–15, 'Appointment (Pötsch)', 12 June 1778–3 March 1779, 211–12.
153 M. M. Thomäe's grandmother was the sworn midwife Maria Magdalena Müller. Tit. (F) XLIV.D.6b, Bd. I, 66–86, 'Beifrau appointment (Thomäe)', 1 September 1767–20 November 1768, 73.
154 KAL, Trau. Thom., 1759, 151 (Johann Heinrich Thomä, Maria Magdalena Bracht).

Alsdorff, Anna Dorothea Braun, worked for her mother for some nine years before Alsdorff died in 1725. Unlike the women mentioned above, Braun's application to replace her mother as Beifrau was unsuccessful.[155] Another Wickelweib, Regina Elisabeth Kühn, was the assistant to her sister, the sworn midwife Juliana Maria Müller. Midwife Müller tried unsuccessfully on two separate occasions to have her sister recruited as her Beifrau.[156] The elderly midwife Anna Catharina Sperling also encouraged her daughter, Hanna Görsch, to accompany her to deliveries and to dispense powders and potions to her clients for a number of years.[157] Despite this experience, Sperling was unable to secure Görsch as her Beifrau.[158]

How may we think about the way midwifery was 'passed on' between family members? How do these practices relate to other occupations in early modern Leipzig? We know, for example, that the transfer of artisan occupations from father to son in sixteenth-century Leipzig was very high (around 70 per cent), although a son only rarely inherited his father's workshop.[159] Occupational continuity amongst artisans was largely due to the legal and social advantages that membership of the father's guild provided, namely a shorter length of apprenticeship and preferential treatment in the allocation of vacant master positions within the guild.[160] Midwifery was not incorporated, yet there are striking similarities between it and the occupational structure of the crafts. Whilst a number of midwives did train both officially and unofficially under female relatives, natural succession or the inheritance of a particular district-bound office was quite rare following the introduction of discrete midwife districts in the early eighteenth century. When a woman related to a midwife was appointed, she was generally placed in whichever district had become vacant once all the Beifrauen and sworn midwives had been promoted according to the principle of the eldest. As the case of midwife Sperling demonstrates, there was a tendency to only appoint the female relatives and protégés of sworn midwives as long as this did not disrupt the established order of entitlement to an office, or provide unwarranted competition for already established Beifrauen and midwives. This meant there had to be a vacant office and the candidate had to be the next waiting 'in turn'.[161] Although

---

155 Tit. (F) XLIV.D.1, 83–118, 'Appointments (Greger and Veiß)', 22 November 1724–4 September 1725, 86.

156 Tit. (F) XLIV.D.6b, Bd. I, 1–8, 37–8, 54–5, 'Stadtaccoucheur reports (Breuer)', 28 May 1757–14 July 1758, 37–38; II. Sekt., M (F) Nr. 670, Bd. III, 50–87, 'Dismissal (Werner)', 19 April 1763–1 March 1764, 61–62, 68.

157 StadtAL, Tit. (F) XLIV.D.1, 'Kindermütter bey hiesiger Stadt betr. ingl. die angenommene Bey Weiber betr. 1673–1756', 64–67, 'Elias Störe complains about midwife Anna Sperling', 31 March–15 June 1720, 67.

158 Tit. (F) XLIV.D.1, 83–118, 'Appointments (Greger and Veiß)', 22 November 1724–4 September 1725, 93–95.

159 Keller, 'Zunft und Familie', 76–77. See also Mitterauer, *Grundtypen*, 113–18.

160 *Grundtypen*, 113, 117.

161 Even Gehler noted in 1785 that he could find no reason for not continuing with the practice of promotion per seniority. Tit. (F) XLIV.D.6c, 54–74, 'Various appointments', 4 October 1782–22 January 1789, 57.

Sperling's daughter Görsch passed Stadtaccoucheur Lischwitz's examination with flying colours, it was not her 'turn' and so her proposed appointment was described as a vexation to the newly instated Beifrauen.[162]

The benefits of such a familial connection with established midwives and the tangible experience and skills that such a relationship might confer continued to find favour with the Council and the Stadtaccoucheurs into the late eighteenth century. Unlike the strict selection criteria applied by Angélique le Boursier du Coudray, who rejected all candidates with an inkling of midwifery experience – in particular 'old matrons' who were already working as village midwives – in Leipzig matrilineal ties and experience remained highly valued.[163] Even Stadtaccoucheur Gehler, with his predilection for blank canvasses, recommended one candidate in 1778 as the daughter of 'one of our most skilful and useful midwives', even though the woman had been assisting her mother since 1775 and had presumably accumulated considerable experience.[164]

Within the system of sworn midwifery, the role of the Leipzig Council was similar to that of the guilds. At least in theory the Council, like the guilds, controlled the number of midwifery offices and determined who was to fill vacancies according to the principle of entitlement. But as we have seen, the Council's influence did not extend to the level of unsworn midwifery. Whereas the *office* of sworn midwife was in general not passed on from one generation to another, the occupation often was.

The social and ideological meaning of midwifery

As Samuel Thomas has argued in the context of late seventeenth-century York, the social meaning and social experience of midwifery varied greatly according to socio-economic status and the types of networks in which midwives operated.[165] For wealthy midwives, whose clientele tended to be socio-economically and geographically varied, midwifery conferred social significance: serving the wealthy demonstrated a midwife's own status within the urban elite and attending the poor was proof of her compassion. Poorer midwives, on the other hand, were more dependent upon the living that midwifery secured, and the social significance of their work, largely amongst the poor and middling classes, was based upon the concept of neighbourliness.[166] Adrian Wilson pursues a similar argument, stressing that early modern midwifery – indeed medicine generally – was characterised by 'richly varied

---

162 Tit. (F) XLIV.D.1, 83–118, 'Appointments (Greger and Veiß)', 22 November 1724–4 September 1725, 99–100.

163 Rattner Gelbart, *The King's Midwife*, 157–58.

164 Tit. (F) XLIV.D.6b, Bd. I, 200–15, 'Appointment (Pötsch)', 12 June 1778–3 March 1779, 211.

165 Thomas, 'Midwifery and Society', 9.

166 Ibid., 9–10.

meanings' which might rest on one or more different types of domestic, charitable or commercial encounter.[167]

The argument both Thomas and Wilson posit for thinking about early modern midwifery, indeed medical occupations in general, is borne out by the data available for Leipzig. As this chapter has shown, some Leipzig midwives were drawn into midwifery by poverty or, at the very least, the desire to bolster the household oeconomy with an additional source of income. For others, midwifery was a family tradition to be passed on through the generations. But these were not the only factors that led women to midwifery. Perhaps more so than many other types of work undertaken by women in the early modern period, the encounter between a midwife and her client involved more than just a financial transaction or the articulation of familial tradition. It was also a demonstration of values. The decision to become a midwife was imbued with social and ideological as well as financial meaning.

Pinning down these social and ideological meanings is not easy. The absence of personal 'ego' documents – diaries, intimate correspondence and the like – means that for Leipzig we must turn to other, less subjective sources. The scores of petitions submitted to the Leipzig Council by aspiring midwives, as well as the petitions of complaint penned by the women in established midwife offices, inform this analysis. Reading these types of document requires great caution. Most petitioners, even when they were literate, employed the services of a scribe to compose their supplications. The petitions of candidacy demonstrate particularly high levels of linguistic and semantic similarity, suggesting that many were based on a *pro forma* text. (It is unclear whether the wording came from the Leipzig Council itself or was the product of textual conventions applied by the scribes and petitioners more generally.) Where petitions are near identical, it must be assumed that candidates were aiming to provide the Council and the Stadtaccoucheur with information they thought their prospective employer wanted to hear. And yet, even if the words and thoughts these women employed were not entirely their own, they cannot have been entirely foreign to them either. The language of these documents is regimented, but this is also indicative of a shared discourse and an appeal to concepts that made sense to both the petitioner and the petitioned.[168]

The chief motivational themes in the late seventeenth- and early eighteenth-century petition letters centre on the concepts of obligation and obedi-

---

167 Adrian Wilson, 'Midwifery in the "Medical Marketplace"', in Mark S.R. Jenner and Patrick Wallis, eds, *Medicine and the Market in England and Its Colonies, c. 1450–c.1850* (Basingstoke: Palgrave Macmillan, 2007), 168–70.

168 On the function of petitioning as a two-way communicative and cooperative process between subject and ruler/government in early modern society, see Rosi Fuhrmann et al., 'Supplizierende Gemeinden. Aspekte einer vergleichenden Quellenbetrachtung', in Peter Blickle, ed., *Gemeinde und Staat im alten Europa* (Munich: R. Oldenbourg Verlag, 1998), 320–21; Andreas Würgler, 'Desideria und Landesordnungen. Kommunaler und landständischer Einfluß auf die fürstliche Gesetzgebung in Hessen-Kassel 1650–1800', ibid. On 'Policey-Ordnungen' and supplication practices in particular, see Holenstein, 'Die Umstände der Normen'; Dinges, '"Policeyforschung"', 342–44.

ence that these women felt as the subjects of the communal authority. Susanna Bähr, midwife at the Rannstädter Tor of ten years, spoke of her desire 'with God's help and assistance, to loyally and diligently prove myself in such an office ... with the best of [my] abilities and in as much as my obligation demands the debt of obedience as a Loyal Subject ... to conduct myself in every way as a loyal and caring midwife.'[169] A midwife's chief duty, as Bähr stated, was to conduct herself so that 'those pregnant women who, in their time of need desire next to God my loyal and [best] possible help, will be content and happy with me.'[170] At least in this kind of discourse, the social meaning of a woman's midwifery work revolved around serving the city's women. It was based on the Christian ideal of loving one's neighbour and the need for support in pain and suffering. Women referred to their desire to 'lend a hand to my suffering neighbour with my little knowledge and experience'.[171] The discourse of obligation was outwardly oriented; a midwife's duty was to assist God by pleasing mothers and, by default, the Leipzig Council. For example, in 1713 Catharina Ehrlich, a born Leipziger but at that time working as midwife in the nearby city of Wurzen, described 'how dearly of spiritual indebtedness I had wished to let myself be used in the service of my Father City' as she petitioned for a midwife office in Leipzig.[172] In Lutheran Leipzig the religious and the civic melded together; this enmeshment was played out in the mingling of patriotic and religious language in petition letters. In the early eighteenth century holding a midwife office entailed serving both God and the civic authority.

These concepts of obligation and obedience fed into the way in which suitability for office was determined. Women had to supply letters of recommendation from the communities within which they lived, from physicians, pastors and the honourable women they had delivered. These *Attestata*, as well as the examination, provided a means of gauging a woman's qualification for the job. Reputation and the medium of recommendation was not just something imposed on midwives from above. It was central to the self-perception of all midwives and was deployed in petitions by candidates to assert their suitability. Incumbent midwives likewise deployed these categories to articulate their status as loyal, obedient and hard-working subjects.[173]

The road to becoming a midwife, however, did not just demand loyalty and obedience; it also entailed hard work. Far from being the type of work

---

169 StadtAL, Tit. (F) XLIV.D.1a, 'Verschiedenes die Kindermütter oder Hebammen betr. 1680–1831', 1r–1v, 'Midwife supplication (Susanna Bähr)', 24 August 1680, 1v.
170 Ibid.
171 Tit. (F) XLIV.D.1, 83–118, 'Appointments (Greger and Veiß)', 22 November 1724–4 September 1725, 98.
172 Tit. (F) XLIV.D.1, 16–43, 'Appointment (Ehrlich)', 10 January–24 July 1713, 16.
173 For example Anna Kirchlöffel claimed that as a Gassenmagd, all of her neighbourhood had been happy with her services. See ibid., 27–28. Regina Meder also stressed that she had observed 'how a knowledgeable midwife acts, that no one has complained about me'. See Tit. (F) XLIV.D.1, Bd. I, 74–80, 'Beifrau application (Meder)', 8 July 1724–25 January 1725, 76–79.

any woman could turn to if the family's financial situation worsened, midwifery was an occupation that normally required a good deal of learning and training. As Chapter Two has shown, almost all midwives could look back on a number of years in which they acquired their knowledge and experience, generally through a type of apprenticeship or as an assistant with a more experienced midwife. Yet many women who aspired to take on midwife offices in the early eighteenth century often looked beyond the traditional apprenticeship to other forms of training – anatomical lessons or self-study – that would equip them with the necessary 'edge' over other candidates.

Candidates wove the act of amassing of knowledge about midwifery, whether through books or physicians, into these concepts of obligation and obedience by reversing the relationship of obligation between petitioner and authority. Learning the art of midwifery through lessons and books involved a good deal of self-sacrifice. Regina Meder claimed to have almost driven herself to financial ruin in the quest to gain the necessary knowledge and experience for a Beifrau office. In several letters of petition to the Council, Meder outlined the steps she had taken to qualify for the job. In addition to taking 'information' from the Stadtphysicus Lischwitz for six months, she had 'procured all the necessary books and equipment, practised in it [midwifery] diligently', watched and observed at several births and finally successfully passed the Stadtphysicus' examination.[174] Having given up her 'regular hand- and wash-work' in order to 'fully satisfy her office', she claimed not to know how she would earn an honest living if she were not conferred the office.[175] It was now the Council who was obliged to appoint her.

From roughly the 1760s onwards, prospective midwives began to employ a new kind of language in their petitions. The rhetoric of neighbourly love and obligation endured, however, women such as Christiana Behnhold began infuse the notion of 'Lust' (desire in a non-sexual sense) into their petitions for appointment. 'Because I have a great yearning and desire for such tasks,' Behnhold wrote, '[I] promise to learn exactly and attentively that which [this work] requires, and that which is conferred upon me as lesson[s].'[176] The deployment of a discourse of 'Lust' as a motivation to work as a midwife found resonance with the Stadtaccoucheurs. Gehler, for example, found it necessary to mention the 'extraordinary desire' demonstrated by one Beifrau candidate in 1763 'to multiply the partial knowledge in the art of midwifery learnt from her mother'.[177] Another candidate he shortlisted could prove not only a good reputation and nature, but also demonstrated, in Gehler's words, an 'uncommon desire for this office'.[178] As Figure 9 shows, 'Lust' did not feature in sup-

174 Tit. (F) XLIV.D.1, Bd. I, 74–80, 'Beifrau application (Meder)', 8 July 1724–25 January 1725, 75.
175 Ibid., 76.
176 Tit. (F) XLIV.D.6b, Bd. I, 154–57, 'Midwife appointment (Westphal)', 2–30 September 1771, 155.
177 II. Sekt., M (F) Nr. 670, Bd. III, 50–87, 'Dismissal (Werner)', 19 April 1763–1 March 1764, 59–60.
178 Tit. (F) XLIV.D.6b, Bd. I, 120–48, 'Appointment (Schultz)', 12 March–28 April 1770, 120.

plications prior to 1740 as a motivation for applying for a midwife office. In the two later cohorts, however, the frequency of this language in the petitions for office ranged between 20 and 30 per cent.

So what exactly did women and the Stadtaccoucheurs mean by 'Lust' and why did women begin to use this kind of rhetoric? Around the same time, women and the Stadtaccoucheurs also began to mention another new concept; the willingness and ability to learn. Maria Porckwitz promised in 1767 'not to fail to learn, through untiring diligence, the necessary sciences'.[179] The Beifrau Maria Herrmann who, as the eldest Beifrau in 1769 was in turn for the next vacant midwife office, qualified her suitability nonetheless by stating that she was 'incumbent in this function, perfected to such a degree not [through] renown [but] through my diligence and craving to learn.'[180] The chronological correlation, albeit with a slight lag, with the introduction of the Stadtaccoucheur and formal instruction for midwives is not incidental. The Stadtaccoucheurs, who were particularly interested in this quality, made the connection between 'Lust' and teachability.

The best kind of midwife was now one who, next to the motivation of obligation and neighbourly love, demonstrated a desire and the capacity to learn the art of midwifery, not just in the traditional manner from midwife to apprentice but within the context of formal instruction at the hands of the Stadtaccoucheur.[181] Instead of merely deploying, as Regina Meder did in 1725, learning endeavours as a means of invoking obligation on the part of the Council, candidates in the latter eighteenth century were using their studies and experience to prove their willingness and ability to learn. From the perspective of the Stadtaccoucheurs, however, it was mostly age and modesty rather than actual skills or experience that determined a woman's teachability. The idea that midwives had to be moulded to be useful was related to the idea that government could intervene in the health of its subjects and that education was the key ingredient. Most of the Beifrau candidates, as Stadtaccoucheur Pohl claimed in 1785, were too old 'and therefore incapable of learning anything else, [whereas] others were so very convinced of their imagined knowledge, that one could [not] hope to rear good midwives out of them'.[182]

As this discourse gained currency in the latter eighteenth century, the social and ideological meaning of midwifery as an occupation changed. Women still understood their work in terms of neighbourliness and obligation. Yet the

---

179 Tit. (F) XLIV.D.6b, Bd. I, 66–86, 'Beifrau appointment (Thomäe)', 1 September 1767–20 November 1768, 76r–76v.

180 Tit. XLIV.D.6b, Bd. I, 112–19, 'Beifrau appointment (Medel)', 2–4 December 1769, 16.

181 See, for example, Maria Rößler's petition from 1 December 1769 in Tit. (F) XLIV.D.6b, Bd. I, 120–48, 'Appointment (Schultz)', 12 March–28 April 1770, 135. Beifrauen were still expected to learn the skills of a midwife and acquire 'familiarity and practice' alongside a sworn midwife. See Tit. (F) XLIV.D.6b, Bd. II, 53–62, 'Appointment (Gentsch)', 12 November–9 December 1785, 58.

182 Tit. (F) XLIV.D.6b, Bd. II, 53–62, 'Appointment (Gentsch)', 12 November–9 December 1785, 61.

emphasis on teachability and the need to educate 'useable' midwives meant that midwives were increasingly inclined to stress the socially and politically crucial nature of their occupation, albeit implicitly, in a language reminiscent of cameralist discourses. These emphasised the importance of health and its correlation to well-trained practitioners: the 'most treasured good of the pregnant woman, health, above all her life, is dependent upon our treatments', claimed the city's Beifrauen in 1800.[183] Hence, Stadtaccoucheur Gehler stated that the 'practice and perfection of the art of delivery that we have yet to learn' should not be prevented.[184] We should not take this argument too far, however. The midwives in Leipzig were no Mme du Coudrays, gadding about the country teaching midwifery to the peasants on a mission of state to save 'future soldiers and cultivators of the earth'.[185] In practice, as Chapter Four will explore, obligation and the rights of those with an office – entitlement – continued to be the primary factor shaping the way the Leipzig Council and the Stadtaccoucheurs organised and managed midwifery, as well as the way midwives both perceived and plied their trade.

Conclusions

As charted in this chapter, the profile of Leipzig's midwives was greatly affected by demographic growth and changing economic circumstances in the city. By the late seventeenth century the socio-occupational background of Leipzig's midwives was already relatively homogeneous, with by far the largest proportion of these women situated within the artisan milieu. Many came from master artisan families where midwifery was more likely to complement the family income and, perhaps just as importantly, family honour and importance within the local neighbourhood. The population and economic pressures of the eighteenth century changed this. Midwives continued to be situated within the milieu of the crafts, yet midwifery was less and less the kind of work that the wives of master artisans might carry out. Instead, midwifery became the preserve of families, both artisan and other, dependent upon wage labour. Midwives' husbands were often journeymen, unincorporated artisans, day labourers and soldiers whose work was precarious and rarely brought home enough to feed and house a family. Poverty, incapacity, unemployment and underemployment were the buzzwords in a large proportion of women's petitions for office. In many cases, midwifery became the central, if not the only financial pillar of the household oeconomy. Some continuity in midwifery as a complementary part of the family oeconomy persisted, perhaps more so in families where the occupation was passed down through the gen-

---

183 Tit. (F) XLIV.D.6b, Bd. I, 158–285, 'Various complaints', 14 July 1772–1810, 279–81.
184 See the collective Beifrau petition against the ban on taking in unwed women during their confinement from 3 February 1800 in ibid. Note, however, that the wellbeing of the mother rather than that of the child, formed the centre of their argument.
185 Rattner Gelbart, *The King's Midwife*, 74–75.

erations. However, commercial midwifery had well and truly become part of the economy of makeshift experienced by the growing urban precariat. The wives of the genteel and educated social groups had long since withdrawn from commercial/official midwifery.

Prior to the 1760s age range at appointment was highly erratic for both midwives and Beifrauen; despite the control exercised by the Stadtphysici and the Stadtaccoucheurs over appointment since the latter seventeenth century, appointment practices demonstrated far more continuity with tradition than innovation 'from above'. From the 1760s onwards, however, we can see a tightening of the age range of new recruits for both sworn midwives and sworn Beifrauen that correlates directly with the informal policy of the city's Stadtaccoucheurs to appoint younger women to office. This did not affect the bottom range of age at appointment nearly as much as it did the top range, bringing the maximum age for midwives down to around sixty and for Beifrauen down to around forty-five years. This fetish with age stemmed from the idea that midwives ought be 'useable' and, most importantly, teachable, with the prospect of a long career ahead of them, a concept that emerged from the encounter between midwives, Beifrauen and the Stadtaccoucheurs in the newly instigated midwifery lessons. The new desirable Beifrau was a blank sheet, or at the very least, too young to have developed any terminally bad habits. She was roughly a decade younger than her historical counterpart. And although the Stadtaccoucheurs managed to reduce the age spread enduringly, they showed little interest in tweaking the system any further.

Prospective midwives were well aware of the new meaning of their occupation and their role in maintaining the health of the population, and they masterfully deployed this late Enlightenment rhetoric of 'Lust' and the ability to learn. Indeed, we see a sharp spike in professions of skill and knowledge in midwifery in supplications between 1770 and 1775 (refer to Figure 9). However, skill, experience and (book)-learning were not new criteria for the office of midwife but, as we have seen, were vital criteria for aspiring midwives to demonstrate from at least 1700 (and most likely earlier). Midwifery was still passed down from mother to daughter or daughter-in-law in many cases, yet economic necessity also increasingly propelled women to either seek office or participate informally in the midwifery landscape, with husband's underemployment cited by well over one-third of aspiring midwives as grounds for appointment during the latter half of the eighteenth century. Thus the emphasis on youth combined with increasing poverty in the city, which necessitated a growing reliance on women's ability to contribute and sometimes uphold the household oeconomy, produced younger midwives who often relied on midwifery more as a source of income than as a source of social capital.

Chapter Four

The Moral Economy of Midwifery

On 14 February 1705 two of the sworn midwives in the Vorstadt, Catharina Köhler and Anna Schmied, sent off a petition to the Leipzig Council to complain about the activities of two unsworn women who they accused of slanderous gossip, attending women during confinement and lying-in, and bringing infants to baptism. Most outrageously, the midwives argued, the guilty women made no attempt to heed previous reprimands from the Council but instead sought to 'insult us and to curtail our bite of bread'.[1] The sworn midwives also claimed: 'As they are engaged [for this purpose] … such tasks must be left to the [sworn] midwives and should not be encroached upon'.[2] Schmied's and Köhler's tirade against other women working as midwives was not unique – the administrative records in Leipzig bulge with disputes over indecorous interlopers and injured livelihoods.[3] As this chapter will demonstrate, the conflicts revolving around encroachment ('Eintrag') and quackery ('Pfuscherei') were those that increasingly came to define the working life of midwives in eighteenth-century Leipzig.

Instead of dismissing these squabbles as examples of unruliness and acrimonious rivalry, I will show here how these conflicts revolved around the demarcation of livelihood and appealed to contemporary ideas about social and moral order. In doing so, I explore a way of understanding the practice of occupational norm-setting in midwifery that goes beyond the paradigm of regulation/resistance. This chapter will trace the way in which the concept of livelihood, together with the attendant concepts of encroachment and entitlement, infused and shaped the behaviour of women working within the midwifery landscape. In doing so, I will draw out the lines of demarcation that were being continually drawn and redrawn between the various groups operating within the midwifery landscape, and explore the practices that provoked this boundary-making.

Taken at face value, the motivations for such conflicts appear strictly economic – a knee-jerk reaction to the prospect of diminished or insufficient earnings through too much or unfair competition. As Chapter Three has shown, the economic pressures of the eighteenth century were felt acutely by many women operating in the midwifery landscape, yet these conflicts boiled down to a great deal more than just economic deprivation. Köhler and

---

1   Tit. (F) XLIV.D.2a, 1–7, 'Midwives vs Hentschell', 14 August–2 September 1705, 1r–2r.
2   Ibid.
3   The earliest example of such a petition by a Leipzig midwife dates from 1680, when midwife Anna Reiche complained about the activities of two Gassenmägde. Further examples survive from 1696 and 1699. See StadtAL, II. Sekt. R (F) Nr. 91, 1–2, 'Beschwerde der Kindermutter Anna Reiche (vs Gassenmägde)', 25 February 1680, 2v–3v; II. Sekt. K (F) Nr. 255, 1–6v, 'Kindermutter gegen Schönwolff', 22–25 January 1696; II. Sekt. P (F) Nr. 175b, 1–5, 'Marie Plessingen', 2 June 1699–17 July 1703. There are numerous such petitions from the eighteenth century.

Schmied were certainly concerned about the threat unsworn midwifery posed to their income, however, their objections were not based upon an exclusively economic rationale. Encroachment disrupted the socio-occupational order that entitled certain women to work as sworn midwives and Beifrauen. Early modern governments (both territorial and communal) were primarily concerned with maintaining orderliness through the practice of Policey, or the triage of administration, economy and social order. Policey – in the form of ordinances – was designed to ensure the stability of social and economic order for both the honour of God and the good of the community (the common weal).[4] In late seventeenth- and eighteenth-century Germany economic order *was* social order: the work a person carried out was defined by his or her estate (Stand) in society. Thus encroachment was an act of economic *and* social-communal impropriety that threw social and economic order as well as customs and traditions into turmoil and threatened the very fabric of society. The midwives Köhler and Schmied lamented, for example, that when unsworn midwives had infants brought to the baptismal font 'there occurred much trouble as the [sworn] midwives present do not even know whether the children sent to them are illegitimate or legitimate'.[5] Worse still, such encroachment could pervert the authority of maturity and turn the most fundamental and serious religious moment in an early modern person's life into a farce when 'servants of fifteen to sixteen years old have to lend a hand at the baptism, whereby the children's clothes are often muddled up, which often gives cause for laughter from both strangers and other persons.'[6]

The moral economy as a dialogue

Such conflicts must be understood as an expression of a 'moral economy', as coined by E. P. Thompson. Just as the eighteenth-century crowd that rioted and ransacked food stores in times of dearth was informed by a 'legitimising notion' based on the belief that it was defending traditional rights and customs, the gripes and squabbles occasioned by late seventeenth- and eighteenth-century midwives were also underpinned by a 'moral economy' grounded in the concept of 'livelihood', which governed occupational interaction and the right to practice.[7] Of course Thompson conceived the 'moral economy' strictly in terms of food riots in eighteenth-century England and was careful not to decontextualise. He defined the 'moral economy' of the crowd in the food riot as a defensive manoeuvre on the part of the people that sought to resist the Smithian 'free market' economy and rearticulate the traditional customs and usages that were in place within a society grounded in

---

4   Dülmen, *Dorf und Stadt*, vol. 2, 223–24; Flügge, *Hebammen und heilkundige Frauen*, 186–98.
5   Tit. (F) XLIV.D.2a, 1–7, 'Midwives vs Hentschell', 14 August–2 September 1705, 2r.
6   Ibid., 2r–2v.
7   E. P. Thompson, 'The Moral Economy of the English Crowd in the Eighteenth Century', *Past and Present* 50: 1 (1971): 76–136, 78–79.

paternalism.[8] He nevertheless accepted that a 'looser' use of the concept was possible, for 'no other term seems to offer itself to describe the way in which, in peasant and in early industrial communities, many 'economic' relations are regulated according to non-monetary norms'.[9] The notion of the 'moral economy' has since been extended as an explanatory framework for large-scale industrial disputes throughout the eighteenth and nineteenth centuries, yielding an even more complex understanding of the ambiguous interplay between paternalism and capitalism throughout modernity.[10]

But what about midwifery? The conflicts between midwives as well as those between midwives and the urban authorities hardly count as riots or even acts of large-scale rebellion. Moreover, eighteenth-century German territories differed both politically and economically from their English counterparts. It is nonetheless useful to translate the conceptual framework of the 'moral economy' to the micro-context of midwifery disputes.[11] The concept of the moral economy entreats us to consider the patterns of behaviour relating to work and occupation displayed by midwives in Leipzig on their own terms, rather than subsuming decisions and actions into the anachronistic rubric of 'rational' economic behaviour. The modern 'rational' economy has little in common with the early modern notion of 'livelihood', which combined both the necessity of subsistence and the idea of occupational propriety based upon the socio-occupational category of the Stand. Mary Lindemann has used the concept of the 'moral economy' to describe the clash of traditional corporate and nascent consumer cultures in the medical world of the eighteenth century.[12] I intend here to explore the characteristics of this moral economy and the types of conflicts it threw up specifically within the midwifery landscape.

---

8   Ibid.
9   See Thompson's chapter 'The Moral Economy Reviewed' in *Customs in Common* (New York: The New Press, 1991), 340.
10   The labour historian John Rule, for example, has demonstrated that in eighteenth-century England the pattern of industrial conflicts between master and journeymen shipwrights and wool-sorters frequently moved from attack to defence of the 'moral economy'. During boom times occupational groups went on a capitalist offensive, demanding higher wages and negotiating themselves a better deal. During periods of economic difficulty, however, they turned coat to defend the principles of paternalism, drawing strongly on the 'language of the moral economy'. See John Rule, 'Industrial Disputes, Wage Bargaining and the Moral Economy', in Adrian Randall and Andrew Charlesworth, eds, *Moral Economy and Popular Protest: Crowds, Conflict and Authority* (Basingstoke: Macmillan Press, 2000), 168–69.
11   For an example of how the concept of the 'moral economy' may be used to survey the micro-politics of class relations and non-violent or disruptive peasant resistance within South-East Asian villages, see James C. Scott, 'The Moral Economy As an Argument and As a Fight', in Adrian Randall and Andrew Charlesworth, eds, *Moral Economy and Popular Protest: Crowds, Conflict, and Authority* (Basingstoke: Macmillan Press, 2000).
12   See Lindemann, *Health*, 61–62 and 181–82. In specific reference to midwifery, see 'Professionals?'.

I argue here that although these disputes and the regulation they invoked were about defending livelihood, we need to think about them as part of a dialogue between women working in the midwifery landscape and the urban authority rather than as a demonstration of resistance and/or repression. As discussed in Chapter One, scepticism about the efficacy of the early modern state and growing criticism of explanatory frameworks that locate the legislative power of early modern states and communal governments in police ordinances has led social and legal historians to revisit the field of early modern legislative practice.[13] I will briefly sum up the points of interest to this discussion explored in Chapter One. Recent research into the practice of petitioning and supplicating, carried out largely by legal historians in the field of *Policey-Forschung* (Policey research, a distinct branch of legal history), has gone beyond the binary conceptualisation of Policey as social discipline emanating from rulers onto the ruled. These historians stress the 'circularity' of early modern Policey legislation, preferring to think about it as a 'learning process' and 'implementing process' in which 'norm-setter, norm-implementer and norm-addressee participate equally'.[14] Social disciplining might only be used to describe the good intentions of rulers in this process, not to describe the overall aim of early modern legislation.[15] It was not the case that early modern legislative practices were ineffective, but that, as André Holenstein argues, these shared structures and means of law-making – principally the practices of petitioning and supplicating – could only be implemented on individual problems, which left subject and ruler a good deal of space for negotiation.[16] In other words, the early modern state had neither the capability nor the intention to deploy legislation to inculcate its subjects on a grand scale. The fact that subjects and communes alike had to seek approval for a vast number of social procedures meant that the act of legislation ultimately remained in the hands of early modern princely rulers; yet a great deal of input came from 'below'.[17] The practice of supplicating, petitioning and mercy-seeking was a collective process and functioned as the main 'channel of information' from subjects to rulers because 'the monarchical-administrative penetration and control on a local [level], as much as this was [something rulers] strove for, had not yet found success.'[18] It was a co-operative rather than strictly confrontational procedure and the 'wish for order' derived as much from subjects as from rulers and ruling administrations themselves.[19]

---

13 See discussion in Chapter One.
14 Dinges, '"Policeyforschung"', 344.
15 Ibid.
16 André Holenstein, 'Bittgesuch, Gesetze und Verwaltung. Zur Praxis "guter Policey" in Gemeinde und Staat des Ancien Regime am Beispiel der Markgrafschaft Baden(-Durlach)', in Peter Blickle, ed., *Gemeinde und Staat im alten Europa* (Munich: R. Oldenbourg Verlag, 1998), 356–59.
17 Ibid.; 'Die Umstände der Normen', 46.
18 Quoted in Fuhrmann et al., 'Supplizierende Gemeinden', 320; See also Holenstein, 'Bittgesuch', 357.
19 Würgler, 'Desideria und Landesordnungen', 206–7.

If we apply this understanding of the early modern legislative process to midwifery petitions, we need to rethink the claims historians make about regulation via oaths, ordinances and instructions as being imposed from above.[20] The petitions midwives made to the Leipzig Council in relation to encroachment were not merely demonstrations of resistance. In laying bare their demands and grievances and insisting on resolution, midwives were entering into a communicative process – albeit a somewhat uneven one – of norm-setting. Their appeals to the moral economy of midwifery were intended to reinforce and shape social, economic and legal norms, rather than undermine them. The petitions that arose from the squabbles and disputes between women operating in the midwifery landscape were thus productive 'legislative' forces. The ever more detailed midwife instructions, which dealt more and more with the nature of the relationship between midwives and mothers, midwives and Beifrauen, and midwives and other women working as inofficial midwives were the result, not the cause, of this culture of petitioning.

We can trace this trend by comparing the versions of the instructions and then comparing their development to the disputes documented in the archival sources. Although between two and three women were working at any one time as midwives-in-waiting around 1700, reference to the midwife–Beifrau relationship is entirely absent in the 1689 oath. By the time the midwife instruction was renewed in 1758, this relationship was the subject of four separate items.[21] Midwives were told to each take on a Beifrau and to use her exclusively. They were to maintain peaceful relations with their Beifrauen, to teach them everything they needed to know and to pay them accordingly. Finally, there were particular guidelines about when midwives might permit a Beifrau to attend a birth on her own.[22] The relationship between midwives was likewise subject to new regulations: 'No midwife should turn another midwife's clients against her through insults and evil libel, less still force herself upon a pregnant woman through coaxing words.'[23] These issues were also dealt with in the Beifrau instructions, albeit from a different perspective. A Beifrau was expressly instructed not to attend a birth without the permission of her midwife.[24] She was not to 'preference one midwife over another, much less preference one Medicum over another or belittle [him or her]', but in-

---

20 Hampe and Flügge, for example, both argue in terms of a process of ever increasing control and regulation by the urban authority over midwives. See Hampe, *Zwischen Tradition*, 133; Sibylla Flügge, 'Die gute Ordnung der Geburtshilfe. Recht und Realität am Beispiel des Hebammenrechts der Frühneuzeit', in Ute Gerhard, ed., *Frauen in der Geschichte des Rechts. Von der Frühen Neuzeit bis zur Gegenwart* (Munich: Verlag C. H. Beck, 1997), 143–44.

21 Ohne Sig., 67v, 'Midwife oath', 1689. See Items 8 to 11 of Tit. (F) X Nr. 23b, Bd. XIII, 58r–69v, 'Instruktion Kinder Mutter N. N.', 14 July 1758, 61r–63r.

22 Tit. (F) X Nr. 23b, Bd. XIII, 58r–69v, 'Instruktion Kinder Mutter N. N.', 14 July 1758, 61r–63r.

23 See Item 3 of ibid., 65v–66r.

24 See Item 3 of Tit. (F) X 23b, Bd. III, 234–36, 'Instruction Beÿweiber', c. 1715 (undated).

stead 'conduct herself in all these [situations] completely impartially'.[25] Likewise, she was forbidden from 'telling anything unequal, [or] … speaking badly about anything'.[26] All of these issues – slander, stealing clients, the use of unsworn midwives, in short the terms of occupational relations between midwives – related to the idea of livelihood and were part of the moral economy of midwifery in early modern Leipzig. As such, these were the issues that provoked sworn midwives and Beifrauen to petition the Leipzig Council. The regulation of these issues by the Council, through ever more elaborate midwife and Beifrau instructions, was a response to the attention midwives and Beifrauen drew to these issues, in particular in the early eighteenth century. Midwifery regulations, which focused largely on these moral-economic issues, stemmed thus in part from midwives and Beifrauen themselves. This chapter will examine in detail the patterns of this moral economy that informed midwifery regulation in eighteenth-century Leipzig.

The central concept of this moral economy – 'livelihood' – was premised upon the idea that economic activity was a matter of entitlement. Everyone in early modern German society was entitled to a means of earning a living. Livelihood, grounded in the concept of *Hausnotdurft* (household necessity), was the idea that each individual household was entitled to provide its own material subsistence, procuring that which it could not produce from others through exchange and bartering. Hausnotdurft was both a value *and* a norm because, according to Renate Blickle, 'the independently productive household was acknowledged as the basic unit of social and political order'.[27] According to van Dülmen, this culture of subsistence was to a large extent the product of natural circumstance. Up until the end of the eighteenth century there existed little opportunity for increasing crop yields and intensifying livestock numbers in order to feed more people. In the absence of any means of increasing production, it was impossible for any Stand other than the nobility to actively accumulate wealth. For the ordinary household, the daily grind continued to revolve around ensuring survival. Surplus of production was not invested in improving production levels, but tended to be deployed in the pursuit of socio-religious meaning through the medium of feasts and festivities.[28] Within this context, the 'economy' was the household. The art of householding and house-husbandry functioned to guarantee morality and the maintenance of the socio-economic-moral status quo.[29] The division of production and services was not based upon individual merit but instead depended upon membership of a corporate group – in the case of midwives, through a municipal office.

25   See Item 4 of ibid.
26   See Item 4 of ibid.
27   Renate Blickle, 'Nahrung und Eigentum als Kategorien in der ständischen Gesellschaft', in Winifried Schulze and Helmut Gabel, eds, *Ständische Gesellschaft und soziale Mobilität* (Munich: Oldenbourg Verlag GmbH, 1988), 83.
28   Dülmen, *Dorf und Stadt*, vol. 2, 277–78.
29   Marion W. Gray, 'Kameralismus: Die säkuläre Ökonomie und die getrennten Geschlechtersphären', *WerkstattGeschichte* 19 (1998): 41–57, 44–45.

The defensive tactics early modern people deployed when their livelihood was under threat were thus grounded in a moral-economic paradigm, for ensuring an independent existence was the only 'honourable' means of socio-economic behaviour.[30] Persons who sought a livelihood outside of their designated occupational or geographical sphere were condemned as quacks and interlopers, an accusation from which no one was immune. 'Mir Eintrag thun' (to encroach on me) – a common parlance in the Leipzig sources – was not just a matter of stolen earnings. Encroachment, however commonplace, constituted economically immoral behaviour in the minds of early modern people. When midwives attempted to manoeuvre themselves into a better situation, either via promotion or the reallocation of better accommodation, or when they defended their entitlement to practise, they commonly deployed the notion of economic propriety and appealed to the paternalist model of governance premised on the principles of privileges and protection. Hence, midwives like Dorothea Plessing would plead with the Leipzig Council to 'protect' them against the activities of interlopers.[31] The quotidian disputes between midwives were tactically defensive and restorative, and they depended upon a language of the moral economy. Conflicts revolved, as Mary Lindemann has argued for the Duchy of Braunschweig-Wolfenbüttel, around this central principle of 'livelihood', which was simultaneously a commonly accepted and hotly contested concept.[32] 'Livelihood' was a value-cum-norm that required constant negotiation and re-negotiation, in particular in the increasingly socially and economically complicated space of the city. Yet as we shall see, these disputes were at the same time productive, forcing the Leipzig Council to regulate the domain of midwifery in increasing detail. It is these constellations of conflict revolving around this moral economy that this chapter will now explore.

Encroachment and the moral economy of early modern work

The concept of the 'medical marketplace', which has been fruitfully deployed as an analytical framework both for exploring and describing the structure of medical interactions in England before 1800, has enjoyed a somewhat subdued reception from historians of continental Europe.[33] Born around the same time as the idea of 'medical history from below', the 'medical marketplace' offered a new way of conceptualising early modern medicine that was 'diverse, pluralistic, pre-professional and commercialised, in which patients

30 Blickle, 'Nahrung und Eigentum', esp. 83–84.
31 II. Sekt. P (F) Nr. 175b, 1–5, 'Marie Plessingen', 2 June 1699–17 July 1703, 3. See also Tit. (F) XLIV.D.1, 11–13, 'Midwives vs Hentschell and Stöps', 1707, 12.
32 Lindemann, *Health*, 203–5.
33 See, for example, David Gentilcore's recent survey of the term and its uses in David Gentilcore, 'Medical Pluralism and the Medical Marketplace in Early Modern Italy', in Robert Jütte, ed., *Medical Pluralism – Past – Present – Future* (Stuttgart: Franz Steiner Verlag, 2013).

were active and promiscuous.'[34] The concept served to deconstruct the tripartite hierarchy of physician–surgeon–apothecary as well as other occupational demarcations, take seriously the role of the 'quack', and place the medical encounter at the centre of the social history of medicine. More recently, however, the 'medical marketplace' as a guiding concept has sustained criticism.[35] The concept was originally deployed to describe very specifically the situation in seventeenth-century England whereby a commercial market for medical skills and services managed to thwart any kind of regulatory clout wielded by incorporated medical practitioners. However, it was the idea – transferable in time and space – of the plurality of medical services of which early modern people availed themselves that would prove so irresistible to historians.[36] It is this latter model that has provoked historians such as Jenner, Wallis and Gentilcore to review the concept and call for greater precision and rigour when deploying the 'medical marketplace', in particular for the Continental European experience.[37] These reservations about the concept have led historians to explore non-monetary 'markets' existing alongside and in communication with the economy of health commodities, such as the oeconomy of the household, the economy of spiritual and magical power, and the economy of social capital, as a means of addressing the social and cultural 'deficit' of the 'economic' reading of the medical encounter.[38]

Whereas historians of the English medical marketplace placed competition and conflict on centre stage, the debates in the German context have tended to focus on the processes of medicalisation and professionalisation 'from above' and the collusion of absolute enlightened rulers and academic medical practitioners. In the area of midwifery, most studies focus on the steady increase in the regimentation and regulation of midwives' knowledge and practice, hand-in-hand with 'professionalisation' and the subsequent loss of midwives' autonomy through the activities of municipal physicians and communal governments.[39] In these narratives, the illegal practitioner and the marginal healer were always those without university-derived knowledge, the

---

34 Roy Porter's essay from 1985 initiated this historiographical reorientation. See Roy Porter, 'The Patient's View: Doing Medical History from Below', *Theory and Society* 14 (1985): 175–98. Quote from Gentilcore, 'Medical Pluralism', 45.

35 See the edited volume by Jenner and Wallis, eds, *Medicine and the Market*. The concept has been even more recently subject to discussion in connection with the concept of 'medical pluralism' across all of Europe in Robert Jütte, ed., *Medical Pluralism – Past – Present – Future* (Stuttgart: Franz Steiner Verlag, 2013).

36 Mark S. R. Jenner and Patrick Wallis, 'The Medical Marketplace', in Jenner and Wallis, eds, *Medicine and the Market*, 3–7; Gentilcore, 'Medical Pluralism', 45–46.

37 See esp. Gentilcore, 'Medical Pluralism', 53–54.

38 In particular the following contributions to the same volume: Leong and Pennell, 'Recipe Collections'; Lauren Kassell, 'Magic, Alchemy and the Medical Economy in Early Modern England: The Case of Robert Fludd's Magnetical Medicine', in Jenner and Wallis, eds, *Medicine and the Market*; Ben Mutschler, 'Illness in the "Social Credit" and "Money" Economies of Eighteenth-Century New England', ibid.

39 Examples of the control thesis: Hampe, *Zwischen Tradition*, 133; Flügge, 'Die gute Ordnung', 143–44.

requisite socio-occupational standing and the necessary incorporation; they were doomed from the outset to ignominy and inferiority. Yet these approaches fail to take into account that early modern people (and this includes governments) did not preference a type of knowledge for its own sake. Firstly, there appears to have been very little difference between the type of medicine practised by quacks and that practised by trained medical practitioners, suggesting that the patients did not necessarily select their health services according to whether practitioners were licensed or not.[40] Secondly, the decisions the authorities made about who was licensed were governed – at least in Germany – not principally by the idea that a certain type of knowledge was effective, but often by the moral-economic imperative of livelihood and the need to maintain occupational order.

A number of studies have since encouraged us to re-evaluate the way eighteenth-century people in Germany defined *Pfuscherei* (quackery). Far from being an expression of incompetence, during the eighteenth century and well into the next, quackery was a synonym for economic impropriety. 'For most people in the seventeenth and eighteenth centuries,' Lindemann argues, 'quackery continued to be cast principally in terms of a deviation from a more traditional division of labour and markets, as well as from an accepted moral and economic ethos'.[41] In other words, the definition of marginal and unauthorised medical practitioners (and indeed their practice) in the eighteenth century had less to do with ideas about improving the health of the nation by ensuring certain levels of 'professional' standards and knowledge. It had everything to do with conserving the 'traditional' means of social and economic survival: livelihood. At the same time, the right to a livelihood was both a process of entitlement *and* a judgement of proficiency.[42]

Mary Lindemann's thesis about quackery and 'economic propriety' rightly placed early modern medical practice back into the broader framework of work and economic life. In eighteenth-century Germany, medical practice was shaped by the exclusive, corporate ethos of the artisan guilds, whose objective it was to uphold the concept of livelihood and the 'fair' distribution of economic activity. This was not just the ethos of a particular social group, but of society as a whole. Even those who transgressed drew upon the language of

40 As already discussed, there is criticism relating to the direct applicability of this thesis for Continental Europe, however, the commonalities are still worthy of mention: For England, Porter finds that regular practitioners were often just as helpless against disease as irregular. Porter, *Health for Sale*, 23–25. Pelling also finds that practitioners labelled 'irregular' often also sported medical degrees just as did licensed practitioners. Pelling, *Medical Conflicts*, 143–46.

41 For a more detailed discussion, see esp. Chapter Three of Lindemann, *Health*, 170–71. See also Alison Klairmont Lingo, 'Empirics and Charlatans in Early Modern France: The Genesis of the Classification of the "Other" in Medical Practice', *Journal of Social History* 19: 4 (1986): 583–603; Pelling, *Medical Conflicts*, 136–88; Porter, *Health for Sale*, 1–20.

42 Lindemann, *Health*, 203.

entitlement.[43] And those people penning petitions played a major role in creating the identity of the quack or the unauthorised healer, not by presenting medical arguments based on efficacy, but instead by appealing to the moral economy of livelihood. Midwives, when they complained about encroachment to the Leipzig Council, were taking part in this exact process.

This 'old-regime' corporatism came under fire during the latter part of the eighteenth century, not only from territorial rulers and governments who sought to diminish the political clout of the guilds, but also from the burgeoning market in (quasi-industrially) produced goods such as medical pills, potions, books and medical contraptions.[44] As Lindemann argues, those 'medical entrepreneurs' – including academic medical practitioners – who peddled and hawked the new medicines and treatments pushed a new language of 'free competition' and 'good provision', redirecting the focus of medical regulation away from the producer and onto the consumer. Yet both the older concept of livelihood and the newer idea of 'provision' existed side-by-side well into the nineteenth century, as governments, practitioners and consumers continued to use both languages to justify the choices they made about their medical activities and physical well-being.[45]

Protecting burghers' livelihoods was writ large in communal politics. In Leipzig assuaging the interests of corporate bodies and maintaining the status quo of livelihood was one of the main preoccupations of the municipal Council. No less than eleven ordinances were published between 1648 and 1765 condemning the practice of quackery, usually as a response to complaints by the barber-surgeons' or chemists' guilds. In 1648 the Council reprimanded a whole swathe of practitioners: foreign barber-surgeons, *Feldscherer* (assistants to military barber-surgeons), foreign stonecutters, oculists, tyriack-hawkers, salve-sellers, midwives and old women. Those 'who have not learnt the craft of the barbers' and had 'wholly improperly treated their patients' were also problematic because 'their crimes could not be punished, but would rip the guild barbers' bread from in front of their mouths and such other disturbances'.[46] In 1728 doctors ('Ärzte') with too few clients or patrons also made it onto the list of suspected interlopers.[47] Of course the discourse of entitlement, rights to practise and encroachment was not specific to the medical crafts and professions, but underpinned the moral-economic understanding of all guilded or incorporated activities.[48] Linen weavers, bakers, furriers and butchers

---

43 'Professionals?', 186–87.
44 On consumerism and medical culture, see Porter, *Health for Sale*, 39–55.
45 Lindemann, *Health*, 175.
46 StadtAL, Tit. LX.B.(F).7, 'Verordnungen und Patente des Rates', 16, 'Ordinance for surgeons (quackery)', 29 August 1648. Further ordinances prohibiting quackery were released in 1660, 1683, 1707, 1712, 1721, 1728, 1735 and 1765. See Tit. LX.B (F) 7; Tit. LX.B (F) Nr. 1a; Tit. LX C (F) Nr. 8.
47 Tit. (F) LX.B.8, 'Verordnungen und Patente des Rates', 287, 'Ordinance for surgeons and barbers (quackery)', 24 August 1728.
48 These kinds of conflicts over encroachment were common to other occupations in eighteenth-century Germany. See Reinhold Reith, *Arbeits- und Lebensweise im städtischen Hand-*

all spoke a common language of livelihood. Indeed in the seventeenth century and for much of the eighteenth, the language of livelihood enjoyed a far broader applicability than this. In a world where economic life was largely determined by the ethos and practices of incorporated craft bodies and craft production, livelihood formed the conceptual basis for all types of economic behaviour, whether incorporated or not; in Saxony it endured with the small-scale artisan production that continued to be a mainstay of the economy throughout the eighteenth century.[49] Midwives, as Chapter Three demonstrated, were linked into this world two-fold; as both municipal officials and the daughters and wives of predominantly artisan men. Neither official nor unofficial midwifery operated within a freely commercial medical market-place regulated by supply and demand. The midwifery landscape functioned instead within a medical market that conflated economic propriety with moral rectitude and the preservation of a particular understanding of economic fairness: what I call here the moral economy of midwifery. This next section will explore the underlying demarcations that governed it.

Patterns of encroachment

Rivalry and conflict between women operating as midwives was a central characteristic of the midwifery landscape in Leipzig. Disputes ranged from catty spats resolved with a petty fine or warning, to conflicts that provoked full-scale council investigations. This is not to say that midwives did not cooperate with one another; a number of examples documented here demonstrate that they did band together when necessary. It is not my purpose here to enumerate instances of collective action. I am interested in how such disputes reveal the conceptual moral-economic framework that informed the behaviour of midwives as well as their relationships to one another and to the Council. Whether a conflict was small or large, it always revolved around the notion of livelihood; everyone (including the Council) accepted the primacy of livelihood. Just as the sworn midwife was entitled to her practice through her office, unsworn practitioners of midwifery also had a right to a livelihood if they were not to fall into the dishonourable chasm of poor relief. For the Leipzig Council, this presented a real conundrum. On the one hand, it had to uphold the rights of those women defending their 'turf'. On the other, it could not afford to curtail the means to a livelihood for women who found themselves accused of improper midwifery. Thus there emerged a messy, makeshift collage of exceptions and compromises that muddied the boundaries of enti-

werk. Zur Sozialgeschichte Augsburger Handwerksgesellen im 18. Jahrhundert, 1700–1806 (Göttingen: Verlag Otto Schwartz & Co., 1988), 173–77 and 225–30.

49   Helmut Bräuer, 'Das zünftige Handwerk in Sachsen und die "Landes-Oeconomie-Manufactur- und Commercien-Deputation" im 18. Jahrhundert', in Karl Czok and Helmut Bräuer, eds, *Studien zur älteren sächsischen Handwerksgeschichte* (Berlin: Akademie-Verlag, 1990), 56–57.

tlement so central to the structure of 'corporate' sworn midwifery. Unsworn midwives were permitted to deliver children in 'emergency' situations, Beifrauen were authorised to attend women on their own or to take children to baptism as long as their midwife-teachers agreed, and the sworn midwives in the Vorstadt maintained a monopoly over the care of indigent women. And, as we shall see in this chapter, the Council pursued a reactive rather than prophylactic policy towards encroachment, usually only taking action when practitioners themselves complained about occupational impropriety.

A close reading of the numerous midwife disputes demonstrates that the accusation of encroachment was *not* restricted to the activities of unsworn women working as midwives. Encroachment was not specifically related to qualifications of skill or knowledge that sworn midwives were supposed to possess and which was absent in all other women. Rather, we can identify three discrete constellations of conflict – relating both to geographical and occupational divides – that characterised the midwifery landscape of late seventeenth- and in particular eighteenth-century Leipzig:

Stadt (city)	vs	Vorstadt (suburbs)
sworn midwife	vs	sworn Beifrau
sworn	vs	unsworn

These conflicts reflected broader socio-economic divisions characteristic of eighteenth-century German cities: the sprawling extramural suburbs housing the poorer and middling sorts, the nascent manufacturing industry as well as the development of large numbers of career journeymen that threatened the authority of the guild masters.[50] Midwives and midwifery operated according to prevailing moral-economic norms, and it was largely within these constellations that contestation of livelihood took place. The next section will explore these forms of rivalry in greater detail.

---

50   This was certainly the case in the printing workshops of mid-eighteenth-century France and Switzerland, where printer journeymen faced stiff competition for work not only from within their own ranks, but also from so-called cheap labour *allouées* (printers without an apprenticeship). These allouées 'personified the tendency of labor to become a commodity instead of a partnership'. The 'Great Cat Massacre', as Robert Darnton has shown, was a cultural expression of these socio-economic circumstances. See Robert Darnton, *The Great Cat Massacre and Other Episodes in French Cultural History* (New York, NY: First Vintage Books, 1985), 79–81. Michael Mitterauer also notes that there was a significant increase in the number of journeymen living within artisan households in Salzburg between 1647 and 1797. This corresponded to a decrease in the number of apprentices that lived-in, suggesting a change in the make-up of the workshop in general as the proportion of wage journeymen increased. As a result, the balance of authority within the workshop was affected as the traditional master–apprentice relationship declined in favour of a looser employer–employee relationship. See Mitterauer, *Grundtypen*, 189–81.

a) Stadt versus Vorstadt

Conflict between midwives stationed within the Stadt (within the city walls) and those in the neighbourhoods at the city gates (Vorstadt) arose not just because a sworn midwife office was tied to a particular neighbourhood. Indeed, conflicts between individual midwives rarely revolved around defending a particular district. Rather, the major demarcation divided the Stadt and the Vorstadt because the terms of entitlement for those midwives living in the city and for those working in the Vorstadt were different. The Stadt/Vorstadt divide was essentially a product of the socio-economic demography of the city. The wealthier burghers tended to live as property-owners within the city walls, whereas the Vorstadt was home to those middling and poorer sorts as well as to itinerant workers.[51] As midwives were largely dependent upon the discretionary fees and gifts they received, an office in the Vorstadt mostly meant a lower income. A further bone of contention was the fact that Vorstadt midwives had no right to expect the Council to provide accommodation free of charge, as was the standard in the city. However, the accusations levelled at interlopers from the city reveal that it was not the discrepancy between gross earnings in the Stadt versus those in the Vorstadt that were at stake, but much more so the peculiar 'customary' rights the Vorstadt midwives had over their district and, in particular, the care of unwed pregnant women and mothers.

In 1728 all three midwives in the Vorstadt petitioned the Council to put an end to the activities of two city midwives, Anna Martha Priebs and Sabine Streller, who they claimed were working day and night in the Vorstadt and 'taking our very livelihood away from us'.[52] The complaint was an amalgam of both indignation at the refusal of Priebs and Streller to keep to the Stadt and concrete accusations of impropriety. The Vorstadt midwives had confronted midwife Streller, but her purported response had been that 'they should adorn and lick her …'.[53] Priebs had been overheard at the baptismal font bragging that she would not stop working in the Vorstadt no matter how high the penalty. The midwives claimed further that Priebs had submitted a fraudulent baptismal certificate to the sexton, and rounded off their petition with a plea to the Leipzig Council to prohibit the city midwives from attending women in the Vorstadt on two counts. Firstly, the clientele was wealthier in the city and, secondly, the city midwives enjoyed free lodgings.[54] Clearly, the Vorstadt midwives were very conscious of the fact that the livelihood to which they were entitled was qualitatively different to the livelihood to which the city midwives could lay claim. Yet their aim in petitioning the Council was not to level the playing field by demanding equal terms of entitlement, such as free

51   Feige provides a detailed breakdown of the economic status of residents in the various intra- and extramural communities. Feige, 'Sozialstruktur'.
52   StadtAL, Tit. (F) XLIV.D.1, 124–26, 'Vorstadt midwives complain about midwives in the city', 29 June 1728, 124–25.
53   Ibid.
54   Ibid.

accommodation. It constituted an attempt to reinforce and restore that to which they were entitled through their office: the sole right to practise in the Vorstadt. The midwives wanted to restore the moral-economic order.

That the terms of a midwife's livelihood differed according to whether she was stationed in the city or in the Vorstadt is even more apparent in the disputes that centred on the right to take in unwed and widowed pregnant women. For seventeenth- and eighteenth-century Leipzigers, the Vorstadt was a particularly suspicious urban space. It was here where those on the social and moral margins – the beggars, the migrants, the prostitutes and the single women – could infiltrate the upstanding burgher society. Indigent 'wanton women', who posed a moral threat to social mores and placed a financial burden on the city's system of poor relief, were considered a particular problem. As early as the sixteenth century, residents in the Vorstadt were strictly forbidden from accommodating single women and female servants. The Council, which had taken an increasingly intolerant stance on beggary since the sixteenth century, carried out annual visitations of the Vorstadt neighbourhoods to weed out those residing without the prior knowledge of the Gassenmeister.[55] 'Illegal' residents not only posed a moral threat to the burgher society and its communal institutions; they also robbed the neighbourhoods of the Vorstadt taxes due.[56]

The emergence of a nascent manufacturing industry, wars and population growth during the eighteenth century brought greater levels of poverty to the city. Yet the measures taken to control immigration, largely via visitations of the numerous inns and guesthouses in the Vorstadt and incarceration in the workhouse, remained largely ineffective.[57] 'Fallen women' who sought assistance from the *Almosenamt* (Alms Office) posed a major problem for the Council because they were costly and soiled the moral-religious fabric of the city. In 1717, for example, the Council lamented the 'large number of wenches who get themselves pregnant in dishonour and have the fruit of their whoredom baptised in our churches'.[58]

Laxity amongst City Court officials, who often pocketed small bribes from such women in exchange for giving permission to deliver babies in the city without the requisite physical examination and interrogation, was rife. The Gassenmeister also turned a blind eye in return for a few pennies, sometimes even taking such women into their own homes so that 'the ordinary appointed midwives are not called upon, [the lay women] deliver the children themselves [and] take them to other places to be baptised'.[59] The problem had escalated so much, that in 1717 the Council moved to provide a strong disincen-

---

55 According to the Vorstadt Ordinance from 1550, as quoted in Bräuer, *Der Leipziger Rat*, 56–57.

56 Ibid.

57 Ibid., 71.

58 Bestimmung des Leipziger Rates über die Behandlung "verdächtiger" schwangerer Frauen und Mädchen, 14 April 1717. Quoted in ibid., 147–48.

59 Quoted in ibid., 147.

tive to women who came to Leipzig with the sole purpose of delivering their illegitimate children in ignominy. Gassenmeister in the Vorstadt were ordered to stop such women from renting lodgings in their districts unless they had supplied the Leipzig Court with details of 'when, where, how often and by whom they [had] gotten pregnant.'[60] These women were then sentenced to corporal punishment, which was naturally postponed if they were 'too close to their time and there [was] a danger for the fruit'.[61]

Despite the amount of revulsion they provoked within the community, cases in which women were accused of infanticide and newborn abandonment were relatively rare.[62] Contrastingly, unwed motherhood and illegitimacy were shameful and undesirable states for both mother and child, but they were commonplace and were integrated into the fabric of the community. Unmarried mothers tended to deliver their children in the community rather than rely on municipal poor and medical relief institutions. Whilst the lazarette at the Rannstädter Tor was known to take in unwed pregnant women in the early 1700s, it was touted by some contemporaries as a fearful space. Stadtphysicus Michael Ernst Ettmüller noted in 1725 that an 'unclean' woman had recently given birth in the lazarette, but that no midwife or Beifrau had been willing to attend for fear of scaring off or even infecting her own clientele.[63]

In Leipzig the 'problem' of unmarried mothers was dealt with in a rather pragmatic fashion. The preoccupation with population growth had led to a gradual shift in attitudes towards illicit sex and its consequences. Whereas earlier generations had insisted on meting out draconian forms of punishment to those whose sexual behaviour failed to conform to Christian law, by the early and mid-eighteenth century many considered this to be ineffectual in halting the incidence of child abandonment, abortion and infanticide.[64] In the late eighteenth century, Enlightenment ideas about the human condition and the need to accept the fallibility of human nature meant that fornication had been downgraded from a crime to a social problem and a human weakness.[65] For the efficiency- and productivity-loving cameralists, it was desirable 'to

60 Ibid., 78–79.
61 Quoted in ibid.
62 Only ten women were tried for infanticide between 1700 and 1800 in Leipzig. Rublack notes that there was strong geographical variation in the trying of women for infanticide. In the region of Württemberg, for example, a total of 182 women were tried between 1600 and 1700. In the city of Constance, on the other hand, a mere six. See Ulinka Rublack, *The Crimes of Women in Early Modern Germany* (Oxford: Clarendon Press, 2001), 191–92.
63 Tit. (F) XLIV.D.1, 83–118, 'Appointments (Greger and Veiß)', 22 November 1724–4 September 1725, 117–18. Schlenkrich notes a similar case for 1721. See Schlenkrich, *Von Leuten*, 113–14.
64 Dülmen, *Frauen vor Gericht*, 98–99.
65 Otto Ulbricht, 'The Debate about Foundling Hospitals in Enlightenment Germany: Infanticide, Illegitimacy, and Infant Mortality Rates', *Central European History* 18: 3/4 (1985): 211–56, 221–22. The same process took place with infanticide. See Dülmen, *Frauen vor Gericht*, 98–108.

make fornication less damaging or even useful to the state'.[66] The Leipzig Council, whose poor relief institutions had to deal first-hand with the consequences of illegitimacy, appears to have recognised that draconian punishments were not solving the problem of illegitimacy even before the open discourse over the causes of infanticide and illegitimacy commenced in the 1760s. The Council was prepared to tolerate illegitimacy only so long as it did not burden the city's coffers, which it achieved by letting the Vorstadt residents do business in unmarried mothers. And so by the mid-eighteenth century at the very latest, a lively 'industry' of lying-in houses accommodating unmarried mothers without familial and social support within the city flourished, providing both a livelihood for many residents and reducing the economic burden of illegitimacy on the city's poor relief.

Unwed pregnant women or, in the case of servants, Hausväter or Hausmütter would usually approach a woman running a lying-in house several weeks prior to delivery to reserve a place.[67] Customarily, the heavily pregnant woman would take up her bed in the lying-in house a few weeks later to await the birth, after which she was supposed to stay on for the full six-week postpartum lying-in period, the so-called *Sechswochen*.[68] Poverty meant that many did not see out the full term of lying-in. The women that midwife Johanna Christina Held took in during 1782 spent a mere nine days lying in, for which Held was paid substantially less than the usual rate of 2 Taler.[69] And whilst pre-arranged confinements were common, some women first sought refuge in a lying-in house or with a sworn midwife or Beifrau at the height of their birthing pains.

Lying-in houses were run by both midwives and lay women (working in collusion with sworn or unsworn midwives) and had been in existence since at least the early eighteenth century. In 1717, for example, Rosina Huth operated such a lying-in house in her lodgings in the Bettelgasse in the Vorstadt. Huth, not a midwife, relied upon the services of both the city midwife Johanna Sabina Netzold and the long-standing Gassenmagd in the Bettelgasse, Maria Lindner, to deliver the women she took in. Midwife Netzold attended daytime deliveries and Gassenmagd Lindner was fetched whenever a woman went into labour at night.[70] Although the activities of women running lying-in houses have by and large gone undocumented, the small collection of

---

66 According to the document 'Über die Wiederherziehung entwichener und entführter Einwohner, Fabrikanten und Bauern' (Dresden, 19 July 1762), quoted in Ulbricht, 'The Debate about Foundling Hospitals', 223.

67 For example, Johanna Defer reserved her place to lie in with the wife of a soldier in the city garrison almost two months prior to the actual birth. Straf. Nr. 708, 'Defer and Reinheckel', 1741, 14r–15r.

68 See witness statement made by lying-in house owner Maria Magdalena Dreßler in ibid., 14–15. One woman's delivery and lying-in had been arranged by her master. See Tit. (F) XLIV.D.6b, Bd. I, 158–285, 'Various complaints', 14 July 1772–1810, 189.

69 Tit. (F) XLIV.D.6b, Bd. I, 158–285, 'Various complaints', 14 July 1772–1810, 239.

70 II. Sekt. W (F) Nr. 332, 1–9, 'Midwives vs Gassenmägde', 30 January–10 March 1717, 5–6.

Schwängerungsacta (registers of illegitimate children fathered by students of the
Leipzig University between 1736 and 1783) kept by the University Court
reveal that both Gassenmägde and sworn midwives routinely earned or augmented their living in this fashion.[71] According to this source, Anna Maria
Rein, the midwife at the Grimmaisches Tor, took a total of three women into
her home in the Neugasse during the autumn of 1736 and the midwife at the
Rannstädter Tor, Regina Mader, also accommodated a woman during lying-in
that same year.[72] In 1783 sworn Beifrau Josephina Regina Popp tended one
Johanna Elisabeth Winckler in her midwife lodgings in the Stadtpfeiffengasse.[73] Council records also reveal the following: Over a period of three
months in 1772 the city Beifrau Johanna Elisabeth Matthes was reported
to have taken in six 'geschwächte Weibespersonen' (morally weakened
women).[74] Rahel Leib took in ten such women, and yet another Beifrau,
Johanna Regina Popp, eight in 1782.[75]

The business of taking in single mothers was not regulated by instruction
or ordinance, but was instead governed by the politics of rights and entitlement. Custom dictated that the right to earn a living off these unfortunate
women was the preserve of those sworn midwives and Beifrauen living and
working in the Vorstadt neighbourhoods. Sworn midwives and Beifrauen located within the city walls who contravened this custom were branded as interlopers. In 1717 city midwife Johanna Sabrina Netzold was the target of
such an accusation levelled by the three sworn midwives in the Vorstadt.
Netzold, they complained, had been living and working in the Vorstadt without permission from the Council. What particularly raised their ire was the
fact that the Vorstadt Gassenmägde, who took in single mothers, engaged
Netzold to take the children they delivered to baptism instead of calling for
the Vorstadt midwives, whose right this actually was.[76] The Council ratified
the Vorstadt midwives' claim, directing Netzold to 'remain in her allocated
area' and not to engage or assist any of the Vorstadt Gassenmägde.[77]

---

71 All but one of the Schwängerungsacta are from 1736–43. See GA IV 205, 1–41, 'Schwän-
    gerungsacta', 1736–83. As the University was not under the jurisdiction of the Leipzig
    City Court, when the illegitimate child of a university student was brought to St Thomas
    or St Nikolai to be baptised, the sexton was obliged to communicate the names of the
    mother, father and child to the University Court (Gerichtsamt), as well as the place where
    the mother was lying-in. Since 1717 all other illegitimate children baptised had to be
    registered with the Leipzig Court (Stadtgericht). The illegitimate mothers were then in-
    terrogated by both courts. See 'Bestimmung des Leipziger Rates über die Behandlung
    "verdächtiger" schwangerer Frauen und Mädchen' from 14 April 1717, transcribed in
    Bräuer, *Der Leipziger Rat*, 148–49. See also Schlenkrich, *Von Leuten*, 112–13.
72 GA IV 205, 1–41, 'Schwängerungsacta', 1736–83, 6–8.
73 Ibid., 41.
74 Tit. (F) XLIV.D.6b, Bd. I, 158–285, 'Various complaints', 14 July 1772–1810, 164.
75 Ibid., 237–38.
76 II. Sekt. W (F) Nr. 332, 1–9, 'Midwives vs Gassenmägde', 30 January–10 March 1717,
    1–3.
77 Ibid., 4.

Midwives and Beifrauen in the Vorstadt, who were permitted to earn money from women lying in, were also quick to denounce city midwives harbouring single pregnant women. Not infrequently, it was the Vorstadt midwives and Beifrauen who notified the Vorstadt Gassenmeister when their rivals did so.[78] Their indignant accusations were couched in a language of entitlement concerning income derived from unwed mothers. In 1782 sworn midwife Maria Catharina Vogel was moved to petition the Council in writing, arguing that the midwives and Beifrauen in the city had several privileges that those in the Vorstadt did not. The midwives in the Stadt enjoyed larger, free lodgings and because of the 'great difference between the city and the gate people [Vorstadt residents] for the purposes of paying for our services ... we must work almost for nothing'.[79] Lying-in might not have been particularly lucrative, however, a steady stream of women could certainly lift a midwife's earnings: a midwife could expect to receive 2 Taler for a woman's lying-in and 1 Taler as the *Kindermutterlohn* (midwife's fee) for the delivery.[80]

The Vorstadt midwives' entitlement to extract a livelihood from fallen women was underpinned by the very same entitlement exerted by the Vorstadt neighbourhoods. For the extramural neighbourhoods, unwed mothers had two uses: they provided a means of lining the local community coffers and ensured an additional source of rental income for landlords. Unwed mothers who gave birth in the lying-in houses in the Vorstadt were expected to pay a *Nachbarschaftsgeld* (neighbourhood levy) of 2 Taler to the neighbourhood in which they chose to spend their confinement. Of these 2 Taler, 1 Taler went into the community coffers and 1 Taler was due in rent to the landlord of the house where the woman resided during lying-in.[81] By the eighteenth century the Vorstadt communities had been granted a monopoly on taking in unwed pregnant women, in part because this removed the problem of immorality to outside the city walls. Yet this was also partly a solution to the financial weakness of the Vorstadt, and neighbourhood elders fought vigorously to protect this particular source of income. Midwives' and the Vorstadt inhabitants' 'entitlement' to this source of income and their right to 'make use' of illegitimate pregnancies was very well established, so much so that when Stadtaccoucheur Gehler submitted his proposal for a lying-in hospital in Leipzig in 1764, he voiced concerns that the midwives and Beifrauen in the Vor-

78 In 1773 both midwife Herrmann and Beifrau Schulz tipped off the Gassenmeister, who subsequently informed the Council about women lying-in with city midwives and Beifrauen. See Tit. (F) XLIV.D.6b, Bd. I, 158–285, 'Various complaints', 14 July 1772–1810, 170 and 76.
79 Ibid., 235–36.
80 Ibid., 189–92 and 239.
81 18 Groschen went to the church where the child was baptised and 12 Groschen were handed over to the Office of the Leipzig Court (Richterstube), presumably as a fine for illegitimacy. See ibid., 189–92.

stadt as well as the Vorstadt neighbourhoods would be displeased about having that aspect of their income curtailed.[82]

In July 1772 the Gassenmeister in the Vorstadt lodged an official complaint on behalf of the Vorstadt neighbourhoods against the midwives and Beifrauen working within the city walls. For several years the midwives in the Stadtpfeiffengasse had been accommodating unwed women in some of the vacant apartments the Council used to house its minor officials. This, they claimed, robbed the Vorstadt midwives and Beifrauen as well as the Vorstadt neighbourhoods of an essential source of income that paid for municipal maintenance works, such as the night watchman's salary and the construction and maintenance of the wells. The Vorstadt neighbourhoods, the Gassenmeister argued, already had to contend with the fact that many of their residents were too poor to pay the Nachbarschaftsgeld. The antics of the city midwives, they alleged, had forced the Vorstadt communities into debt. The Council responded by rounding up the Stadt midwives and Beifrauen and reprimanding them for taking in unwed mothers.[83] The Vorstadt Gassenmeister mounted further collective attacks in 1773 and again in 1789, arguing once again that it was the Vorstadt neighbourhoods' right to take in unwed mothers for a fee citing, once again, that the infrastructure of the Vorstadt depended upon this income. These complaints sparked off further Council investigations and more punitive fines for those midwives and Beifrauen who persisted in contravening the rules of entitlement.[84]

As the case of the Stadt Beifrau Regina Pötsch in 1790 demonstrates, the Vorstadt neighbourhoods were more interested in obtaining their Nachbarschaftsgeld than ensuring the Vorstadt midwives maintained their entitlement to earn an income in this fashion. Together with another Beifrau, Pötsch petitioned the Council in 1789 for permission to take in women to supplement her meagre income and bolster her midwifery experience, promising in return to pay 1 Taler per woman housed to the Vorstadt neighbourhoods.[85] Problems arose when one of the Gassenmeister accused Pötsch of taking 2 Taler in Nachbarschaftsgeld from the women she housed but only passing on a part of that money to the Gassenmeister. During the course of the Council's investigations, it came to light that Pötsch had a covert 'agreement' with the Gassenmeister in the Bettelgasse at the Grimmaisches Tor. Of the 2 Taler Pötsch paid to the neighbourhoods, the Gassenmeister returned 12 Groschen because, if the woman stayed in the city with Pötsch, the 1 Taler rent paid to a Vorstadt landlord was no longer due. Women residing with Pötsch thus earned

---

82　StadtAL, Tit. (F) XLIV.D.2a, 'Varia, die Hebammen und das Hebammeninstitut betr. 1705–1812', 10–13, 'Stadtaccoucheur Dr Johann Carl Gehler's proposal for a midwifery institute', 19 March 1764, 111r.

83　Tit. (F) XLIV.D.6b, Bd. I, 158–285, 'Various complaints', 14 July 1772–1810, 158–59.

84　In 1773 the Council fined midwives 20 Groschen. By 1782 the fine had risen to 5 Taler, and in 1789 to 10 Taler (more than a midwife's annual salary retainer). Ibid., 159, 73–74, 243, 248.

85　Ibid., 249–50.

the neighbourhood in the Bettelgasse 20 Groschen more than when they were confined with one of the midwives or Beifrauen in the Vorstadt.[86] The Leipzig Council, however, construed the deal between Pötsch and the Gassenmeister in the Bettelgasse as bribery, fined both, and prohibited the midwives and Beifrauen in the city yet again from taking in fallen women, except in an emergency.[87]

Hence, as far as the Council and the rules of entitlement were concerned, taking in a woman in an emergency was tolerated, but keeping a woman for lying in within the city walls was not. A servant living in the Brühl had come to Beifrau Christina Bauer's house one night in 1774 and, seeing that she was in labour, Bauer had taken her in and the servant gave birth the following morning. After the child had been christened, the woman left for one of the Vorstadt neighbourhoods to lie in. The ruse of 'emergency' enabled midwives to circumvent the moral economy of midwifery without injuring the established norms. It was consequently the most popular excuse city midwives and Beifrauen employed to escape punishment when they were discovered to have women lying in in their homes.[88]

b) Sworn midwife versus sworn Beifrau

In 1715 the Leipzig Council appointed the first sworn Beifrauen and so commenced an open conflict between sworn Beifrauen and the city's sworn midwives lasting most of the eighteenth century. Whilst the introduction of sworn Beifrauen was intended as an official extension of the relationship that had existed between a midwife and her informal apprentice, this development curtailed somewhat the formal autonomy sworn midwives had previously exercised over the selection and training of their protégées. At the same time, the instruction and office invested Beifrauen with more status and a greater degree of independence. Conflicts that arose between midwives and Beifrauen were about entitlement to a livelihood, but they also revolved around the question of authority and status underpinning the notion of livelihood.

From the Council's point of view, Beifrauen were subordinate to the sworn midwives. They were to 'assist the midwives to the best of their ability, to take instruction from them and to carry out their orders without neglect or delay'.[89] Only in the height of an emergency was a Beifrau permitted to act without the knowledge or permission of one of the sworn midwives. If a Beifrau was asked to provide her assistance independently and was unable to turn down the request, she was instructed to first seek permission from the

---

86   Ibid., 261–63.
87   Ibid., 263–68.
88   Ibid., 185.
89   See Items 3 and 4 of Tit. (F) X 23b, Bd. III, 234–36, 'Instruction Beÿweiber', c. 1715 (undated).

burgomaster.[90] Yet it was this 'emergency' clause which gave sworn Beifrauen leeway to attend a woman outside the teacher–apprentice framework. Beifrauen exploited this loophole readily, so much so that their instruction had to be amended in 1723 to regulate their activities in emergencies. Now Beifrauen were required to register all such emergency births that they had attended without the consent or knowledge of a midwife with the Council.[91] By 1758 the opportunity for Beifrauen to operate independently of their allocated midwives had been reduced even further. The 'emergency' clause had all but disappeared from the Beifrau instruction and Beifrauen were instructed 'never to attend a birth without the knowledge of [their] … allocated midwi[ves]'.[92]

There is little known about the dynamics of the relationship between midwives and their apprentices prior to the eighteenth century. In the midwifery manuals of Justine Siegemund (1690) and Anne Horenburg (1700) the 'chatty' question-and-answer interaction between the apprentice and the midwife depicts the idyll of a suitably subordinate novice eager to learn from the wiser, experienced, patient and motherly midwife.[93] Yet it should be noted that neither Siegemund nor Horenburg learnt the art of midwifery in the traditional manner; both were self-professed autodidacts who claimed to have acquired their initial knowledge of childbirth by reading contemporary midwifery manuals.[94] The relationship between a midwife and her apprentice could be positive and enduring, but it might also be modelled on the relationship between a mistress and her servant.[95]

90   See Items 3 and 4 of ibid. This was the wording of an instruction from around 1715. A later instruction with amendments from 1758 lacks this paragraph and instructs the Beifrauen instead to attend, but in the case of a difficult birth, to immediately consult either the midwife or the Stadtaccoucheur. See Item 7 of Tit. (F) X 23b, Bd. VIII, 70–76, 'Instruktion Beÿfrau N. N.', 14 July 1758, 72r–72v.

91   See Item 3 of Tit. (F) X.23b, Bd. V, 'Instruktionen (1676–nach 1800)', 36–39, 'Instruction geschworenen Beÿweibern', 10 June 1723.

92   See Tit. (F) X 23b, Bd. VIII, 70–76, 'Instruktion Beÿfrau N. N.', 14 July 1758.

93   Justine Siegemundin, *Die Chur=Brandenburgische Hoff=Wehe=Mutter* (Cölln an der Spree: Ulrich Liebperten, Churfl. Brandenb. Hofbuchdrucker, 1690); Anna Elizabeth Horenburg, *Wohlmeynender und nöhtiger Unterricht der Heeb=Ammen* (Hannover and Wolfenbüttel: Gottfried Freytag, 1700).

94   Whilst serving the Duchess of Anhalt, who had a particular interest in medicine and healing, Horenburg began to study the collection of midwifery manuals in the Duchess' library. She later married a corporal in the army and worked as a midwife to wives in the regiment before she was finally, several years later, called to an office of sworn midwife in Mansfeld and Eisleben (Thüringia). See *Nöhtiger Unterricht*, 2v–3v. A terrible experience at the hands of her local midwives prompted Siegemund to study various manuals and sketches 'in order to learn a thing or two about my condition'. Some of the town midwives began to call for her assistance in difficult births and she came to be known in the area as a highly proficient midwife. Some years later she was eventually called to the town of Liegnitz to take on a midwife office. See Siegemund, *Court Midwife*, 48–49.

95   In France, for example, some midwives used their apprentices for other domestic and clerical tasks as well. See Rattner Gelbart, *The King's Midwife*, 47.

Sworn midwives dispatched their apprentices as it suited them, for example, to carry out the menial tasks of swaddling or to attend a delivery or baptism on their behalf. Moreover, as we have seen in Chapter Three, women frequently entered into midwifery through some type of familial, household or kin connection, which suggests that 'apprentices' were largely selected from the ranks of the known and trusted: sisters, sisters-in-law, daughters and female servants (often from within the midwife's own household). This meant that the relationship between a midwife and her 'apprentice' was built upon pre-existing social hierarchies based on both maturity and the micro-politics of household authority that dictated the subordination of the daughter, the daughter-in-law or servant to the female head of household.[96] Similarly, the politics of progression within the ranks of sworn midwifery was based on a hierarchy of age; the eldest Beifrau was almost always promoted to fill a vacant office when one of the sworn midwives died.[97] Many Beifrauen continued to be drawn from families with a background in midwifery. However, they were often allocated to midwives outside their immediate social and familial sphere. As it became less common for a Beifrau to inhabit the same house or the same neighbourhood as her midwife-teacher, social and physical dislocation became the norm. And even though Beifrauen were becoming younger towards the end of the eighteenth century, the hierarchy of age did not remain stable. As the eighteenth century progressed, for many Beifrauen midwifery became a crucial component of the family income, at times the only source of a livelihood. Armed with their 'entitlement' to practise, these women often demonstrated a level of occupational tenaciousness that ruptured the confines of the midwife–Beifrau relationship and upset its traditional structures of authority.[98]

Resistance amongst the city's sworn midwives towards the newly appointed Beifrauen in 1715 was substantial. The arguments that midwives presented rested upon the concept of entitlement and the establishment of a subordinate relationship. Midwives refused to acknowledge the existence of the Beifrauen, claiming (in the words of the Beifrauen) 'they would rather relinquish their office than use the Beifrauen, they refused to have such Bei-

96 On the importance of life-cycle as a variable of social relations, see Pam Sharpe, 'Disruption in the Well-Ordered Household: Age, Authority, and Posessed Young People', in Paul Griffiths et al., eds, *The Experience of Authority in Early Modern England* (Basingstoke: Macmillan Press, 1996), esp. 187–90. On the authority of the wife over household, servants and children in England, see Bernard Capp, 'Separate Domains? Women and Authority in Early Modern England', ibid., 126–27.

97 Stadtaccoucheur Gehler noted this practice, which appears to have been generally followed, in 1785. See Tit. (F) XLIV.D.6c, 54–74, 'Various appointments', 4 October 1782–22 January 1789, 57.

98 This situation demonstrates parallels with developments in the artisan world where the glut of career journeymen also put pressure on the authority of the master over the worker, see Mitterauer, *Grundtypen*, 63–64.

frauen imposed upon them'.[99] They also employed collective tactics to avoid relying on sworn Beifrauen, such as carrying infants to baptism in person, even when their busy work schedules delayed this by two to three days, just so that the Beifrauen 'would have nothing from them'.[100]

In 1715, only days after the Beifrauen had sworn their oath, the sworn midwives submitted an angry petition to the Council on account of two discrete incidents. Unbeknown to the midwives, one Beifrau, Christina Lorend, had delivered twins. Another Beifrau, Sabine Lehmann, had caused an unseemly fuss at the baptismal font as she had attempted to wrestle a child from the arms of another woman on the grounds that only she, as Beifrau, was entitled to replace a midwife who was too busy to attend a baptism.[101] In doing so Lehmann and Lorend had trespassed on the traditional occupational-economic territory of the city's sworn midwives. The Beifrauen, the midwives argued, 'encroach indiscriminately upon us sworn midwives, who carry such heavy responsibility, in our duties and snatch the little [fees], which amount these days to little or nothing from those lowly and poor people, from out of our mouths'.[102] Yet in acting independently, Lehmann and Lorend had also upset the traditional balance of authority and subordination between a sworn midwife and her 'apprentice'. Eventually the sworn midwives begrudgingly accepted the introduction of the sworn Beifrauen. Yet they were unwilling to have their authority truncated any further, promising acquiescence on condition that the Beifrauen remained completely subordinate to the midwives.[103] Only 'if none of us eight midwives be available', they continued, should the Beifrauen be permitted '*to help us* [my italics] to assist in a childbirth or to swaddle or take the children to church for holy baptism.'[104]

For the sworn midwives, the Beifrauen presented direct competition, not because their existence augmented the pool of women actually practising midwifery in Leipzig, but instead because the sworn Beifrauen could not be clearly subsumed and subordinated within the traditional framework of authority and hierarchy. The sworn midwife had traditionally been distinguished from her lay peers through the office of midwife. Yet with the introduction of the sworn Beifrauen, this simple marker of entitlement (and authority) necessitated renewed differentiation between the 'full' and the 'trainee' midwife. If both were under oath and in possession of an instruction, how was one to demarcate their areas of activity and their occupational status?

The matter of who was 'qualified' to deliver a child also became an issue in 1715. Yet these contests did not revolve around experience and knowledge

99 StadtAL, Tit. (F) XLIV.D.1, 'Kindermütter bey hiesiger Stadt betr. ingl. die angenommene Bey Weiber betr. 1673–1756', 48–53, 'Midwives complain about the Beifrauen', 24 April–6 May 1715, 50–53.
100 Ibid.
101 Ibid.
102 Ibid., 49.
103 Ibid., 48–49.
104 Ibid., 49.

as 'qualifiers' but rather hinged on the idea of entitlement. From both the perspective of the community and the Council, the act of delivering a child was not the sole preserve of a sworn midwife. As we have seen in Chapter Two, there were places and times where unsworn women and Gassen-mägde could practise relatively freely. Indeed sworn midwives often used un-sworn women to assist or act of their behalf and justified their actions with arguments about occupational propriety. In 1715, for instance, the sworn mid-wives spread rumours amongst their clients and neighbours that the new Bei-frauen had sworn under oath never to deliver a single child. According to the Beifrauen, the midwives continued to use unsworn women 'without any ex-perience and without obligation' to assist them. The Beifrauen claimed fur-ther that 'it did not mean anything' for such women to deliver babies as they 'had not sworn against it, [and] no one would reprimand them for it'.[105] As this example suggests, for the sworn midwives the factor that qualified a woman to deliver a child was either a midwife office or a subordinate position as 'apprentice' or 'assistant' with a *willing* sworn midwife. The unwillingness of many of the sworn midwives to take the newly appointed Beifrauen under their wings meant that these Beifrauen had neither a sworn midwife office nor the authority afforded through an apprenticeship with a sworn midwife based upon mutual consent. Thus these early Beifrauen stood outside of the tradi-tional hierarchy of midwifery which, in the eyes of the midwives, disqualified them to practise midwifery officially on any level.

Over the next decades open defiance on the part of the sworn midwives towards the sworn Beifrauen waned, yet the relationship between the two groups remained tense. A persistent point of contention between the Bei-frauen (in particular those in the Stadt) and the sworn midwives was the prac-tice of taking in unwed women to deliver. As already discussed, the cost of bearing an illegitimate child in a lying-in home in the Vorstadt was consider-able (around 5 Taler). The only way unwed pregnant women could circum-vent this cost without running the risk of being accused of concealing a birth was to feign an emergency and spend confinement and lying in with a mid-wife or Beifrau in the city.[106] Yet by the latter eighteenth century it was not just demand that fuelled this illicit activity. Many Beifrauen still had a poor rela-tionship with their midwife-teachers, which threatened, firstly, the substance of their livelihood and, secondly, their ability to gain the experience and knowledge of childbirth required and cultivate a clientele. The Beifrauen Johanna Maria Werther and Johanna Elisabeth Matthes both argued that they had been forced to take in unwed women because, except in the greatest emergency or if the midwife was otherwise indisposed, none of the midwives would call either Beifrau out to attend an 'honourable woman'. Unwed women, both Beifrauen claimed, provided them with their sole opportunity

---

105 Ibid., 50–53.
106 Tit. (F) XLIV.D.6b, Bd. I, 158–285, 'Various complaints', 14 July 1772–1810, 239–43.

to learn their chosen occupation.[107] This was the first explicit association of moral-economic entitlement (not aptitude) with some kind of discrete knowledge of midwifery.

In 1789 a new generation of Beifrauen came up against the same barrier. 'None of the real midwives take us with them to deliveries, nor does any lady of status or wealth let us touch her', Beifrau Rahel Regina Pötsch, whose story has just been discussed, complained in her supplication to the Council:

> I consider myself therefore forced, most particularly as a widow with three young children ... to turn to Your Excellency the Leipzig Council to humbly request that You would want to consider our paltry income and not prohibit us the exercises and experience accomplished through such people [unwed mothers], but instead generously permit us to take such women in.[108]

Pötsch's practice was improper on two counts. Firstly, it contravened the 'moral' monopoly of the Vorstadt over unwed mothers. Secondly, it contravened the Beifrau instruction. Yet the Beifrauen still turned to the moral economy of entitlement to combat the dearth of work they experienced at the end of the eighteenth century:

> Both the Alms Office and the midwives in the Vorstadt send poor women, from whom [the midwives] would not earn anything, to the *Beifrauen*. And so that these people would not become a burden to the Almosen Amt, they [the Beifrauen] cared for them without payment and let them lie in within their homes *because they considered it only proper that they be granted an income in another way* [my italics].[109]

They couched their transgressions in the language of entitlement, rendering encroachment as a moral-economic imperative as long as it ensured a person's moral 'right' to extract a living.

c) Sworn midwives and Beifrauen versus unsworn midwives

Complaints from sworn midwives about the activities of Gassenmägde and other unsworn women working as midwives also invariably revolved around the issue of livelihood. The clash between official and unofficial midwifery was greatest in the latter seventeenth and early eighteenth centuries, waning somewhat towards the latter eighteenth century. For sworn midwives such as Maria Plessing, intrusion brought financial crisis, but it also posed an affront to the honour of the sworn midwife, for it was this livelihood that maintained a midwife's social status: the Gassenmägde who 'scold me most horribly [and

---

107 Tit. (F) XLIV.D.6b, Bd. I, 'Acta, Die Einrichtung der Kindermütter und Beÿweiber betr.', 109–13, 'Midwife Maria Westphal complains about the Beifrauen', 10–16 January 1769, 109v–11r.

108 See Pötsch's supplication from 18 June 1789 in Tit. (F) XLIV.D.6b, Bd. I, 'Acta, die Einrichtung der Kindermütter und Beÿweiber', 245–55, 'Gassenmeister complain about Beifrau Rahel Regina Pötsch', 17 June 1789–11 April 1790, 249–50.

109 See the statement made by the Beifrauen in Tit. (F) XLIV.D.6b, Bd. I, 158–285, 'Various complaints', 14 July 1772–1810, 159.

who], on the other hand, boast of their skill and who desire to be used in my place during confinements' stood in direct contrast to the sworn midwife Plessing, who had 'behaved with propriety and administered the task of baptism faithfully for some twenty years'.[110]

Keeping face and status did not entail stamping out all unsworn midwifery. Not all women practising midwifery without an office were considered rivals by sworn midwives and Beifrauen. Up until the mid-eighteenth century the activities of so-called Wickelweiber (swaddling women), female relatives and domestic servants were generally tolerated by sworn midwives as long as these women held a subservient role. And the Leipzig Council usually only pursued unofficial midwives if their activities had clashed with those of the sworn midwives and Beifrauen. Gassenmägde, on the other hand, often operated independently of any sworn midwives and were not so easily subsumed into the web of authority surrounding sworn midwives. They drew their status from within the community and, as we have seen in Chapter Two, from their Gassenmagd office. Often a tacit agreement existed between a Gassenmagd and a sworn midwife, enabling the former to attend births or care for mothers during lying-in. In return, the sworn midwife might insist that the Gassenmagd call on her exclusively for taking the child to baptism. Midwives often only voiced accusations of encroachment when such an arrangement went awry. In 1717, for example, the Gassenmägde Mrs Pech and Mrs Lindner felt the wrath of the midwife at the Grimmaisches Tor. They had delivered infants in the Vorstadt but called upon the city midwives to carry out the baptism, thus failing to 'grant us [the Vorstadt midwives] the absolute least'.[111] The disputes between sworn and unsworn midwives operating in Leipzig were in fact extensions of the divisions that existed between the Vorstadt and the Stadt on the one hand, and between midwives and their apprentices on the other. It was these divides, and not the sworn/unsworn divide *per se,* that really mattered. After all, as discussed in Chapter Two, many sworn midwives could look back onto a good deal of midwifery experience gained in such an informal capacity.

From the perspective of the Leipzig Council, unsworn midwifery posed a threat to the livelihood of its sworn midwives. Yet it was cognisant of the impracticality of ensuring that women only used sworn midwives. Rather than banning unsworn midwifery outright, the Council merely reminded women accused of encroachment to seek the assistance of a sworn midwife as soon as possible.[112] As well as needing to protect the occupational propriety of its sworn midwives, the Council harboured concerns about the trustworthiness of the Gassenmägde, in particular with respect to baptism.[113] The possibility that unsworn midwives might deliver the illegitimate children of unwed mothers

---

110 II. Sekt. P (F) Nr. 175b, 1–5, 'Marie Plessingen', 2 June 1699–17 July 1703, 2.
111 II. Sekt. W (F) Nr. 332, 1–9, 'Midwives vs Gassenmägde', 30 January–10 March 1717, 1–3.
112 Ibid., 5.
113 Ibid., 4–6.

and arrange for these infants to be smuggled out to the surrounding villages to be baptised was an ever-present anxiety and one that continued to be of greater concern than their level of obstetric skill.[114] Christina Hentschell, for example, incurred several bans on practising in 1704, 1705 and 1707, despite accusing one midwife of having 'an unskilled finger' and having 'damaged five women in a short space of time'.[115] The Council did not pursue Gassenmägde and unsworn midwives prophylactically. The activities of these women only came under the scrutiny of the Council when sworn midwives and Beifrauen levelled accusations of encroachment against them. Unsworn midwifery was thus only really a 'problem' when a Gassenmagd transgressed the Stadt/Vorstadt divide or subverted the authority of the sworn midwives and, in so doing, injured the moral economy governing the midwifery landscape.

Conclusions

In mapping out the patterns of conflict that persistently characterised the midwifery landscape in eighteenth-century Leipzig, it has become clear that disputes between midwives revolved in the main around two issues: the demarcation of rights across the Stadt/Vorstadt divide and the problem of ensuring internal occupational hierarchies. Both these issues were aggravated by developments peculiar to the eighteenth century: the growth and impoverishment of the Vorstadt communities and the institutionalisation of the traditional midwife–apprentice relationship. Underpinning these battles was the moral-economic framework of 'livelihood'.

Conflict occurring between sworn and unsworn midwives revolved around the same two issues. In all cases, the accusation of encroachment was not specifically directed at unsworn women operating independently in the midwifery landscape. It was deployed more often against women – both sworn and unsworn – whose activities undercut the traditional entitlement of the Vorstadt midwives to income from illegitimate births or challenged the authority of the sworn midwives in their role as teachers. The threat of encroachment did not come from the fringes of the midwifery landscape but from within the very core of official midwifery and, in particular, from within the relationship between a sworn midwife and her Beifrau-apprentice. This insight suggests that throughout the eighteenth century, the notion of 'quack' or 'interloper' was not coupled with practitioners on the 'medical fringe', but was a label brandished at any individual or group who strove to undermine the

---

114 Ibid., 6. See, for example, Stadtphysicus Petermann's report on a case of negligence brought against a sworn midwife, in which the character and behaviour of the midwives took up most of the page, whereas anatomical knowledge consumed a mere paragraph. See II. Sekt. W (F) Nr. 319, 1–27, 'Beschwerden (Willendorf)', 8 May–14 August 1717, 13–16b.

115 Tit. (F) XLIV.D.2a, 1–7, 'Midwives vs Hentschell', 14 August–2 September 1705, 1r and 5r; See also Tit. (F) XLIV.D.1, 11–13, 'Midwives vs Hentschell and Stöps', 1707.

very specific moral economy of livelihood upon which both the practice and the organisation of midwifery in Leipzig rested.

Finally, the regulation of livelihood was not something imposed upon midwives by the Leipzig Council in an act of legislative violence. Impetus for regulation came from within the ranks of sworn midwives. Through the medium of petitions and complaints, midwives and Beifrauen were able to communicate their interests and 'entitlements' to the Council and effect regulatory enforcement. Until now, midwives have been cast largely as the victims of ordinance and oath, as mere subjects of the power and will of communal and territorial governments. This study of conflict and the moral economy of livelihood suggests that this assumption requires reassessment. Legislative procedure in early modern societies was a two-way street. Norms were the product of communication and negotiation between the ruling and the ruled. This was equally apparent in the process of legislating matters relating to livelihood, the contours of which midwives and Beifrauen, through their supplicating activities, helped to draw themselves.

Chapter Five
Midwives, Clients and Trust

Early modern midwifery operated within a culture of trust. Sworn midwives and Beifrauen were expected to build up a clientele and embed themselves in a particular community; in so doing, the melange of the social and the occupational shored up their economic livelihoods. However, the structural changes introduced by the Leipzig Council, in particular the introduction of Beifrauen as a means of guaranteeing the constant supply of capable, oath-bound midwives, altered the practice of allocating midwives to a particular district. Where she had previously enjoyed a long-term association with a single neighbourhood, often the one in which she was born and bred, a midwife might now be forced to inhabit one or more 'foreign' offices over the course of a lifetime. This threatened to dislocate the figure of the midwife from her social milieu and de-personalise her services.

The process of social estrangement was not a strategic act of professionalisation or bureaucratisation on the part of the communal government, but was rather a pragmatic attempt on the part of the Council to adjust existing midwifery provision to the changing demands of the growing city. The system of allocation was in fact both an effort to ensure social consistency between a midwife and her neighbourhood and an attempt to guarantee this consistency in all areas of the city, not just where rich pickings were to be had. Leipzig was divided up into districts: the city within the fortified walls formed one such district, with a further four at the communities at each gate (the Grimmaisches Tor, the Peterstor, the Rannstädter Tor and the Hallisches Tor). Between three and four midwives were appointed to the city district and one midwife was posted to each of the Vorstadt neighbourhoods (see Figure 1, Chapter 1). The resulting social dislocation was an unfortunate by-product of which the Leipzig Council and its Stadtaccoucheurs were well aware. To counter this problem, the Council assumed a rather relaxed attitude to midwives' client-building practices. It turned a blind eye to midwives who overstepped their practice boundaries, as long as their actions did not provoke cries of encroachment from other office holders. It also made every attempt to keep its midwives in familiar territory because it recognised the importance of trust for both mothers and midwives. As this chapter will demonstrate, this culture of trust was a persistent characteristic of the relationship between a midwife and her clients throughout the eighteenth century and it continued to inform the decisions affecting midwifery made by both the Council and the Stadtphysici/Stadtaccoucheurs.

The wealth of normative sources for midwifery in the cities has led to the general assumption that midwifery was already 'professionalised' by the beginning of the eighteenth century.[1] As a result there has been little attention paid to the precise dynamics of the midwife–client relationship in the urban

---

1   See Labouvie, 'Frauenberuf'; 'Sofia Weinranck', 225–28.

context. This chapter suggests that midwifery in Leipzig, a bustling, international city, remained surprisingly 'parochial' throughout the eighteenth century *in spite of* the reforms instituted by the Leipzig Council and its municipal
medical officers. As I will show here, personal trust continued to be the essential ingredient in the midwife–client relationship – one that no amount of professionalisation and standards could replace. To paint the persistence of trust
as a mere mark of resistance on the part of midwives against the 'medicalis-
ing' and 'bureaucratising' programmes of an enlightened communal government would be a misreading of the intentions and actions of those in power.
The Leipzig Council was not concerned with rationalising midwifery services
and standards but ensuring instead that the existing midwifery structure continued to function within a community that was rapidly growing in size and
changing its socio-economic make-up.[2] As this chapter will demonstrate, midwives continued to build their clientele through the medium of trust during
the eighteenth century, and this practice was supported and encouraged by
the Council.

    This chapter will first examine the social and geographical patterns of
midwives' client networks before exploring the notion of trust between a midwife and her clients. Finally, it will analyse the written and unwritten codes of
behaviour that underpinned client-building practices over the course of the
eighteenth century. It will become apparent that the way midwives demarcated individual practice and individual clients suggests that client-building
methods were shaped by the concept of trust, which then informed the notion
of entitlement to a livelihood, as discussed in Chapter Four. The right to a
livelihood was, in turn, both an element of entitlement *and* a judgement of
proficiency.[3]

The social and geographical patterns of client networks

The casebooks that have been so useful for tracing the social and geographical
spread of midwives' client networks in early modern Holland and North
America are not available for early modern Leipzig (or indeed any urban
centre in the Germanies prior to the nineteenth century).[4] Nevertheless, two

---

2   As has been argued by Lindemann, *Health*, 139 and 143. See also Loetz, *Vom Kranken
    zum Patienten*, 146.
3   See also Lindemann, *Health*, 203; Blickle, 'Nahrung und Eigentum', 84.
4   These detailed studies reveal how the geographical spread of clients could be influenced
    by factors such as age and urban or rural settings. The Frisian midwife Catharina
    Schrader, for example, served a much more limited geographical area after moving to
    the town of Dokkum and restricted her practice substantially in later years. See M.J. van
    Lieburg, 'Catharina Schrader', 9–13. The rural Maine midwife Martha Ballard served a
    very wide area and was often away from home for days at a stretch. See Thatcher-Ulrich,
    Midwife's Tale. English Quaker midwives' employment opportunities, in contrast, were
    dictated by religious networks rather than geographical boundaries. This meant that
    Quaker midwives travelled widely. See Hess, 'Community Case Studies', 34.

administrative sources – the reports submitted by the Amtsphysicus/'certain medicus' Benjamin Benedict Petermann (1715–20) and an investigation into the use of Wickelweiber (swaddling women) in 1756 – provide an insight into the breadth and geographical scope of sworn midwives' client networks in Leipzig.

The reports produced by Petermann were first and foremost an inventory of cases in which Petermann had intervened in a birth, frequently operatively. They also functioned as a general report about the comportment of the city's sworn midwives and Beifrauen.[5] Each spring and autumn Petermann presented the Council with a list of 'difficult births' he had attended, including details of the mother's husband (name, profession and address) and of the main midwife in attendance. Petermann named only one midwife per birth, suggesting that he left out details of any other midwives who might have been called upon to provide second or third opinions. Although Petermann was technically 'in charge' of midwifery, his degree of involvement in day-to-day obstetrics was quite limited (as Chapter Six will show). In the early eighteenth century midwifery was still firmly in the grasp of women: sworn midwives attended the full social spectrum of expectant mothers, from the 'gefallenes Mensch' (fallen person) to the wives of councillors and other members of the urban elite. In turn, the consequences of a 'difficult birth' in early eighteenth-century Leipzig – that is, treatment by the Stadtphysicus/Stadtaccoucheur – was likewise socially indiscriminate.

But how reliable are these reports? Is it possible that the dominance of certain midwives in Petermann's register derives from a particular incompetence on the part of these women? I suggest not. More plausible is the argument that those midwives who feature repeatedly were simply popular (and thus attended a higher number of women) and enjoyed a reputation for dealing with difficult births. For example, one of most frequently mentioned midwives in Petermann's list, Christina Hempel, was noted in 1725 as having 'the best knowledge and experience of how to treat women in labour' on her appointment as midwife in the city.[6] As such, Petermann's reports provide a reasonably accurate sample of the types of clients a well-established Leipzig midwife might have.

According to the births attended by the four most prolific midwives (Johanna Sabina Netzold, Christina Lorend, Christina Hentschell and Christina Rosina Hempel), sworn midwives did not work exclusively within their allocated districts. The tendency to operate in other neighbourhoods was far greater amongst midwives positioned in one of the extramural districts (Rann-

5   Petermann produced the reports at the behest of the Council immediately following his appointment as 'certain medicus' in 1715, in which he assumed direct responsibility over midwifery in the city. The reports are complete with the exception of 1719. Tit. (F) XLIV.D.3, 1–33, 'Petermanns erstattete Berichte', 23 January 1715–19 October 1723.

6   According to Stadtphysicus Dr Michael Ettmüller's examination attest. See Tit. (F) XLIV.D.1, 83–118, 'Appointments (Greger and Veiß)', 22 November 1724–4 September 1725, 117.

städter Tor, Grimmaisches Tor, Peterstor or the Hallisches Tor) than it was for midwives stationed within the city walls. This is hardly surprising given that the Vorstadt neighbourhoods were generally less affluent and, crucially, formed a holding pen for the penniless masses of seasonal workers, servants, immigrants, vagrants, wandering journeymen, and indigent women who came to Leipzig to deliver their illegitimate children.[7] Christina Hempel, for instance, held the sworn midwife office at the Rannstädter Tor from 1719 to 1725, yet attended only half (5/10 no.) of 'difficult births' in her allocated district during that time.[8] Of the remaining cases, one took place in another Vorstadt district, three in the city itself and one in one of the villages surrounding Leipzig. In contrast, one of the sworn midwives stationed in the city, Johanna Sabina Netzold, performed two-thirds (8/12 no.) of deliveries within the city walls. Despite being a native of the Peterstor, the Stadt midwife Dorothea Seidel appears to have also largely kept her practice intramural. The fact that two of her 'difficult births' were the wives of two brothers from one of Leipzig's illustrious merchant-families suggests that Seidel had earned herself a reputation as a particularly skilled midwife, so much so that she had less of a need to seek clients in her home neighbourhood in the Vorstadt.[9] There are also a few examples of sworn midwives attending women outside of Leipzig, in particular serving women of the landed aristocracy on their estates for several weeks at a time.[10]

Economic pressure was not the only reason midwives operated outside of their allocated districts. A more rigorous geographical analysis of these four individuals reveals that sworn midwives maintained strong ties, firstly, to neighbourhoods where they had worked previously and, secondly, to neighbourhoods in which they had formerly resided.[11] Christina Lorend provides the most comprehensive example of this socio-geographical pattern of work. Between 1709 and 1713 Lorend assisted her mother, the sworn midwife Christina Hentschell, at the Peterstor, where both also lived. In 1716, she was appointed sworn midwife and allocated to the Rannstädter Tor / Hallisches Tor. Until she was 'promoted' to sworn midwife in the city in 1719, Lorend was recorded as being present at a mere 37 per cent (3/8 no.) of 'difficult births' in the neighbourhoods within her district. Whenever she operated away from the Rannstädter Tor, Lorend demonstrated a preference for attending mothers at the Peterstor (3 out of 5 non-district births), followed by women within the city walls (2 out of 5 non-district births). Lorend's association with the

---

7   Bräuer, *Der Leipziger Rat*, 77–80.

8   The midwife at the Rannstädter Tor also served the community at the Hallisches Tor.

9   These were the wives of Paul and Hartmann Winckler, whose family was also part of the political elite and the Leipzig Council.

10   Beifrau Herrmann attended the local lord in Brandis, a town some 18 km east of Leipzig, for several weeks in 1769. See II. Sekt. M (F) Nr. 670, Bd. III, 96–98, 'Beifrauen vs midwife Westphal', 29–30 March 1769. The midwife Maria M. Müller worked in the village of Petersberg (10 km north of Halle) for one year in 1740, see Tit. (F) XLIV.D.1, 173–89, 'Müller (leave) and Beifrau appointment (Lorend)', 17 May 1740–20 January 1741.

11   Sometimes the one and the same neighbourhood.

community at the Peterstor was strongly familial. She was the daughter of a Leipziger burgher and a sworn midwife with property in the Klitschergässgen (Peterstor) and she had grown up in the neighbourhood. Moreover, the close working relationship Lorend maintained with her mother had endured despite her allocation to another district, providing Lorend with plenty of opportunities to step in for her mother during her illness and even share her clients.[12] Once appointed as a city midwife, Lorend's popularity appears to have permitted her to restrict her practice largely to within the city walls (9 out of 12 'difficult births' took place within the city). The fact that she attended the archdeacon of St Thomas' wife – a Carpzov no less – suggests that Lorend's practice was quite successful.[13] A similar pattern of district preference is demonstrated by the midwife Hempel, who, following appointment as a sworn midwife to the Rannstädter Tor in 1719, continued to practice for a year thereafter in the Hallisches Viertel (intramural) where she had lived and worked as an informal apprentice since at least 1713.

The investigation into the use of Wickelweiber in 1756 provides a rare insight into the number and geographical spread of the 'normal' clients of one of the Vorstadt midwives, Johanna Rosina Krämpff. Faced with the prospect of a month's suspension after repeatedly using a Wickelweib, Krämpff scrawled a list of the sixteen women that she had 'at the time' and submitted this to the Council in the hope of reducing her penalty to a fine.[14] In 1756 Krämpff lived on the Rannstädter Steinweg and had been recently appointed sworn midwife at the Rannstädter Tor. Prior to this she probably occupied a sworn Beifrau office at the Rannstädter Tor.[15] The bulk of Krämpff's practice was concentrated around the neighbourhoods of the Rannstädter Tor and the Hallisches Tor, which for the purposes of midwifery belonged to the same district (see Figure 10). Krämpff clearly favoured the Hallisches Tor, with families in the Gerbergasse and the Hallisches Pförtgen making up five of Krämpff's seven clients in her allocated district. Nevertheless, half of Krämpff's clients lived outside her allocated district. Krämpff had two further women in the Gerbergasse (Grimmaisches Tor), as well as the wife of an organ maker in the city and an additional three women in villages to the north of Leipzig.[16]

---

12 Lorend had replaced her mother during a long illness. Tit. (F) XLIV.D.1, 16–43, 'Appointment (Ehrlich)', 10 January–24 July 1713, 25.
13 The Carpzov family (largely lawyers, doctors, clerics and councillors) was one of the most powerful urban dynasties in early modern Leipzig.
14 II. Sekt., M (F) Nr. 670, Bd. II, 1–41, 'LC investigation swaddling women', 30 January–16 March 1756, 37.
15 I have no precise record of where she was stationed, however, the only vacant posts at that time were the Beifrau office at the Rannstädter Tor and one Beifrau office in the city.
16 II. Sekt., M (F) Nr. 670, Bd. II, 1–41, 'LC investigation swaddling women', 30 January–16 March 1756, 19–20, 25, 37.

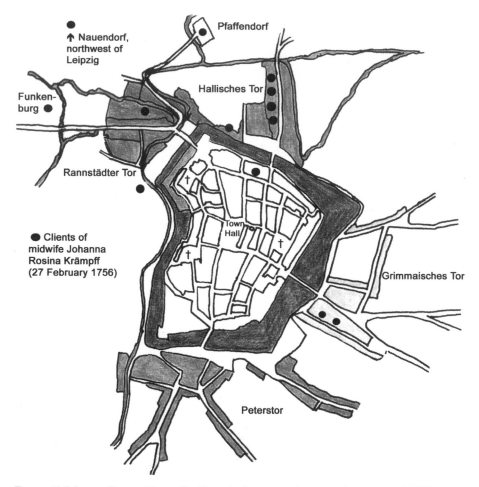

Figure 10 Johanna Rosina Krämpff's clients in Leipzig and surrounding region, 27 February 1756

Source: StadtAL, II. Sekt. M (F) Nr. 670, vol. II, 'Hebammen. Verschiedenes', 37.

Krämpff's client patterns reinforce the trend in client networks noted in Dr Petermann's reports that midwives operated both within and without the boundaries of their allocated district. This suggests that up until the middle of the eighteenth century at least, a sworn midwife's allotted district played a subordinate role in determining clientele *in the Vorstadt*. For as we have seen, midwives practised discrete patterns of client-building depending on whether they were stationed in the city or in the extramural suburbs. Social embeddedness, whether through prior work or through family networks or residency, was just as important in securing and maintaining a clientele in the Vorstadt as the rights afforded by an office to a particular geographical space. Within the city walls, conversely, where almost no midwife could claim a birthright or afford to live without the free accommodation from the Leipzig Council, the ties of family and neighbourhood in the midwives' client networks were less visible. Nevertheless, once a family had used a midwife, she appears to have remained the midwife of choice for members of the household. When, for example, the widower Johann Weber feared that one of his servants had given birth in secret in 1751, he did not fetch the midwife appointed to his neighbourhood at the Grimmaisches Tor, but instead sought out the midwife stationed in the city who had attended his deceased wife during her confinements.[17] For families, the bond forged with a midwife through repeated experience was of greater value than the particulars of office.

Thus for an urban midwife, whether sworn or unsworn, the cultivation of a long-standing clientele of families was both necessary and desirable; clients, not the Leipzig Council, contributed most of a midwife's income. An office conferred an entitlement to derive a living from midwifery, yet this living depended very much on the strength of a midwife's clientele. However, it was not only economic rationale that encouraged midwives to build up a clientele that crossed the geographical boundaries of office. The axis upon which the relationship between a midwife and a mother or her family turned was trust. In the words of Stadtaccoucheur Gehler, 'the laud and trust of many persons' earned by one of the city's Beifrauen was the marker of particular expertise.[18] Undermining the trust between a midwife and her clients was one of the surest means of ruining a midwife's practice. The newly introduced Beifrauen felt the full force of such an attack on their reputation in 1715, shortly after the creation of the office of Beifrau. The sworn midwives, they complained bitterly, spread evil rumours about them 'by which not only all the trust in us amongst [the women] extinguishes, but also that we are stripped of our honourable name through this disgrace'.[19] Trust secured both an independent economic existence as well as honour and status within the community.[20] In short, trust – not just medical or occupational standards ordained and upheld by communal government – secured a livelihood.

Midwifery: a matter of trust

So what exactly was this thing midwives, mothers and the urban authority called 'trust' ('Vertrauen'), and why was it so central to midwifery practice in the early modern period? For Labouvie, the trust vested by women in a particular midwife was largely social or functional. Women trusted a midwife because she was known in the community; mistrust, on the other hand, grew

---

17   StadtAL, Straf. Nr. 718, 'Erdmuth Augusta Schab', 1751, 3r.
18   Tit. (F) XLIV.D.6b, Bd. I, 193–98, 'Appointment (Leib and Küchler)', 19 February–4 March 1776, 193–94.
19   Tit. (F) XLIV.D.1, 48–53, 'Midwives vs Beifrauen', 24 April–6 May 1715, 50–53.
20   See also Blickle, 'Nahrung und Eigentum', 84.

out of inappropriate behaviour or negligence in the birthing chamber.[21] In her study of surgeons in early modern Italy, Sandra Cavallo identified a complex mechanism that created professional trust, the main part of which was geographical embeddedness within the community. 'Professional credibility', Cavallo argues, 'had more to do with the place, the shop and its history, than with the family tradition and the persons involved.'[22] The 'transfer of trust' was also achieved by surgeons holding minor non-medical offices.[23] Yet, whilst these approaches describe to some extent the relationship between trust and occupational identity and activity, they do not tell us what 'trust' actually was and why it was so important in the client–practitioner relationship. As I argue here, in the late seventeenth and eighteenth centuries 'trust' was not just something produced by social relations or the credentials of office. As this next section will explore, in the early modern period 'trust' was something corporeal, something tangible.[24]

According to the eighteenth-century encyclopaedist Johann Heinrich Zedler, 'trust' was 'a higher level of hope' that developed when, under the assurance of another person, someone hoped or expected something good.[25] Moreover, trust was an essential element of successful medical treatment:

> An example of well-founded trust is … when patients have great trust and confidence in their doctor, that is [a trust] which greatly expedites the cure, because one sees on a daily basis that through composed delirium and good trust in the doctor, in particular when he [the doctor] is happy, the sick people in turn regain their prior health.[26]

Trust, therefore, had a physical effect on the health of a patient, but not just because it encouraged good spirits in the sick person. Trust could be in itself curative. Early modern theories of health and illness were based upon the idea that 'imagination and impression have a strong effect in the body and its condition'.[27] Such an 'imagination' could 'bring forth such a trust to a doctor and his medicines … and have such an effect in the body of the patient that [this trust] achieves more than the best remedy'.[28] Trust, therefore, was *the* essential component in the early modern medical encounter because it func-

---

21 Labouvie, *Beistand*, 48–49. Gleixner argues that trust was characteristic of the normal relationship between a midwife and a mother. However, this trust was absent when the midwife assumed a medico-legal role. See Gleixner, 'Hebammen als Amtsfrauen', 96.
22 Cavallo, *Artisans of the Body*, 232–33.
23 Ibid., 237–38.
24 Labouvie indeed mentions the physical consequences mistrust could have on a pregnancy but does not conceptualise trust in corporeal terms. See Labouvie, *Beistand*, 48–49.
25 See entry for 'Vertrauen' in Zedler, *Zedler's Universal-Lexicon (online)*, vol. 21, 23.
26 Ibid.
27 According to Johann Heinrich Zedler. See ibid., 24. The impressionistic notion of health and illness and the idea of the body as bound up in and affected by the cosmos has been the subject of a large body of research. See, for example, Barbara Duden, *Geschichte unter der Haut. Ein Eisenacher Arzt und seine Patientinnen um 1730* (Stuttgart: Klett-Cotta, 1987), esp. 24–30; Ulinka Rublack, 'Erzählungen vom Geblüt und vom Herzen. Zu einer historischen Anthropologie des frühneuzeitlichen Körpers', *Historische Anthropologie* 9 (2001): 214–32, 214–17.
28 Zedler, *Zedler's Universal-Lexicon (online)*, vol. 21, 23.

tioned as a sort of switch in the body which enabled the doctor's treatment to work. A lack of trust, Zedler asserted, would 'disturb the disposition and cause certain disorders in the body itself' whereby 'the efficacy of the remedy is inhibited greatly'.[29]

Just as trust could cure, a lack of trust could have dire corporeal consequences and upset the patient's humoural balance. Mistrust, according to Zedler, was 'a variety of fear [that] one will not have help from the other [person]'.[30] Thus, for early moderns 'trust' was not some ethereal, emotive or social concept. It was a powerful, curative and tangible force that could physically affect the body. Trust was not merely something that existed; it was something to be deployed in the same manner as pills and advice.[31] The midwife Louise Bourgeois, for example, appears to have understood 'trust' between a midwife and a client as the relationship that arose when a mother conferred control over the medical encounter, that is, the process of interpreting and treating maladies, to the midwife.[32] According to Bourgeois, it could be deadly if a woman refused to heed her advice and Bourgeois had no qualms about allowing her clients to seek assistance elsewhere.[33] Trust was, therefore, an essential part of the medical armoury deployed by medical practitioners. The paramount importance accorded to the presence of trust between a midwife and her client was, therefore, a visceral one. Trust, as a physical and medicinal force, had to be present if childbirth was to be successful.

This tangible understanding of trust meant that trustworthiness was something one could see on the body of the healer. Far from being merely a trait of personality knowable through a person's actions, trustworthiness was embodied in the person of the healer. In midwives, trustworthiness resided in the hands and general appearance as well as in a woman's comportment. Midwifery was referred to as a 'craft', the German word for which was quite literally 'hand work' ('Handwerk') or simply 'work' ('Arbeit'). In the early modern period both these terms evoked the use of the hands.[34] Women spoke of their midwife as serving them with a 'faithful hand'.[35] Prospective candidates spoke of their experience in terms of how many women they had had 'under their hands'.[36] Physicians examining midwives spoke about the 'Handgriffe' (man-

29 Ibid., 24.
30 Ibid., 268.
31 On the central role that the dispensing of medical advice (rather than actual remedies) played in the occupational understanding of early modern physicians, see Harold J. Cook, 'Good Advice and Little Medicine. The Professional Authority of Early Modern English Physicians', *Journal of British Studies* 33 (1994): 1–31, 13–14.
32 Perkins, *Midwifery and Medicine in Early Modern France*, 97–98.
33 Bourgeois' nonchalance may, however, have been due to her particularly high-level status as a royal midwife to Marie de Medici. See ibid., 91–92.
34 Tit. (F) XLIV.D.1, 173–89, 'Müller (leave) and Beifrau appointment (Lorend)', 17 May 1740–20 January 1741, 188–89.
35 II. Sekt., M (F) Nr. 670, Bd. III, 50–87, 'Dismissal (Werner)', 19 April 1763–1 March 1764, 69.
36 Ristu, Akten Teil 1, Nr. 185, Bd. I, 408–41, 'Ansuchungs-Schreiben (Zschachin)', 1775, 410r.

ual manoeuvres) that a midwife needed to master in difficult births and also described a midwife's self-professed experience in terms of how many women she had had 'under her hands'.[37] By the 1740s the connection between a woman's hands and her skill became more explicit when the Stadtaccoucheur began to employ the physical condition of candidates' hands as a criterion for office. Stadtaccoucheur Johann Valentin Hartrauff noted that all of his short-listed candidates had 'good hands' and in 1760 Stadtaccoucheur Breuer preferred two candidates because both had 'more skilled hands and longer fingers' than the other women who had petitioned for office.[38] A good midwife now had concrete physical characteristics: supple, smooth hands and long fingers, not hands that had been 'disfigured and hardened too much through rough work'.[39]

The fact that both midwives and the Stadtaccoucheurs shared a common understanding of trust as something physical means that we need to rethink the notion that tactile knowledge and visual knowledge were two discrete and oppositional epistemological things. In her study of male midwifery in early modern France, Lianne McTavish argues that historians such as Lynne Tatlock, who claim male obstetric practitioners objectified and institutionalised knowledge about the female body via the male gaze and their use of instruments, overestimate the power of the 'gaze' in the seventeenth-century lying-in chamber.[40] McTavish claims instead that 'childbirth was part of the visual culture of early modern France, a period when authority was largely determined by the precarious act of putting oneself on display'.[41] The moral dilemmas that surrounded the surgeon man-midwife's (*chirurgien accoucheur*) place in the birthing chamber in France meant that male practitioners who claimed authority in the area of practical obstetrics during this period had to emphasise their competence, appropriateness and trustworthiness. One of the major signs they deployed was that of the hands, a motif that was also established in the midwifery manuals produced by the two most famous female midwives

---

37   Tit. (F) XLIV.D.5, 1–12, 'Kindermütter Attestata', 1727–28, 2r–3r.

38   Tit. (F) XLIV.D.1, 173–89, 'Müller (leave) and Beifrau appointment (Lorend)', 17 May 1740–20 January 1741, 188; Tit. (F) XLIV.D.6b, Bd. I, 56–66, 'Appointment (Held and Plau)', 26 April–16 May 1760, 63v.

39   StadtAL, Tit. (F) XLIV.D.6b, Bd. II, 'Acta, die Einrichtung der Kindermütter und Beÿweiber de anno 1782', 79–84, 'Beifrau appointment (Maria Mehmel and Dorothea Ulrich)', 27 April–7 July 1789, 82.

40   Lianne McTavish, *Childbirth and the Display of Authority in Early Modern France* (Aldershot: Ashgate, 2005), 219; Tatlock, 'Speculum Feminarum', 759. In a similar vein to Tatlock: Waltraud Pulz, 'Zur Erforschung geburtshilflichen Überlieferungswissens von Frauen in der frühen Neuzeit', in Christine Loytved, ed., *Von der Wehemutter zur Hebamme. Die Gründung von Hebammenschulen mit Blick auf ihren politischen Stellenwert und ihren praktischen Nutzen* (Osnabrück: Universitäts-Verlag Rasch, 2001), 16–17.

41   McTavish, *Childbirth*, 219. This visual early modern culture was common to all aspects of identity. In her study of old age in women Lynn Botelho has, for example, also found that 'age was assigned, like status, on the basis of visual clues and physical signifiers'. See Botelho, 'Old Age and Menopause', 60–61.

Louise Bourgeois and Justine Siegemund.[42] Amidst criticism of the use of instruments, widespread in the discourses of both male and female practitioners, depictions and descriptions of the hand demonstrated trust.[43] The inability to see into the womb meant that surgeon men-midwives readily took up the motif of the hands in both the textual and visual parts of their treatises. By emphasising tactile knowledge they thus 'affirmed that touching the female body was more meaningful than looking at it'.[44] Traditionally associated with denigrated manual labour, surgeon men-midwives re-signified the motif of the hands by elevating obstetrics as the trickiest and most skilled aspect of medicine and surgery because it was dependent on touch only.[45]

In the selection of midwives, overall physical appearance provided an equally important means of seeing whether a woman would make a good midwife or not. Midwife to the Queen of France, Louise Bourgeois for example, was chosen by the Queen in a wordless, momentary encounter. As McTavish argues, 'the midwife's body was the medium of communication verifying her skill' and outward appearance was of no lesser importance in eighteenth-century Leipzig.[46] Of Anna Magdalena Kirchlöffel, the Council scribe noted favourably that one 'senses … a certain cleanliness on her self as well as in her lodgings'.[47] Johanna Sabina Netzold, he noted further, had a drawn face and a fat body stemming not from illness, but instead from healthy and natural circumstances.[48] In the latter eighteenth century, the Stadtaccoucheurs began to mention traits of character in their recommendations. However, traits of character were not an aspect of the mental condition, but belonged instead to the physical constitution of a person. What we today separate into two distinct categories of 'mental' and 'physical' was a single, fused concept.[49] Stadtaccoucheur Johann Karl Gehler examined candidates on two criteria. Firstly, 'physical qualities required in the execution of this office' and secondly, 'prior comportment'.[50] Gehler's 'physical qualities' included the appearance of the face, the body and a woman's character. In contrast to 'comportment', which relied on the written testimony of mothers, these 'physical

---

42   McTavish, *Childbirth*, 179–80.
43   The forceps were the object of much criticism in eighteenth-century England. See Wilson, *Making*, 79–90. McTavish argues that the 'desire to re-signify the hands of the obstetrical surgeon, and to downplay his use of dangerous instruments' was the only common visual display strategy deployed in the portraiture of seventeenth-century male Accoucheurs. See ibid., 115.
44   McTavish, *Childbirth*, 217.
45   Ibid., 137 and 186.
46   Ibid., 82. See also McTavish's analysis of the link between appearance and competence in male obstetric treatises in ibid., 119–37.
47   Tit. (F) XLIV.D.1, 16–43, 'Appointment (Ehrlich)', 10 January–24 July 1713, 22–25.
48   Ibid.
49   Thus 'socially delivered shocks' might directly and physically cause a miscarriage. See Ulinka Rublack, 'Pregnancy, Childbirth and the Female Body in Early Modern Germany', *Past and Present* 150 (1996): 84–110, 86.
50   II. Sekt., M (F) Nr. 670, Bd. III, 50–87, 'Dismissal (Werner)', 19 April 1763–1 March 1764, 59.

qualities' could only be gauged through a face-to-face examination. Gehler's knowledge of a woman's constitution was visual and he described the genesis of his knowledge about the character of prospective midwives in visual terms.[51] Susanna Maria Hornung, for example, 'seems relaxed and content' and her fellow candidate 'seems sober, modest and polite'. Maria Stor 'appears quiet and relaxed'.[52]

As a physical property, trust was highly visual and could therefore only be forged and evaluated through visual means, for example, through face-to-face contact or portraiture.[53] Likewise, because trust was curative, it was of great consequence for the success of the treatment or medicine that the healer called upon was trusted. Midwives, early modern people understood, were not interchangeable. It was thus essential for midwives (and other healers and medical practitioners) to operate within a particular locale in which the midwife could put her body 'on display' to be 'read' by potential clients.

Once this trust had been won, women were loath to engage the services of another midwife, and went to great lengths to secure their midwife of choice. The pattern cutter and burgher Christian Knaubs, for example, even requested the Council override sworn midwife Christina Lorend's refusal to permit her Beifrau from attending his wife. Mrs Knaub, he appealed, had 'set her trust in the sworn Beifrau Mrs Müller, who attended her faithfully the previous time, so that she would like her to assist her now'.[54] The petition was turned down and the Council instructed Mr Knaub to seek the services of a sworn midwife, not because Beifrau Müller was incapable of delivering a child, but rather because of the need to ensure the midwife's livelihood and her authority over her Beifrau; the Council's concern for maintaining moral-economic propriety overrode, in this instance, the needs of the family. What this incident demonstrates, however, is that midwives were not readily interchangeable for contemporaries. What 'qualified' a midwife in the eyes of mothers and their families was not her office, the type of knowledge and breadth of skill she possessed or her social reputation *per se*. Rather it was the presence of 'trust' between a midwife and her client. Trust was both visual and social, requiring the gaze as well as constant re-articulation. Midwives had to

51 This is consistent with Duden's argument that early modern people also described their illnesses in sensual, including visual, terms so that experiences of illness were 'bound up with the embodied mode of experience of daily gestures, actions, and orientations'. See Barbara Duden, 'Medicine and the History of the Body: The Lady of the Court', in Jens Lachmund and Gunnar Stollberg, eds, *The Social Construction of Illness: Illness and Medical Knowledge in Past and Present* (Stuttgart: F. Steiner, 1992), 49.

52 II. Sekt., M (F) Nr. 670, Bd. III, 50–87, 'Dismissal (Werner)', 19 April 1763–1 March 1764, 59–60.

53 Visual 'texts' were just as important as written texts in this period. On the role of portraiture and early modern medical identity, see Chapter Four of McTavish, *Childbirth,* 113–42.

54 StadtAL, II. Sektion W (F) Nr. 332, 'Acta, Die inn: und vor der Stadt wohnende Wehmütter; und Beÿweiber, auch deren Amt und Verrichtung betr. (1717–37)', 85, 'Petition from Christian Knaubs to Leipzig Council re: Beifrau Maria Magdalena Müller', 11 January 1730, 85.

therefore be both geographically and socially omnipresent figures in the neighbourhoods that held them in trust. The allocation of midwives to a particular neighbourhood by the Leipzig Council in the late seventeenth and eighteenth centuries echoed this very tangible necessity in midwifery practice.

Of course, as we have just seen, this requirement for trust could at times conflict with the moral economy of midwifery. The mobility generated by the practice of allocating midwives to a particular neighbourhood and shifting them around as and when needed in a city as large as Leipzig had a questionable side effect; it was counter-productive to a culture of clientele cultivation based on the medium of trust. Both the Council and the Stadtaccoucheur realised this problem and sometimes overturned decisions to reallocate a midwife or Beifrau where the move threatened to curtail a practitioner's ability to retain her carefully tended clientele. In 1770, for instance, the death of one of the Beifrauen necessitated a rigorous shake-up of the current order. Unhappy about her impending reallocation, the midwife at the Peterstor, Maria Dorothea Westphal, petitioned the Council to move instead to the Grimmaisches Tor because, she explained: 'I have gained much trust and clientele in the city and in particular in front of the Grimmaisches Tor'.[55] Old age and the difficulty of passing through the Rannstädter Tor at night, she continued, meant that 'if I move to the Rannstädter Tor it will become very difficult for me to tend these [clients] as obligation and duty requires'.[56] Westphal suggested instead that midwife Hein take on the office at the Rannstädter Tor 'as her trust and clientele is mostly in the Gerbergasse'.[57] The Council agreed some days later.[58] Neither the Stadtaccoucheur nor the Council was entirely convinced that a midwife could (or should) function without the 'trust' of her clientele and sometimes sought to compromise so that this culture of trust could be upheld.

Mistrust: midwives, illegitimacy and infanticide

Midwives operated outside this relationship of trust only when they performed medico-legal examinations on women convicted of crimes. In these kinds of situations, fear of the midwife was morally and socially sanctioned. Laura Gowing argues that childbirth was a public ritual in seventeenth-century England which served to embed women in their families and communities. Hence, conflicts in the birthing chamber revolved around women censoring each other's morality and behaviour according to prevailing gender norms.[59] Whilst the female collective in the birthing chamber afforded seclusion and protec-

---

55 Tit. (F) XLIV.D.6b, Bd. I, 120–48, 'Appointment (Schultz)', 12 March–28 April 1770, 143r–v.
56 Ibid.
57 Ibid., 143–45.
58 Ibid.
59 Gowing, *Common Bodies*, 150.

tion for honourable wives, it brought regulation and punishment for unwed and poor women.[60] The midwife, in particular the sworn midwife, was part of this female collective and, hence, part of this mechanism of social censure. She, more than any other woman, embodied this split identity of 'good' and 'bad'.[61]

Gowing's argument certainly holds for the behaviour displayed by many Leipzig midwives in physical examinations of women accused of infanticide or illicit sexual activity. Concealment of bearing a child was subject to particularly harsh censure by the entire community (both male and female) and the midwife often played a leading role in these situations.[62] When sworn midwife Regina Meder was instructed in 1730 to examine a domestic servant who 'kept sitting on the pisspot', her conduct was far from sympathetic.[63] Arriving at the house, Meder was greeted by two servants, the cook and the master's fisherman, who showed her the way to the suspect. Sighting fresh blood on the chair, midwife Meder asked the girl what was wrong, to which the latter replied that she 'had done much purging during the previous night'.[64] The midwife, who 'saw the bloody matter flowing so strongly from under the maid', grabbed the girl to examine her vagina and, seeing that the maid had 'a complete opening just as would a woman who had borne a child', began her interrogation.[65] It is clear from this incident that the sworn midwife operated within a moral code shared with the rest of the community (including the communal authority). She provided an interface between community morality and the female criminal because of her ability to touch and interpret areas of the female body that were otherwise kept out of sight. This status permitted the midwife to be rough of hand and deploy harsh words; the very opposite behaviour expected by a 'client'.

Although Gowing's and Rublack's claims apply to the role of midwives in medico-legal situations, it does not necessarily follow that this mistrust characterised the relationship between midwives and poor, unmarried mothers more generally. Certainly most of the women brought before the courts on counts of infanticide were poor and single. However, it was the women's criminality, not their social or marital status, which enabled midwives and other women to slip into the role of surveillant and censor. In Leipzig concerns that midwives

---

60   Ibid., 176.
61   According to Ulrike Gleixner's study of rural midwives in Brandenburg, the midwife's 'bad' identity stemmed from her status as an official of the local authority (not from socio-moral pressure of the community per se). See Gleixner, 'Hebammen als Amtsfrauen', 96.
62   Rublack also advances the argument that midwives were the 'chief agents of control' in policing deviant sexuality and motherhood in seventeenth- and eighteenth-century Germany and rejects the idea that reproductive processes were the exclusive domain of a subversive female culture extinguished in the eighteenth century. See Rublack, 'Public Body', 58.
63   StadtAL, Straf. Nr. 693, 'Rosina Elisabeth Uhlrich', 1730, 2r–3r.
64   Ibid.
65   Ibid.

colluded with women to get rid of an unwanted 'fruit' were always present, despite the status sworn midwives enjoyed as moral police. Not reporting a suspicious situation immediately to the City Court officials, not binding the woman's belly as custom dictated, and neglecting to physically examine a suspect's vagina as well as her breasts and belly: these all counted as omissions that alerted the authorities to the possibility that a midwife had entered an arrangement with a woman to conceal a birth, or at the very least acted negligently.[66] Yet whilst midwives acted harshly and roughly towards women suspected of concealing a birth, their moral stance regarding unwed women who came to them for assistance during their confinement was more accommodating. The midwife Johanna Werner, for example, claimed in 1751 that she had told a pregnant young servant that 'she should bear her child in the proper manner, so one would be able to provide her with a lovely job as a wet nurse.'[67]

As discussed previously, unwed mothers were considered socially and morally problematic. At the same time midwives, Beifrauen and the Vorstadt communities were financially dependent on the income they derived from providing accommodation and care to these women during their confinements. For midwives like Werner, the unwed mother was a reality that had to be dealt with practically if the crime of infanticide were to be avoided. Some midwives also recognised the need for a relationship of trust to exist between a desperate unwed mother and a midwife. The guarantee of secrecy and anonymity for the unwed mother-to-be was given a high priority by some midwives, as a petition filed by midwife Johanna Schulz in 1782 against her landlord reveals. Schulz complained that her landlord insisted on locking the front door at night, thus preventing her from carrying out her 'urgent and mostly nocturnal duties'.[68] Moreover, Schulz argued, it was an untenable situation for a midwife that 'pregnant women, often also of status, who come to us in secret, should be expected to let themselves be seen by an unknown doorman'.[69] Schulz was a woman of her time and the sentiments she expressed about unwed motherhood would not have been ignored. The 1770s had witnessed a paradigm shift in the interpretation and punishment of deviant motherhood and infanticide from an evil act worthy of death to a crime explicable through socio-economic status, psychological condition and familial relationships.[70]

---

66 Straf. Nr. 718, 'Schab', 1751, 13r–14r; Straf. Nr. 735, 'Peinick', 1769, 35v–36v.
67 Straf. Nr. 718, 'Schab', 1751, 75v. Of course, most of the data we have comes from court cases of infanticide, etc.
68 II. Sekt. S (F) Nr. 2068, 1–20, 'Acta, Die von Johannen Sybillen Schulzin, wider Conrad Peter Melken Seidenfarbern alhier angebrachte Beschwerde, den freyen, Ein= und Ausgang in des letzten Hauß betr.', 14 January–26 March 1782, 3r.
69 Ibid.
70 Wessling argues this paradigm shift was the result of the legal and intellectual debates over the use of torture in the legal process and the pressure this debate brought to bear on material evidence. See Mary Nagle Wessling, 'Infanticide Trials and Forensic Medicine: Württemberg 1757–1793', in Michael Clark and Catherine Crawford, eds, *Legal Medicine in History* (Cambridge: Cambridge University Press, 1994), 131. See also Dana Rabin, 'Bodies of Evidence, States of Mind: Infanticide, Emotion and Sensibility in

And indeed, Schulz's sentiments had been voiced some fifty years earlier by members of the Leipzig Council during discussions on how to prevent infanticide.[71] Midwives, the Council and the community more generally took a relatively pragmatic approach to illegitimacy and the examples discussed here suggest that even unwed mothers placed their 'trust' in a midwife.

Defending a clientele, defining a client

As I argued in Chapter Four, 'encroachment' was painted in moral-economic terms: what upset both the authorities and the sworn midwives was the moral-social 'disorder' that ensued when other midwives and Beifrauen overstepped the bounds of their office and poached each other's clientele. One aspect of this moral 'disorder' was the subversion of gender roles. The 1758 instruction ordered that 'no midwife should use insult or evil libel to poach the clients of another, much less impose herself onto a pregnant woman by coaxing means'.[72] Good midwives would attract women as clients 'with the acquired skill, with goodly diligence and a sensible comportment' without the least bit of 'false trust and mistrust'.[73] Aggressive and assertive clientele-building tactics were considered an unseemly and improper activity for a midwife. Passivity, on the other hand, was highly desirable and the instruction ordered midwives to 'wait for whomever demands her help and services'.[74] These codes of practice sought to reinforce eighteenth-century gender ideals of the subservient, genteel female onto a group of women whose occupation, as we have seen, took them outside the boundaries of the household. The disorder occasioned by client-poaching and encroachment was also an affront to religious order. Spats between midwives at the baptismal font were of particular concern to the authorities, firstly, because these occurred in a sacred environment and, secondly, because baptisms were public affairs.[75] In all these situations, midwives were on display, submitting their bodies to the scrutiny of mothers, the Council and the general public. This trust was on display in her appearance,

---

Eighteenth-Century England', in Mark Jackson, ed., *Infanticide: Historical Perspectives on Child Murder and Concealment, 1550–2000* (Ashgate: Aldershot, 2002), 74. Fuhrmann, on the other hand, sees the leniency towards infanticide as resulting from fears about depopulation and the relaxation of marriage restrictions. See Fuhrmann, *Volksvermehrung*, 72–107.

71   StadtAL, Tit. (F) XLIV.D.6, 1–17, 'Acta, Die wieder die vielen Abortus und Wegsetzung auch Ermordung unehelicher Leibes=Früchte vorzukehrende Anstalten betr.', 20 February–7 May 1732, 4–11.

72   See Item 18 of Tit. (F) X Nr. 23b, Bd. XIII, 58r–69v, 'Instruktion Kinder Mutter N.N.', 14 July 1758, 65v–66r.

73   Ibid., 66r.

74   Ibid.

75   See the Leipzig council minutes from 14 July 1758 in Tit. (F) XLIV.D.6b, vol. 1, 'Stadtaccoucheur reports (Johann Gottfried Breuer)', 1757–58, 54–55.

when a midwife used her hands to deliver a baby or to pass a newborn to the pastor at the baptismal font.

Once a woman vested her trust in a particular midwife, there were certain 'rules' that governed her entitlement to that woman as a client. This right was based upon the midwife's physical presence and her hands-on treatment. In 1720, for example, Mr Elias Störe lodged a complaint with the Leipzig Council against the sworn midwife Anna Catharina Sperling. His wife, fourteen weeks pregnant, had experienced pains one night. The next morning Elias called his wife's mother, who immediately went out to fetch the midwife Sperling. Upon learning of the daughter's state, Sperling told the mother that the 'fruit' could not be saved and refused to examine or treat Mrs Störe on the grounds that she was of no use. Sperling then sent the mother out to purchase a 'powder'. After some cajoling, Sperling eventually accompanied the mother to the house but refused to go inside. On seeing her daughter's situation had worsened, the mother called for a doctor, who ordered the mother to fetch a midwife without delay. This time, however, the mother called for another sworn midwife, Christina Rosina Hempel. Later that day, midwife Sperling stopped past the Störe family's house to check on the ill woman but, seeing midwife Hempel, left saying once again that she was of no use.[76]

Although midwife Sperling was the first midwife to be consulted, and indeed provided treatment in the form of a medication, these actions 'by proxy' did not turn Elias Störe's wife into Sperling's client. Midwife Hempel, however, took on the task of assisting the woman, from whom by now 'the blood was running thickly'.[77] Midwife Sperling, who quickly left the scene once she realised another sworn midwife was in attendance, did not contest Hempel's claim to Mrs Störe. Once it had been decided that a midwife's services were required, what counted was the attendance and assistance at the delivery. Being 'under the hands' of a midwife conferred this precise relationship.

This way of defining a client remained current well into the late eighteenth century. In 1783 Mrs Gundermann, the wife of a printer's journeyman, had given birth under the assistance of the Beifrau Christiana Dorothea Behnhold. Fourteen days later, the young mother had 'fallen into a heavy illness' and the family requested Behnhold's sworn midwife-teacher, Johanna Sybilla Schulz, to examine Mrs Gundermann. Schulz's diagnosis, which was later backed up by the university surgeon Dr Eckholdt, was that Behnhold had failed to remove all of the placenta. Behnhold, who felt that both Schulz and Eckholdt 'could be very disadvantageous to her good reputation and clientele', approached the Council to request the matter be examined by the Stadtaccoucheur Johann Ehrenfried Pohl.[78] This set off a flurry of examinations and depositions and a lengthy report from Pohl, who declared the accusations of negligence against Behnhold to be fabricated. On the matter of midwife

76   Tit. (F) XLIV.D.1, 64–67, 'Störe vs midwife Sperling', 31 March–15 June 1720.
77   See Elias Störe's deposition from 31 March 1720 in ibid., 64–65.
78   Tit. (F) XLIV.D.6b, Bd. II, 11–20, 'Negligence (midwife Behnhold)', 26 June–17 September 1783, 11–14.

Schulz's behaviour, Pohl remarked that she was 'highly careless to so readily examine a woman who called her up from the street, as she [Schulz] had not even assisted her [Mrs Gundermann] during her childbirth travails'.[79] Here Pohl clearly articulates a code of practice that resonates strongly with the preceding sources. Firstly, a woman only became a midwife's client ('Kundin') when that midwife attended her in childbirth and not by any other means. Secondly, this relationship between a midwife and her client was binding. And, thirdly, no other midwife had the right to impinge upon this relationship without the permission from the 'treating' midwife.

Even in cases of physical neglect of duty ('Verwahrlosung'), midwives recognised each other's claims to particular women. In such cases, claim turned into obligation. In 1717 Maria Elisabeth Schipgen submitted a lengthy complaint to the mayor and Council of Leipzig regarding the so-called Wittenberg midwife, Rosina Willendorf. The Wittenberg midwife had handled her delivery so incompetently that Schipgen now suffered 'great damage to the uterus' and, because the midwife 'tore me down there, and [the vagina] is now completely knotted and swollen', she was now 'completely unfit for marriage'.[80] Sometime after the birth, Schipgen became uneasy as the bloody matter flowed out of her 'very shockingly and supernaturally in copious pieces ... so that [she] ... thought nothing other than that [she] ... must be on death's door'.[81] Collecting the bloody evacuations, Schipgen sought out the midwife at the Rannstädter Tor (Christina Lorend). Midwife Lorend recognised the bloody matter as pieces of a retained placenta and told Schipgen that her midwife had 'ruined her completely'.[82] Schipgen returned home, but on her way she continued to expel more bloody pieces. In her panic she collected them and called upon the Amtsphysicus Dr Petermann. Petermann applauded the diagnosis of midwife Lorend and sent the poor Schipgen to be examined by another sworn midwife, Anna Catharina Sperling. Sperling agreed with both midwife Lorend's and Dr Petermann's diagnosis and sent Schipgen to be examined further by her Beifrau Heinzell, who also confirmed this opinion.[83] Midwife Sperling then sent Schipgen back to the Wittenberg midwife so that she could 'tell her once more of my miserable condition, into which she has put me and, in addition, to request her [the Wittenberg midwife's] advice'.[84] Schipgen obeyed Sperling's instructions but the Wittenberg midwife refused to treat her, arguing that the bloody matter was a *Monatskind* (mole) and that this was a matter for the 'Doctores'.[85]

---

79 See Pohl's report in ibid., 15–16.
80 See Schipgen's initial petition to the Council from 12 May 1717 in II. Sekt. W (F) Nr. 319, 1–27, 'Beschwerden (Willendorf)', 8 May–14 August 1717, 3v.
81 Ibid., 2r–2v.
82 Ibid., 3a.
83 Ibid.
84 Ibid.
85 Ibid., 3r–3v. A *Monatskind* (mole) was 'an unformed, imperfect, thoroughly faulty foetus that aborts spontaneously in the first few months [of a pregnancy]; otherwise known as a *Mondkalb* [moon calf]'. See entry for 'Mondkalb' in *Grimms Wörterbuch*.

The exhausting trail of examinations in this narrative exemplifies the code of practice that guided the division of responsibility over a client. Although no less than three midwives and Beifrauen examined Schipgen, not one of these women attempted treatment. Their role was restricted to the matter of providing a diagnosis and apportioning blame for Schipgen's sorry state. Although Schipgen had sought their advice, examination and consultation, this did not suffice as grounds to claim the right to and the obligation towards a woman as a client. Midwife Sperling even examined Schipgen in an official capacity at the behest of the Stadtaccoucheur. We might consider midwife Sperling's order for Schipgen to go back to the midwife who 'ruined' her for treatment as bizarre, yet for all those concerned, it was the Wittenberg midwife's prerogative and her obligation to treat her own client. She could only attempt to escape this obligation by providing a counter-diagnosis absolving her from all responsibility. In this case, the purported miscarriage required operative extraction which, as midwives were prohibited from using instruments, shifted the responsibility for treatment onto surgical practitioners.[86]

Although the terms of cultivating a clientele outlined here were largely accepted, they were by no means inviolable. In fact, over the course of the eighteenth century, they were hotly contested. An ongoing dispute between the sworn midwife Regina Mend and the Beifrau Juliana Müller demonstrates that there was a tension between the idea that a woman became a client by virtue of where she lived, and the notion that a midwife could only claim a woman who actively sought out her services as a client. In 1751 Mend accused Beifrau Müller of 'interfering' with her office by poaching her clients. To Mend's great displeasure, Beifrau Müller had delivered two women, a widow and the wife of a gardener, in her neighbourhood (Peterstor) and stolen one of Mend's clients, Mrs Liebig. Mrs Liebig had sent for Mend, but Mend was indisposed. Mend's servant instead fetched Beifrau Müller, who also lived at the Peterstor. But that was not all. Even more devious, claimed Mend, was the fact that Müller had communicated to a friend of Mrs Liebig that, should Mend be unavailable when labour began, Liebig should immediately fetch Beifrau Müller.[87]

Mend's claim to these women was linked, on the one hand, to her right as a sworn midwife to be the first port of call for a woman expecting a child. On the other, it is clear that Mend was staking her claim on a geographical basis; all three women lived within the neighbourhood at the Peterstor. Mend did not appeal to a relationship of trust to bolster her claim and, in the course of Beifrau Müller's response to Mend's accusations, we learn that this relationship probably did not even exist. The gardener's wife had not wanted Mend to attend in the first place, argued Müller, pointing out that the woman's pre-

86 Chapter Six deals with the matter of how the body, disorders, illnesses and treatments were divided up between midwives and other medical practitioners.
87 See Mend's petition to the Council in StadtAL, II. Sekt. M (F) Nr. 670, Bd. II, 'Hebammen. Verschiedenes 1748–59', 6–11, 'Midwife Regina Mend complains about Beifrau Juliana Müller', 20 January 1751.

vious delivery had been attended by the Gassenmagd in the Sandgasse (Peters-tor). Mend eventually conceded that her claim to the gardener's wife was based on the fact that the woman's sisters (who both lived at the Peterstor) had promised that Mend could attend the birth.[88] As for Mrs Liebig, Müller admitted that she was in fact a client of Mend's. However, she intimated this was disputable because another midwife had attended Liebig's last confinement.[89] Müller claimed further that she had already been to see the expectant woman twice throughout her pregnancy, thus implying that she too could justify her claim to deliver Liebig. Beifrau Müller received a reprimand from the Council, yet she had managed to undermine Mend's claims to these women. Likewise, Mend's attempt to define her clientele in terms of her office, that is to render the pool of potential clients residing within her allocated district as actual clients, failed to carry weight. Müller had revealed that Mend's claims to have the trust of these women were rather spurious. This was an example of where the moral economy of midwifery, which sought to uphold the stability and propriety of the community, could also at times be at odds with a culture of trust underpinning the general relationship between a midwife and her clients.

Conclusions

The reforms that restructured midwifery in the early eighteenth century – the introduction of the Stadtaccoucheur and sworn Beifrauen, as well as the increase in the number of sworn midwives and sworn Beifrauen – were motivated by the desire on the part of the Leipzig Council to ensure a steady supply of able midwives. They were also intended to combat the problem of 'neglect' and 'ignorance' on the part of the city's midwives that the Council felt threatened both the health and the life of Leipzig women and their children.[90] Old habits, however, die hard and, in spite of the apparently more 'bureaucratic' structure, the traditional basis of midwifery provision, that of the client–midwife relationship based upon trust, persisted through to the end of the century at least. Women and their families continued to engage a midwife because she was known and trusted within that particular neighbourhood. Midwives continued to define their clients as women who gave them their trust, and they continued to lay claim to their accumulated clientele on the basis of entitlement to a living.

The reformers – the Council and the Stadtaccoucheurs – had no intention of upsetting this status quo. For them, just as for midwives, mothers and their families, the idea of estranging the figure of the midwife from her social and familial surrounds was undesirable – and economically untenable. It was in-

88   See Müller's deposition in ibid.
89   See Müller's deposition in ibid.
90   Tit. (F) XLIV.A.1a, 19r–21r, 'Amtsphysicus appointment (Petermann)', 22 August 1715, 19r.

conceivable for contemporaries to think of midwives as interchangeable 'service providers'. Without distinctive occupational standards, skill and suitability had to be based on social relations as well as visual markers. A midwife's livelihood rested on her ability to build up a particular clientele through the medium of trust, not wholly on her status as a sworn midwife and her allocation to a particular district. The Council was relatively lax about midwives operating outside of their designated district. It was similarly concerned about keeping alive the culture of trust in urban midwifery against all odds, which suggests that the geographical allocation of midwives was intended to support, not destroy this tradition. The Council did this for moral-economic reasons, that is, in order to sustain the livelihoods of midwives and Beifrauen. Allocation was, however, also informed by the fact that 'trust' in early modern Leipzig was a physical phenomenon. Women might only have a successful birth if they could 'trust' the midwife. Trust was not something merely engendered by a particular type of training or an office. It was gained by being present and 'on display' within a particular community. Dislocation from client networks proved to be a tricky side effect of allocation, demanding the Council constantly weigh up the disadvantages to the community versus those to the individual.

Chapter Six

Midwives, Medical Men and Clients: Demarcating the Parameters of Midwifery Practice

Whereas childbirth was a female ritual, in late seventeenth- and eighteenth-century Europe women's health and the female body were not exclusively women's business. As Helen King and Monica Green have demonstrated, men had been active in the arena of women's health/gynaecology since Antiquity.[1] Physicians began to take an interest in the problem of sterility, for example, as early as the twelfth century and this was a theme that preoccupied learned medicine well into the seventeenth century.[2] Following the discovery of the Hippocratic writings on the diseases of women in the sixteenth century, both surgeons and physicians developed a fascination for menstruation that went hand-in-hand with demands from the law, political institutions and society more generally to understand the relationship between menstruation, conception and pregnancy in order to interpret 'ambiguous bodies' and thus determine illegitimacy.[3] Well into the eighteenth and nineteenth centuries, menstruation was widely considered in (overwhelmingly male) medical circles as the single most important female bodily function and, mostly crucially, one that regulated both health and illness.[4] By the early eighteenth century at least, the involvement of male medical practitioners in matters of the female body also extended into the practical sphere: in eighteenth-century Germany, women routinely sought out the services of physicians for illnesses that we might consider relevant to the modern practice of gynaecology, for instance a missed menses.[5]

Early modern women consulted a variety of different practitioners and healers depending on their complaint: there was no discrete practitioner for women's medicine, nor was there an exclusive link between competence in childbirth and female maladies. The body, its signs and their meanings were

---

1   Helen King, *Midwifery, Obstetrics and the Rise of Gynaecology. The Uses of a Sixteenth-Century Compendium* (Aldershot: Ashgate, 2007), 40–42; Monica Green, *Making Women's Medicine Masculine: The Rise of Male Authority in Premodern Gynaecology* (Oxford, 2008), 246–87.

2   King, *Midwifery*, 59–60. Green notes a particular moment in this trajectory as a shift from mere interest to actual practice: the sudden claim made by physicians associated with the Montpellier medical school in the fourteenth century to be able to diagnose and treat infertility. See Green, *Making Women's Medicine*, 71.

3   McClive, *Menstruation*, 21 and 230. On how legal and political controversies over determining how women died in childbirth made the 'secrets of women public' in Rome, see Silvia de Renzi, 'The Risks of Childbirth. Physicians, Finance, and Women's Deaths in the Law Courts of Seventeenth-Century Rome', *Bulletin of the History of Medicine* 84: 4 (2010): 549–77.

4   Michael Stolberg, 'Deutungen und Erfahrungen der Menstruation in der Frühen Neuzeit', in Barbara Mahlmann-Bauer, ed., *Scientiae et artes. Die Vermittlung alten und neuen Wissens in Literatur, Kunst und Musik* (2 vols, Wiesbaden: Harrassowitz in Kommission, 2004), vol. 2, 213–14.

5   Duden, *Geschichte under der Haut.*

accorded different categories and physiological understandings. For example menstrual bleeding, a bodily process that we now link to reproduction, was associated more generally with overall internal health in the early modern world; menstrual blood was thought to issue from any orifice, indeed even from those in the male body.[6] Problems of 'congestion', therefore, could just as easily be the preserve of a physician or irregular healer known for treating these kinds of complaints as they might have been a midwife's. Yet it was not merely a matter of early modern people assigning different meanings to bodily functions. Cathy McClive has suggested that 'early modern bodies – male, female and ambiguous – were unstable signifiers' and, using the case of menstruation, argues that these bodies were thus wide fields of interpretation.[7] I suggest then that these epistemologically unstable bodies could not elicit stable occupational boundaries between healers because there was little that could be known about the body that did not derive ultimately from the subjective experience of the sufferer.

Historians of medicine have been sensitive to the role of subjectivity in the early modern medical encounter now for at least three decades. This subjectivity appears to correspond to descriptions of the 'medical marketplace' in England in which, as Roy Porter observed, the 'passive patient, accustomed to place implicit trust in medicine, was a rare bird in pre-modern times.'[8] Illness and health were subjective categories in the eighteenth century and in Germany, as Mary Lindemann has argued, people were 'medically promiscuous', picking and choosing between an eclectic mix of healers without regard for the anachronistic categories of 'professional' and 'folk' medicine.[9] Yet did this 'promiscuous' culture of health also apply to midwifery? I would argue that we need to conceive of childbirth as discrete from other health matters experienced by early modern women because childbirth was perhaps the only area of early modern medicine in which gender and custom so rigidly defined the type of healer a woman might use. Hence, although there were many different actors in the midwifery landscape, the 'marketplace' was heavily circumscribed by the cultural parameters of gender. In Leipzig, as elsewhere, childbirth was a collective female cultural institution and remained so for most of the eighteenth century and beyond.[10] As we shall see, the ubiquitous

---

6   Galenic plethoric and later also iatrochemical medical theories construed evacuation as a necessary component of maintaining humoural balance. See Gianna Pomata, 'Menstruating Men: Similarity and Difference of the Sexes in Early Modern Medicine', in Valeria Finucci and Kevin Brownlee, eds, *Generation and Degeneration: Tropes of Reproduction in Literature and History from Antiquity to Early Modern Europe* (Durham, NC: Duke University Press, 2001), 133–42; Michael Stolberg, 'The Monthly Malady: A History of Premenstrual Suffering', *Medical History* 44 (2000): 301–22, 304–9; McClive, 'Bleeding Flowers', 3–4.

7   McClive, *Menstruation*, 231.

8   Porter, *Health for Sale*, 31.

9   Lindemann, *Health*, 305.

10   As reflected in work on England. See Cody, *Birthing the Nation*, 31–38; Wilson, *Making*, 25–45.

practice of self-diagnosis and the reliance on the sufferer's narrative meant that the authority enjoyed by midwives, indeed any practitioner, was far from absolute.

Although childbirth took place within a female realm, male medical practitioners could and did participate under very specific circumstances. Surgeons in particular had a long history of involvement in childbirth, especially in urban settings.[11] A strict division of labour defined their activities; male surgical practitioners were generally only called upon when the midwife, who was not permitted to use instruments, conceded she could help no further. The premeditated use of surgeons was rare.[12] Of course, mothers and midwives might also turn to certain local midwives who had amassed a reputation as particularly skilled in the art of difficult deliveries, such as Justine Siegemund and Sarah Stone.[13] The arrival of a male practitioner often occurred after several days of labour, when hope of delivering a live child had faded and, by this stage, both bystanders and practitioners were primarily focused on saving the life of the mother. In such emergencies the surgeon or Accoucheur's role was generally limited to craniotomy, hook extraction or sometimes caesarean section.[14]

This chapter will explore the development of this division of labour between midwives, medical practitioners and Accoucheurs from the late seventeenth to the end of the eighteenth century from a division based on the emergency to one grounded in the distinction between 'natural' and 'unnatural' births. It will examine the nomenclature of midwifery in certain widely used midwifery manuals of the period and trace the lived boundaries of midwifery practice within the context of the birthing chamber. It will also explore which bodily signs and which situations prompted early modern people to call upon the assistance of a midwife and which did not. Unlike in England, where in some regions from around 1750 encroachment by male practitioners into the frontier of natural births led to a steep decline in female midwifery practice, midwives in many continental countries continued to hold a monopoly over childbirth or at the very least 'natural' births.[15] Using data gleaned

---

11   In her study of postpartum caesarean section, for example, Park argues that there was already a strict division of labour between midwives, surgeons and physicians in urban sixteenth-century Italy. See Park, 'Death of Isabella Della Volpe', 174–75.

12   Although Wilson notes mothers occasionally called on the services of the surgeon prior to the birth if difficulty was expected or feared. See Wilson, *Making*, 49.

13   See Siegemund's own account of how she came to her reputation as a midwife skilled in difficult births. Siegemund, *Court Midwife*, 48–52; Wilson, *Making*, 57–59.

14   Men were regularly depicted performing caesarean sections from the fifteenth century onwards in European iconography. See Renate Blumenfeld-Kosinski, *Not of Woman Born: Representations of Caesarean Birth in Medieval and Renaissance Culture* (Ithaca, NY: Cornell University Press, 1990), 73–77. On the activities of male practitioners in England, see Wilson, *Making*, 47–55. In seventeenth-century France, calling a senior practitioner during a difficult birth was enshrined in midwifery statutes. See Perkins, *Midwifery and Medicine in Early Modern France*, 102–3.

15   For instance in Sweden midwives were authorised to use instruments, which Romlid argues was symptomatic of their occupational strength well into the nineteenth century.

from the Stadtphysicus and Stadtaccoucheur reports, this chapter will also analyse the obstetric practice of these early (municipal) surgeon-obstetricians, of which we know next to nothing for the period prior to 1750 and only very little thereafter.[16]

In Leipzig the split between natural and unnatural births and the accompanying newer division of labour was already present by the beginning of the eighteenth century, as the obstetric operational activities of Gottfried Welsch and Benjamin Petermann suggest. As I argue here, the policies of providing formal training to midwives served to reinforce and encourage this division of labour between midwives and male practitioners. In so doing, they served to cement the occupational status and practice of midwives in Leipzig. This very division of labour based on 'natural' versus 'unnatural' births was only disrupted when male practitioners began to transcend unnatural births and extend their practice into pre-arranged 'normal' births (non-operative and non-manual intervention) in the middle to late nineteenth century.[17]

Defining midwifery in medical discourses

Helen King has noted that English sixteenth- and seventeenth-century medical writers, medical practitioners and midwives defined 'midwifery' as a broad field of practice encompassing 'all that women experienced, from the diseases of virgins to the processes of childbirth, including the health of young babies'.[18] Contrastingly, in German medical discourses, the definition of 'midwifery' appears to have been narrower. German midwifery manuals and obstetric texts written both by midwives and male practitioners focus demonstrably (and often exclusively) on the process of childbirth. One of the earliest popular-vernacular works on midwifery, Eucharius Rößlin's *Der Swangern Frauwen vnd hebamen Rosengarten* (1513), begins with a chapter on 'how the child moves and rests in the mother's belly'. The next five chapters focus on the birth itself before addressing postpartum complications, problems with the newborn, and the diagnosis and extraction of a dead foetus. The final

See Romlid, 'Swedish Midwives', 49–55. Educating female midwives in mid-eighteenth-century France became state policy when the King sent the midwife Mme du Coudray into the French provinces to train country women in midwifery. See Rattner Gelbart, *The King's Midwife*, 91–100.

16   On hospital-based man-midwifery from c. 1750, see Schlumbohm, *Lebendige Phantome*. On late eighteenth-century private practice, see Jürgen Schlumbohm, 'Als Mann in der Sphäre der Frauen: der schwierige Start einer geburtshilflichen Praxis im späten 18. Jahrhundert', in Michaela Fenske and Carola Lipp, eds, *Alltag als Politik, Politik im Alltag: Dimensionen des Politischen in Vergangenheit und Gegenwart: ein Lesebuch für Carola Lipp* (Berlin: LIT Verlag, 2010). On the end of the eighteenth and principally the nineteenth centuries, see Seidel, *Neue Kultur*.

17   Seidel, *Neue Kultur*, 343.

18   King, *Midwifery*, 65. Wilson also notes that some English midwives appear to have pursued healing practices that took them outside of midwifery. See Wilson, *Making*, 36–38.

three chapters deal with the care of the newborn, breastfeeding and 'of some incidents and illnesses in the newborn child/ and how one should help'.[19] A century later in 1616, Severin Pineau translated the celebrated work of the French court midwife Louise Bourgeois into German 'for all honour-loving matrons, housewives, sworn and other [mid]wives'.[20] Just like Rößlin's text, the Bourgeois translation dealt with women's health only in in relation to pregnancy and childbirth. Likewise the care of children was limited to the newborn infant and breastfeeding.[21] Gottfried Welsch's 1634 translation of *La Commare del Scipione Mercurio Kindermütter oder Hebammenbuch* similarly branched out into a vast array of postpartum problems in both mother and the newborn.[22]

In the late seventeenth century midwifery manuals increasingly focused on the procedure of birth itself, jettisoning extraneous subjects such as conception, care of the infant, breastfeeding and childbed illnesses. Johan Hoorn's midwifery manual was one of the most widely used texts in many parts of Europe, including Leipzig. Hoorn, municipal physician in Stockholm and personal physician to the King of Sweden in the late seventeenth and early eighteenth centuries, had revolutionised midwifery practice in his native Sweden by introducing formal instruction for Stockholm's midwives in 1708.[23] First published in Swedish in 1697, the manual was translated into German in 1726 and underwent some eight editions until 1784. Designed expressly for midwives, it consisted of two parts dealing with 'natural' births and 'difficult and unnatural births' as well as an appendix of some thirty cases detailing complicated labours.[24] Care of the infant or the mother before or after the birth did not feature in his manual.

Although the authors of most early modern medical-midwifery texts were male, the tendency to reduce midwifery to the techniques of delivery was not strictly a masculine phenomenon. Justine Siegemund and Anna Horenburg, who both authored midwifery manuals in 1690 and 1700 respectively, dealt exclusively with the female generative anatomy, the mechanics of childbirth, difficult births and how to 'turn' them.[25] Horenburg, for example, described which 'techniques' a midwife might employ in order to ascertain whether or not the cervix was dilated or how to discern 'the true [childbirth] pains from the wild pains'.[26] Siegemund, who enjoyed a reputation for great skill in 'diffi-

---

19   Eucharius d. Ä. Rößlin, *Der Swangern Frauwen vnd hebamen Rosengarten* (Straßburg: Martin Flach, 1513), Biii, v–r. Rößlin's text went on to have a phenomenal European career lasting more than a century. See Fissell, *Vernacular Bodies*, 14–52.
20   As noted in the long title on the frontispiece of Louise Bourgeois, *Hebammen Buch*, trans. Severin Pineau (4 vols, Frankfurt am Main: Matthaei Merian, c.1644), vol. 1.
21   Ibid.
22   Scipione, *Commare*.
23   Romlid, 'Swedish Midwives', 38–39.
24   Johan von Hoorn, *Die zwo um Ihrer Gottesfurcht und Treue willen von Gott wohl belohnte Weh=Mutter, Siphra und Pua* (Stockholm and Leipzig: Johann Heinrich Rußworm, 1726).
25   Siegemundin, *Hoff=Wehe=Mutter*; Horenburg, *Nöhtiger Unterricht*.
26   *Nöhtiger Unterricht*, 18–20.

cult' births, focused largely on abnormal presentations and procedures such as versions and the artificial puncturing of the waters.[27] Topics such as the care of infant and mother during childbed, breastfeeding or resuscitating a child are entirely absent from their narratives.

Siegemund's advice on prescribing medicines is a telling comment on the theoretical and legal boundaries of a midwife's practice:

> Do not rely too much on remedies. Practice your profession faithfully and assiduously and if you pay attention to everything that comes to pass, you will see and hear a sufficient amount about remedies, but in the end you will find that no clever midwife is so legally privileged that she would not be subject to lawsuits as others are.[28]

Siegemund was issuing a veiled warning to midwives about where the supposed and real boundaries of midwifery practice lay. The corporate structure of medicine in early modern Germany foresaw internal treatments as the preserve of the physician. We know, however, that midwives continued to use various medications and compresses during confinement and lying-in: in 1716 the Stadtaccoucheur Petermann complained that the midwives were:

> still making use of forbidden and dangerous internal curatives, in that they obtain of their own accord powerful abortive medicines from the apothecaries without the prior knowledge of a Medici, and through this, when the child lies wrongly in the mother's birth, often difficult births must develop.[29]

Attempts to outlaw 'cavalier' use of internal medications by midwives was unsuccessful, so much so that the Leipzig Council was forced to legalise the use of certain treatments by sworn midwives in a *Specification* in the early to mid-eighteenth century. Thus midwives were permitted to give women suffering from 'wild pains' at the end of a pregnancy '2 *Lot* of verbena water, by the spoon bit by bit'. For women whose bleeding after the birth was 'not proper or not at all', the midwife might order '30 to 40 drops of balm or rosemary essence'.[30] As Chapter Two showed, midwives (as well as their Beifrauen, Wickelweiber and servants) carried out all the other non-mechanical tasks: bathing and dressing babies, binding mothers, healing 'bad breasts', applying special bandages, changing clysters and vaginal pessaries, and taking infants to baptism.[31] With the exception of emergency baptism, which elicited increasing interference from both the Church and the Council during the period, these auxiliary and non-medical tasks were not contested by practitioners or others outside of the midwifery landscape.

---

27 Siegemund, *Court Midwife*, 89–121 and 60–66.
28 Ibid., 185–86.
29 Tit. (F) XLIV.D.3, 1–33, 'Petermanns erstattete Berichte', 23 January 1715–19 October 1723, 6r–6v.
30 See Items 1 and 7 of the 'Specification' appended to the midwifery instruction from 1758. Tit. (F) X Nr. 23b, Bd. XIII, 58r–69v, 'Instruktion Kinder Mutter N.N.', 14 July 1758. The Specification was introduced before 1758.
31 Compare du Coudray's instruction on antenatal and postnatal treatments. Rattner Gelbart, *The King's Midwife*, 68–69.

Within many late seventeenth-century medical-midwifery discourses, 'midwifery' was thus very narrowly defined. It encompassed the mechanics of childbirth, but not the care of the mother or the newborn infant. It involved the hands to probe the cervix and, if required, to turn a child presenting incorrectly. It did not entail the prescription of medicines or other internal treatments. Similarly, the instruction midwives received from physicians and the Stadtaccoucheur revolved largely around determining the stage of labour and the actual delivery of the child. By the early eighteenth century, medical discourses authored by both genders on midwifery had distilled a whole range of medical, religious and socio-cultural tasks carried out by midwives into a very narrow remit. Physicians and surgeons who authored the midwifery texts of the period had little interest in the non-mechanical aspects of midwifery, either as practitioners or teachers. As a result, on a discursive level midwifery became synonymous with the process of childbirth – it was this aspect of childbirth *that was at stake* in the eighteenth century. Yet to what extent did this apply to the midwifery practices of Leipzig midwives? And what of the physicians and surgeons that practised obstetric surgery? What were the actual parameters of midwifery practice where treatment and care of the female body was concerned?

Childbed maladies and childbed practitioners: the parameters of midwifery practice

One January day in 1756, one of the sworn midwives called on the Stadtaccoucheur Johann Gottfried Breuer to relate the suspicious death of a domestic servant Miss Köhler, who had been living with her brother since her release from service.[32] The point of the brief investigation that followed was to determine whether Miss Köhler had been giving birth at the time of her death. It put the activities of both the family and the midwives under the microscope and, in so doing, articulated the bounds of a midwife's work.

Fearing the child was on its way, Köhler had persuaded her sister-in-law (who did not think it was time) to fetch the Beifrau Maria Dorothea Westphal. According to her deposition, Beifrau Westphal arrived at the Köhlers' house to find Miss Köhler 'in a very bad state' and 'issuing a strong death rattle'.[33] The sister-in-law then recounted to the midwife the genesis of the woman's illness: Köhler had been bled the previous Sunday by the barber. After no blood had poured forth, the barber informed the women gravely that 'if no sweating should occur, the [woman] would die'.[34] Beifrau Westphal then examined Köhler, 'who complained very much about a pain in her side'. Unable to feel either the child in the birth canal or any cramps, the Beifrau assumed

32   StadtAL, II. Sekt. M (F) Nr. 670, Bd. II, 'Hebammen. Verschiedenes 1748–59', 39–43, 'Investigation into suspected case of abortion', 11 January 1756, 39–41.
33   Ibid., 40.
34   Ibid., 43.

that 'the child must still be sitting up high'.[35] Armed with the knowledge of the absent blood – a sure sign of humoural dysfunction and illness – Westphal confirmed the barber's diagnosis of a congestion of the blood ('Stöck=Fluß').[36] Under suspicion of aiding and abetting Köhler, Westphal was questioned repeatedly by Council investigators about signs of an imminent birth, namely whether or not she had seen the woman's waters break and whether 'the fruit as well as the cervix was ready for the entrance [of the child]'.[37] However, Westphal was adamant that the woman 'was not at all ill with child[bed], rather her illness must have had other causes and, according to her circumstances, she would have probably had many weeks to go'.[38] The next day the woman was still ill so the sister-in-law sent for the sworn midwife Regina Mend, who also found the woman 'in the death throes' with a 'cooking' breast, eyes closed, almost unable to give 'any signs of life' so that 'all senses were gone'. Mend felt for the child but was unable to 'sense any life from it' and concluded that it was dead. Having decided that Miss Köhler was not giving birth and was indeed 'lying ill from another illness', Mend claimed that 'she was of no use'. However, she stayed anyway until just before the woman died.[39]

The purpose of the Council's investigation was to determine whether an abortion or infanticide had occurred. It was crucial to establish whether or not the woman had been in childbed because this dictated the culpability or complicity of the midwives in the affair. Unsurprisingly, both Beifrau Westphal and midwife Mend were at pains to extricate themselves from the business. And yet their narratives were credible for all involved in the case. As far as the Beifrau and the midwife were concerned, the health of Miss Köhler lay beyond their responsibility – but not just because they thought death was inevitable. This case suggests that midwives did not treat illnesses such as Stockfluss, which was not a childbirth or childbed malady, even in pregnant women. In the absence of vital signs from the child, the midwives could further absolve themselves of responsibility for attending and treating Köhler. Retrieving the child was not a matter for a midwife but, as midwife Mend advised the family on her departure, 'if Miss Köhler should die, one should fetch the Rats-Barbier Breuer and have her opened up'.[40] That neither Beifrau nor midwife considered Köhler's illness or death to lie within the field of midwifery is supported even further by the fact that it was Köhler's sister-in-law who registered the death with the *Leichenschreiberei* (Council burial registry office). Had Köhler died during childbirth, law required the *midwife* to alert the authorities.[41]

35   Ibid., 40–42.
36   Ibid., 40.
37   Ibid., 40–42.
38   Ibid.
39   See Mend's statement in ibid., 42–43.
40   Ibid.
41   Ibid., 43.

Serious illness involving fevers setting in during lying-in also lay outside the midwife's field of practice. In 1733, shortly after her confinement, Johann Gottfried Seÿdler's wife fell ill. The birth had been long and difficult, but had ended happily following the intervention of medical practitioner Johann Michael Backe. When his wife fell ill, Seÿdler called for Dr Backe who diagnosed 'kalter Brand' (necrophy or gangrene) caused by the midwife 'grabbing about in the uterus with the greatest violence'.[42] Another woman, the wife of a journeyman printer, 'fell into a hard illness' following the birth of her child in 1783.[43] After the pains became unbearable, the family sought the assistance of the University surgeon Eckholdt, who attended the woman for several days without success. Eventually Eckholdt pronounced the probable cause of the woman's suffering as something that had been retained in the uterus. The family only then turned to another midwife, who confirmed that the cervix was not 'properly closed' and that 'something was still sitting in there.'[44]

In contrast, bloody secretions issuing from the area of a woman's vulva – in particular when accompanied by pains in the belly – lay firmly within a midwife's medical jurisdiction. Midwives were expected to be able to diagnose the origins of blood and to determine whether it was parturient, abortive, mole or menstrual – a key duty in the medico-legal context.[45] Pregnant women who suffered from vaginal bleeding before, during or after the birth, tended to first seek the advice of a midwife. Elias Störe's wife was in the early stages of her pregnancy when she began to experience pains one night, and later became 'unconscious once or twice and bloody matter was exiting her strongly'. Störe first fetched his mother-in-law, who immediately went to find a midwife. When this midwife refused to attend her daughter, the mother sought out the services of a sworn Beifrau.[46] Similarly, when Jacob Gumbiß's heavily pregnant wife fell ill with a 'great flow of blood and fainted', he too embarked on a desperate search for a midwife.[47] Not all cases of vaginal bleeding, however, required action on the part of the midwife. There was little that midwives thought they could do other than let nature take its course in the case of a 'premature fruit' or so-called moles (false lumps).[48]

Even when physicians and surgeons did become involved in the diagnosis and treatment of a woman afflicted with vaginal bleeding, they often still deferred to the knowledge of midwives. Maria Schipgen, from whom the 'water [urine] exits day and night' together with 'large pieces of bloody matter from the retained afterbirth', consulted two sworn midwives before she finally

---

42 II. Sekt. W (F) Nr. 332, 'Acta, Die inn: und vor der Stadt wohnende Wehmütter: und Beÿweiber, auch deren Amt und Verrichtung betr.', 165–66, 'Negligence (Midwife M. M. Müller)', 14 June 1737, 165–66.
43 Tit. (F) XLIV.D.6b, Bd. II, 11–20, 'Negligence (midwife Behnhold)', 26 June–17 September 1783, 11–12.
44 Ibid., 12–14.
45 See Chapter 5 of McClive, 'Bleeding Flowers'.
46 Tit. (F) XLIV.D.1, 64–67, 'Störe vs midwife Sperling', 31 March–15 June 1720, 64–65.
47 II. Sekt. W (F) Nr. 332, 13–16, 'Gumbiß vs Stäps', 14–19 November 1722, 13–14.
48 Tit. (F) XLIV.D.1, 64–67, 'Störe vs midwife Sperling', 31 March–15 June 1720, 64–65.

sought out the Stadtaccoucheur Benjamin Petermann.[49] The midwife Rosina Willendorf, who had 'ruined' Schipgen, was her first port of call. Willendorf diagnosed a new pregnancy or 'many Monatskinder' (month-children or moles) that were now 'evacuating from her'.[50] Dissatisfied with this explanation, Schipgen sent a bottle of the bloody matter via one of her female friends to a second midwife, Christina Lorend, for inspection and some 'good advice'. According to her deposition, Lorend interpreted the bloody matter as a new pregnancy, but conceded to the messenger that 'if it was as she [Schipgen] says that the midwife treated Schipgen thus, it could be probable that an artery in the uterus was damaged and the woman ruined for no reason'.[51] Only as the bloody matter was draining from her 'very shockingly and supernaturally in copious pieces ... so that [she] ... thought nothing other than that [she] ... must be on death's door', did Schipgen take a sample of her bloody evacuations to the physicians Dr Petermann and Dr Etmüller. Etmüller's response was cautious 'because all manner of causes may give occasion to ... [such] complaints' and because he possessed no knowledge of what had happened during the birth (which now lay six months back). Neither physician sought to examine Schipgen but instead entrusted the task of determining the cause of the woman's suffering to yet a third midwife.[52]

Thus the question of whether or not a midwife was required when a woman took 'ill' hinged on the presence or absence of vaginal bleeding, but it was also contingent on how bleeding was interpreted. As Cathy McClive has argued for early modern France, 'uncertainty' was not just a socially constructed guise employed by unmarried women, but a medical and physical reality experienced by early modern women in general and recorded by their medical practitioners.[53] Whereas women who thought themselves to be with child might immediately seek out a midwife when bleeding occurred, it was just as plausible for an unmarried or widowed woman to construe blood issuing from her nether regions as some other illness unrelated to childbirth. According to early modern Galenic medical theories, secretions of all varieties, including blood, faeces and pus, formed the basic mechanism of maintaining humoural equilibrium within the body. Evacuative crises such as vomiting, bleeding and sweating were understood not as a symptom, but instead as part of the body's attempt to restore the balance between the body's four humours by expelling excess bad humours.[54] Vaginal bleeding was therefore not necessarily a sign of childbirth, but might also be interpreted as a curative evacuation attributable to all manner of illness. The uncertainty of pregnancy meant that the status of bleeding was unstable and highly susceptible to other narra-

---

49   II. Sekt. W (F) Nr. 319, 1–27, 'Beschwerden (Willendorf)', 8 May–14 August 1717, 1v.
50   Ibid., 2r.
51   Ibid., 9v–10r.
52   Ibid., 12r.
53   'The Hidden Truths of the Belly: The Uncertainties of Pregnancy in Early Modern Europe', *Social History of Medicine* 15: 2 (2002): 209–27, 211.
54   Pomata, 'Menstruating Men', 124–30.

tives of illness. Thus a show of such bloody matter, even when symptoms like cramping or an enlarged belly were present, provided a plausible basis for women to believe that their bodies were afflicted with a malady, rather than in the throes of giving birth. When the widow Maria Bohn, for example, was 'in a terrible state down about [her vagina] in full blood', her neighbour urged her to send for the midwife.[55] Bohn refused, explaining that the bleeding was a 'Blutsturz' (haemorrhage) caused by medicines she had ingested to reinstate her menses.[56]

In 1722 Catharina Günther, a domestic servant, gave birth to a dead child in the presence of her sister, her mistress and a neighbour.[57] An investigation into the cause of death followed, in which Günther stood under suspicion of attempting to abort the 'fruit' or causing the death through improper birthing techniques. As the child was 'very fresh' with neither 'a single trace of decomposition' nor 'a single indication of a violent act', the attention of the Leipzig Court (Stadtgericht) turned to ascertaining whether or not Günther had known she was pregnant.[58] In vehement denial of any knowledge of her condition, Günther admitted she had once had sex with a student of the University but had neither 'suspected less still believed' that she could have become pregnant through this encounter because 'she had not had anything to do with him more than a single time'.[59] As her belly 'became high and grew fat', she took her urine to be inspected anonymously by a shepherdess and one Dr Külbeln. Külben told her she suffered from the 'blehe sucht' (bloating disease) and that she would 'take her high belly with her to her grave'.[60] The shepherdess, on the other hand, advised her to take 'Schafgerbe' and 'Hunderiebe' so that 'if she had busted something in her belly, this should so heal it'.[61] She then turned to Dr Paul Christian Stahl, a physician under the jurisdiction of the University who diagnosed a slipping of the uterus and prescribed 'a small glass jar of uterine drops'.[62] When she began to feel unwell, she had called for her sister and Dr Stahl, who arrived just as she 'had the greatest pains'. Günther told him 'that bloody matter had gone from her' but stressed that the amount had been negligible.[63]

Günther's insistence that she was not pregnant in spite of the bleeding meant that those present did not send for a midwife until just prior to the birth. Those around her suspected a pregnancy, but in the absence of any ex-

---

55   Straf. Nr. 654, 1–97, 'Bohn, Heÿdenreicher, Schacher', 1711, 5r–8r.

56   Ibid., 18r–23r.

57   StadtAL, Straf. Nr. 674, 'Catharina Günther', 1722, 28r.

58   According to sworn midwife Christina Lorend's report to the Leipzig Court. Ibid., 1v.

59   Ibid., 8v–9r.

60   Ibid.

61   Ibid., 26v–27r. *Schafgerbe* is a flowering weed that was used for healing wounds, preventing bad breath and stemming bleeding. See entry for 'Achillea' in Krünitz, *Oekonomische Encyklopädie*, vol. 1(i), 275–82. I was unable to discover what 'Hunderiebe' is.

62   See both the deposition of Anna Maria Günther (25 July 1722) and the interrogation of Catharina Günther (30 July 1722). Straf. Nr. 674, 'Günther', 1722, 22v, 26v–27r.

63   Ibid., 29r–30r.

ternal means of knowing about the body 'under the skin', Günther's own interpretation of her body's suffering determined the course of events. As a number of historians have shown, the eighteenth-century body – in particular the female body – was not the subject of external biological norms, diagnostic tests and ways of 'seeing' the body's workings beneath the skin that characterise modern medical culture. In the absence of an externalised form of diagnosing illness, it was the sufferer's own perception of her body and its signs that informed any kind of diagnosis or therapy.[64] Attempts to determine and treat a condition that ran contrary to the sufferer's own corporeal narrative were at best considered suppositions or suspicions, not matters of fact. Günther's sister, for example, examined her 'birth' and, suspecting a pregnancy because 'everything was soft', left to find 'a woman ... who knew about the conditions of pregnant women'.[65] Yet it was not until the child, the *corpus delicti*, was born that the uncertainty about Günther's ills vanished, and her own body narrative of bloating and colic might have been dispelled. And yet the strength of a woman's own body narrative could also trump the physical signs. After persisting with her story of ignorance through several ordeals of torture, Günther was eventually found not guilty of infanticide by the Schöppenstuhl.[66]

As we have seen, women were not willing to blindly follow a midwife's diagnosis, indeed any practitioner's diagnosis, if it did not fit into their own subjective narrative of illness. A midwife's authority depended greatly on her ability to curry favour with a client. The primacy of the sufferer's own body narrative correlated with the sufferer-centred culture of healing and medical consumption. As Barbara Duden argues, early modern healers were not 'specialists of the body' because they were not associated with particular forms of knowledge.[67] Midwives were instead associated with a cultural event – childbirth – which incorporated the physical, the social and the religious all at once. For women and their families in early modern Leipzig, the midwife was not a generalist healer of female and infant maladies. During illness women sought the medical assistance from a variety of healers, from physicians, surgeons and midwives to 'fringe' healers. Whether a pregnancy was clandestine or not, a midwife was usually only called when birth was believed to be imminent by the mother herself.

---

64   On the 'baroque body', see Duden, *Geschichte unter der Haut*, 24–25; Maren Lorenz, '"... als ob ihr ein Stein aus dem Leibe kollerte ...". Schwangerschaftswahrnehmungen und Geburtserfahrungen von Frauen im 18. Jahrhundert', in Richard van Dülmen, ed., *Körper-Geschichten* (Frankfurt am Main: Fischer Taschenbuch Verlag, 1996), 101.

65   See Dorothea Elisabeth Petschmann's deposition from 27 June 1727 in Straf. Nr. 674, 'Günther', 1722, 4r.

66   Günther was found guilty of 'negligence' ('Fahrlässigkeit') and her sentence reduced to six months in the workhouse. See the Schöppenspruch from c. 11 October 1722 in ibid., 60v–62r.

67   Duden, *Geschichte unter der Haut*, 40.

Midwives, Accoucheurs and the power of the 'patient'

Although the remit of the sworn midwife was perhaps the most clearly defined amongst the municipal medical personnel, throughout the latter seventeenth and eighteenth centuries women and their families determined who provided them with assistance in childbirth and how. This was characteristic of a medical culture in which even poor men and women might seek out several channels of medical advice and treatment in the quest for the 'right' solution to ill health. In 1699, for example, farm servant Dorothea Heh consulted her local pastor, a physician, a woman doctor and 'knowledgeable women' in the hope of curing her 'high belly' and 'congestion'.[68] Even amongst the late eighteenth-century educated burgher estate, where a veritable plethora of 'experts' might be called upon during childbirth, it was mothers who remained at the centre of the decision-making process. Ruth Dawson's extrapolation of the childbirth of Luise Boie is a case in point: although attended by a doctor and an Accoucheur, the only surgical intervention attempted was an incision carried out at Boie's own insistence.[69] As we have seen, within the realm of childbirth sworn midwives did not hold an exclusive monopoly over childbirth but regularly competed with their Beifrauen, Wickelweiber, Gassen-mägde and other female healers working within the midwifery landscape. These women could operate as midwives, in one capacity or another, precisely because they existed within a medical culture which was client-centric, domestically based and in which the incorporated and officially organised medical occupations did not dominate health and healing on either a practical or epistemological level.[70]

Unwanted intervention on the part of the authorities through either a sworn midwife or the Stadtaccoucheur could thus be easily averted. In 1722, for example, a travelling hawker's wife, Mrs Träger, gave birth attended by Dorothea Schröder, a local woman known to 'let herself be used by women in their confinement'.[71] The local sworn midwife heard of the birth and went to see the new mother. Seeing signs of 'Friesel und Flecke', the midwife advised

---

68   StadtAL, Straf. Nr. 624, 'Dorothea Madigt', 1699, 17r, 39v, 76r, 126v.
69   Ruth Dawson, 'The Search for Women's Experience of Pregnancy and Birth: Eighteenth-Century Accounts', in Katherine M. Faull, ed., *Anthropology and the German Enlightenment: Perspectives on Humanity* (Lewisburg, PA: Bucknell University Press, 1995), 117–18.
70   In his discussion of the shift from medical plurality to medical pluralism, Dinges conceptualises the position of physicians until WWI as 'hegemonic', i.e., physicians considered themselves specialists in diagnosis but did not claim expertise in all aspects of healing (medical plurality). Their increasing role in public health meant that they did attempt to 'define the space for the other medical professions, without necessarily considering them as competitors'. The shift to a dominant position was only made possible through legal confirmation and institutions with enough clout to enforce this medical dominance and shun competing bodies of knowledge (medical pluralism). See Martin Dinges, 'Medical Pluralism – Past and Present: Towards a more precise concept', in Robert Jütte, ed., *Medical Pluralism – Past – Present – Future* (Stuttgart: Franz Steiner Verlag, 2013), 197–99.
71   Tit. (F) XLIV.D.4, 1–21, 'Schröderin betr.', 1722, 1.

the family to fetch the Stadtphysicus Benjamin Benedict Petermann.[72] Instead of heeding her advice, the family continued to let Dorothea Schröder treat the mother with her own medicine. On the fifth day the woman's situation had worsened to the point that Dr Petermann was finally called to the house. He prescribed some medicines which the new mother took. However, Mrs Träger soon reverted to the care of Mrs Schröder and passed away a few days later.[73]

Dorothea Schröder was implicated around one month later in the death of another woman in childbed, known as the Speckfrau. Following a short report submitted by Stadtphysicus Petermann, the Leipzig Council began investigating the circumstances surrounding both deaths. We know from the sworn midwife who attended the Speckfrau during her confinement, Christina Lorend, that Mrs Schröder had administered two powder mixtures in order to induce the pains. The Speckfrau was dissatisfied with Schröder's treatment, claiming that it had provoked 'much retching and pressure which held the child too much'.[74] The baby was eventually born alive but midwife Lorend was certain that 'the powder was wholly contrary to the woman's condition' and caused 'a strong uterine cramping'.[75] Stadtphysicus Petermann then prescribed the new mother additional medicine and the Speckfrau 'felt well again twelve days in a row and was able to walk around the room'.[76]

In this story the midwife and the Stadtphysicus only make an appearance towards the end and then only on the periphery. In the eyes of the Speckfrau and her family, Petermann's medication held no greater legitimacy than Mrs Schröder's powders and potions. What sealed the relationship between a client and a medical practitioner was not occupational status; what was important was whether a practitioner could satisfy the expectations the client placed on the medical encounter. In this case, Mrs Schröder's culture of care catered best to the Speckfrau's convictions about what would restore her to good health. Conversely, the Stadtaccoucheur and the midwife lost their standing and authority at the woman's sickbed. As midwife Lorend surmised, because Stadtphysicus Petermann 'did not come every day several times [to see her], she [the Speckfrau] became unwilling, I [the midwife] had abdicated and [the Speckfrau] took on [the services of] … Mrs Schröder again'.[77] As this example shows, the power exerted by early modern people to avoid the hand of the urban authorities could be considerable, even amongst those of lesser social status and wealth. The Council pursued its investigation and collected various witness statements relating to both incidents, but the families and witnesses closed ranks around Dorothea Schröder. Whether out of conviction that

---

72 'Friesel' and 'Flecke' were contemporary terms for diseases involving a rash. 'Friesel' was frequently associated with childbed ('Wöchnerinnenfriesel'), especially when death occurred. See Hermann Metzke, *Lexikon der historischen Krankheitsbezeichnungen* (Neustadt an der Aisch: Verlag Degener & Co., 2005), 62–64.

73 Tit. (F) XLIV.D.4, 1–21, 'Schröderin betr.', 1722, 1–4.

74 Ibid., 10–12.

75 Ibid.

76 Ibid.

77 Ibid.

Schröder's practice was legitimate and effective, or because the community was unwilling to draw attention to its preferred use of irregular medical practitioners: not one of the witnesses called to the Town Hall was willing or able to provide evidence against Dorothea Schröder. Many had requested they not be troubled with the further expense of stopping work and travelling into the city to give evidence.[78] Stadtphysicus Petermann was finally forced to recommend the inquiry be closed unresolved.

As these examples have demonstrated, what constituted 'good medicine' and 'good midwifery' in early modern Leipzig was largely dictated by the recipient of medical care: the client. Bedside manner, diligence and thoroughness – these categories certainly featured in the midwife oaths and instructions, but they were also categories determined and upheld by clients. As Chapter Five demonstrated, where childbirth and childbed were concerned, the bond between a client and a practitioner was strong and enduring, even when deliveries went awry. 'Bedside' etiquette was a crucial criterion through which clients could be both procured and lost by physicians, midwives and 'empirics' (unofficial healers) alike: the community did not appear to have greatly diverging expectations as far as official and unofficial medical practitioners were concerned. As we have seen, in a world with a rather ineffective state encumbered by the patchwork of legal jurisdictions all jockeying to retain their autonomy, medicalisation and professionalisation 'from above', either through governments, doctors or the collusion of both, could be at best billowing rhetoric.[79]

The practice of municipal man-midwifery

Around 1700, male practitioners had yet to transcend the threshold of unnatural birth. No system of municipal or territorial obstetric licensing for physicians or surgeons existed and there were few places in Europe where obstetric knowledge might be acquired. The widespread inclusion of surgery as a sub-discipline of medicine in many European universities during the second half of the seventeenth century no doubt played a role in the growing interest in surgical obstetrics.[80] However, the first German lying-in hospital was a long way off and until the Strasbourg maternity hospital opened in 1728, medical students wishing to acquire skills in obstetrics typically undertook grand study

78   Ibid., 20–21.
79   Dinges, 'Medical Pluralism', 199; Lindemann, *Health*, 289–368. Recent studies have also looked at the way medical consumers shaped medicalisation on an institutional level, for example in voicing their need for hospitals and health insurance programmes. See Iris Ritzmann, 'Der Faktor Nachfrage bei der Ausformung des modernen Medizinalwesens', in Bettina Wahrig-Schmidt and Werner Sohn, eds, *Aufklärung, Policey und Verwaltung. Zur Genese des Medizinalwesens 1750–1850* (Wiesbaden: Harrossowitz Verlag, 2003), 163–65; Eberhard Wolff, 'Medikalisierung von Unten? Das Beispiel der jüdischen Krankenbesuchgesellschaften', ibid., 179–90.
80   Also in Leipzig.

tours of a handful of medical faculties known for anatomical study relevant to obstetrics, in particular Leiden.[81] Many also spent a period of time undergoing 'practical' training at the Parisian Hôtel Dieu's famed maternity ward.[82] From the mid-eighteenth century onwards, students flocked to London, where private clinical education such as that offered by William Hunter flourished, and to the universities of Edinburgh and Glasgow.[83] Private instruction was also available in many other centres of learning.[84] Leipzig would have to wait a lot longer than most university cities in Germany for its own maternity hospital, the Triersches Institut, which opened its doors in 1810 following a very protracted 'birth'.[85]

Designed to keep the Leipzig Council abreast of all aspects of midwifery in the city from instruction through to the general behaviour of the midwives, the petitions and reports filed by Leipzig's Stadtphysici and Stadtaccoucheurs from the late seventeenth to the middle of the eighteenth century provide a rare opportunity to gauge the level of these practitioners' physical involvement in obstetrics. The data is far from seamless: Andreas Petermann's term of office (1680–1703) is missing entirely, leaving a large gap between Gottfried Welsch's death in 1690 and Benjamin B. Petermann's appointment in 1715. The manner in which office holders communicated their information, moreover, lacks uniformity, ranging from Welsch's haphazardly filed petitions and reports to the semi-regular, tabulated reports submitted by Benjamin Petermann in the 1720s. From 1731 onwards the Stadtaccoucheurs were expected to file a report to the Council every six months detailing complicated births attended, notable incidents, what they had been teaching the midwives, and attendance levels at the midwifery lessons, although these often excluded a comprehensive inventory of deliveries. Not all complied with this demand, and there is a notable absence of reports during Johann Karl Gehler's time as Stadtaccoucheur (1759–1781/82): he simply refused to teach the midwives altogether, considering non-clinical teaching a waste of time.

An undated report to the Leipzig Council suggests that Gottfried Welsch did deliver babies with his own hands, but that his practice was restricted to so-called 'difficult births'. In this report Welsch claimed to have 'had 56 *partus*

81 On Johann Jakob Fried's school for midwives in Strasbourg, see Karenberg, 'Lernen', 901–3.

82 Christopher Lawrence, 'Ornate physicians and learned artisans. Edinburgh medical men 1726–1776', in W. F. Bynum and Roy Porter, eds, *William Hunter and the Eighteenth-Century Medical World* (Cambridge & London: Cambridge University Press, 2002), 153–76; Roy Porter, 'William Hunter: a surgeon and gentleman', ibid., 7–34.

83 Illustrated nicely by Göttingen surgeon man-midwife Friedrich Benjamin Osiander's career trajectory in Schlumbohm, *Lebendige Phantome*, 55–72.

84 Mary Lindemann, *Medicine and Society in Early Modern Europe*, (2nd edn, Cambridge: Cambridge University Press, 2010), 148–51.

85 The Triersches Institut will be dealt with in the next chapter. Planning began in the 1760s. See Sabine Fahrenbach, 'Johann Christian Gottfried Jörg und das "Triersche Institut". Zum 150. Todestag am 20. September 2006 und zum 200. Jubiläum der Trierschen Stiftung', *Jubiläen 2006. Personen/Ereignisse* (Leipzig: Universitätsarchiv Leipzig, 2006).

difficilies under his hands' – the period of time he refers to is unclear.[86] He bitterly lamented earning a paltry 120 florin; the women he attended were largely poor, their fee accordingly low or non-existent. However, Welsch did pocket fees from nine families, amongst which one was particularly wealthy, suggesting that he was reporting his actual level of involvement in deliveries, rather than just those he was obliged to tend for free.[87] Although obliged to serve the poor in particular, in late seventeenth-century Leipzig the Stadtphysicus clearly served families from all social estates as and when the need arose. As for Andreas Petermann, we know from his public dispute with the midwife Justine Siegemund that he claimed to have delivered around ninety women in total by the early 1690s.[88]

Table 3 Deliveries attended per month 1715–23, Stadtaccoucheur Benjamin Benedict Petermann

Report start	Report end	Months*	Deliveries	Average deliveries per month
10.10.1715	23.01.1716	3.50	4	1.14
24.01.1716	06.09.1716	7.50	9	1.20
07.09.1716	08.04.1717	6.00	2	0.33
09.04.1717	15.07.1717	3.25	4	1.23
16.07.1717	15.03.1718	8.00	7	0.88
16.03.1717	19.04.1718	Gap in records	–	–
20.04.1718	10.08.1718	3.75	6	1.60
11.08.1718	17.08.1719	Gap in records	–	–
18.08.1719	04.04.1720	7.50	6	0.80
05.04.1720	08.03.1721	10.00	4	0.40
09.03.1721	21.10.1721	7.50	7	0.93
22.10.1721	14.04.1722	5.75	7	1.22
14.04.1722	19.11.1722	7.25	9	1.24
20.11.1722	14.05.1723	5.75	6	1.04
15.05.1723	19.10.1723	5.25	7	1.33
Total			78	13.35
Monthly Average				1.03

*Months rounded up to nearest quarter month

Source: StadtAL, Tit. (F) XLIV.D.3, (1715–23), 1–33 (Benjamin Benedict Petermann's reports to Leipzig Council).

86   Tit. (F) XLIV.A.1a, 14r–16r, 'Stadtphysicus Welsch to LC', Undated (post 1659).
87   84% (47 of 56) of his clients were poor and contributed only 15% of Welsch's total income mentioned. The remaining 85% of his fee income consisted of a single fee of 40 florins from a 'wealthy person' and fees from eight further families ranging between 4 and 8 florins each. See ibid.
88   Siegemund, 'The Court Midwife', 9.

Reports from Benjamin Benedict Petermann are extant for his entire term of office (1715–23), with the exclusion of two periods of around twelve and thirteen months each in 1717/18 and 1718/19. Although filed at irregular intervals, his term of office provides one of the most comprehensive data sets. On average, Petermann recorded attending 1.03 births per month (see Table 3). He does not appear to have suppressed cases ending in the death of either mother or child, however, he went out of his way to justify each individual death; reducing infant and maternal mortality was, after all, the reason why his office had been created in the first place.[89]

Petermann was probably present and active (in some capacity) at many more births than this figure suggests: in his report from August 1721, he successfully 'delivered' many women using medications alone but did not include these cases in his official report.[90] Yet like his predecessor Gottfried Welsch, Petermann's practice concentrated on difficult births – births that had gone so wrong that the midwives and/or families felt compelled to call for operative intervention, knowing full well that saving the life of the child was unlikely. Petermann described one such situation thus:

> Thus it was not possible to free these women from their fruits without operating. Hence I was forced, in the presence of the above-mentioned midwife and, in particular [in the case of] Mrs Bormann, the surgeon Gießen, to carry out a surgical embryotomy, witherto it was finally brought to pass [with the help of] God that under such conditions the children, due to their bad position, [had to be] removed piece by piece because they were already dead anyway.[91]

As this case demonstrates, Petermann was careful to note his reluctance at having to surgically intervene. Petermann deployed the word 'delivery' very loosely to denote medicinal, surgical and obstetric interventions, so that when he writes 'delivery', we cannot be certain whether he was referring to non-surgical techniques sometimes used by midwives (for example versions) or operations requiring surgical instruments. Interestingly, he does not mention versions, a technique favoured and mentioned by later Stadtaccoucheurs in their reports. Either this technique was considered to belong to the midwife's arsenal, or Petermann was providing instruction to midwives when such techniques were required, but did not think it necessary to report deliveries at which he merely gave advice.[92]

According to reports submitted between 1732 and 1737, Stadtaccoucheur Johann Valentin Hartrauff's obstetric practice maintained similar levels, with Hartrauff intervening surgically on average 1.54 times per month during this

---

89   Tit. (F) XLIV.D.3, 1–33, 'Petermanns erstattete Berichte', 23 January 1715–19 October 1723.

90   Ibid., 20r. This probably meant that he prescribed medications during a delivery rather than actually delivering the women.

91   Ibid., 5–6.

92   Ibid. In the latter eighteenth century the practice of providing advice came to be ridiculed by man-midwives as a waste of precious time. See Peter Gottfried Joerdens, *Von den Eigenschaften des aechten Geburtshelfers: eine Skizze; zur besonderen Berherzigung für meine Landesleute* (Leipzig: Dykische Buchhandlung, 1789), 21–22.

period, performing versions, embryotomies, caesarean sections, or delivering twins (see Table 4).

Table 4 Deliveries attended per month 1732–37, Stadtaccoucheur Johann Valentin Hartrauff

Date of report	Period (months)*	Total deliveries over period	Average deliveries per month
29.11.1732	6	20	3.33
08.07.1733	7	6	0.86
c. March 1734**	9	20	2.22
08.03.1735	12	8	0.67
15.03.1736	12	14	1.17
13.03.1737	12	12	1.00
Total		80	1.54

* Months have been rounded up or down to nearest whole month.
** No individual report available for 1733–34. Hartrauff mentions in 1735 report that he had carried out twenty deliveries in that year (see pp. 138–39).

Source: StadtAL, Tit. (F) XLIV.D.1 (1673–1756), 123–60 (Johann Valentin Hartrauff's reports to Leipzig Council, 1732–37).

Like Petermann, Hartrauff prescribed and administered medicines, yet he only included this in his reports when this began eating into his salary.[93] In his bid for a pay rise, he argued that he had more work than his predecessor due to the unusually high number of 'difficult deliveries … given the size of the city'.[94] The fact that he considered twenty 'difficult' deliveries in a year (excluding those involving only medicines and/or advice) to be onerous and unusual warrants our attention. It demonstrates that the category of 'difficult birth' was not confined to the use of instruments or to the active involvement of the Stadtaccoucheur. Whilst the Council's appointment of a specialist for surgical obstetrics elevated the male domain of surgery and male surgeons as experts in difficult births, in practice the field was still open to midwives. With a paltry maximum of 20 hands-on deliveries a year, the Stadtaccoucheur was a numerically minor player on this field, and he became statistically less significant over the course of the eighteenth century. The data leads us to assume that midwives continued to handle many, if not most 'unnatural' and difficult births in the city. The city's Stadtaccoucheurs in the latter eighteenth century left little trace of their individual obstetric activities in their reports to the Council and it appears that this detailed inventarisation was no longer required by the Council. A single report from Johann Gottfried Breuer, the

93   See report from 29 November 1732 of Tit. (F) XLIV.D.1, 132–60, 'Stadtaccoucheur reports (Hartrauff)', 29 November 1732–13 March 1737, 123–25.
94   On population, see Blaschke, *Bevölkerungsgeschichte*, 140. See report from 29 November 1732 of Tit. (F) XLIV.D.1, 132–60, 'Stadtaccoucheur reports (Hartrauff)', 29 November 1732–13 March 1737, 135.

Stadtaccoucheur and *Lazarett-Chirurg* (lazarette surgeon) from 1756, suggests that the Stadtaccoucheur continued to attend and actively participate in only a handful of deliveries each year. Breuer recorded performing an operation or actively delivering a mother only three times over a period of six months. This implies a much lower monthly delivery rate (0.5 births per month) than any of his predecessors.[95] And if we fast-forward to the latter eighteenth century, this pattern appears to have continued. Johann Karl Gehler, an inspired deployer of forceps for both 'natural' and 'unnatural births', had amassed experience of only 426 births during the eighteen years he held the office of Stadtaccoucheur (1759–1781/82): an average of just 23 difficult births per annum (and as such, not much more than his predecessors).[96] Even if we do treat these early eighteenth-century figures as minimums, it remains that the Stadtaccoucheur attended only a very small, very technically specialised share of deliveries – one reason why the introduction of this office had no major quantitative impact on the day-to-day workload of midwives in Leipzig throughout the eighteenth century.

'Natural' and 'unnatural' births

As we have seen, midwifery in early modern Leipzig was a very narrowly defined field. By the middle of the eighteenth century, there was an understanding shared by both the community and medical practitioners that midwives (in particular sworn midwives) dealt with birth only. Furthermore, there were regulatory and customary limits to what a midwife could and could not do. At the end of the seventeenth century medical discourses began focusing on the mechanics of childbirth and this redefined the older division of labour between midwives and surgeons, which had afforded the surgeon a role in the birth on the basis of the 'emergency'. Births were now categorised into 'natural' births, which might be carried out by the midwife exclusively, and 'unnatural' births, many (but not all) of which would require the instruments or expertise of an Accoucheur. This distinction provided the epistemological undergirding for the new role of the obstetric surgeon and, most importantly, gave him the opportunity to act rather than merely react: with the classification of births, emergencies began to be foreseeable and, at times, even controllable. The point of drawing such a distinction was to further delimit the midwife's sphere of activity within the birthing chamber. A midwife had to know what kind of delivery to expect, as well as if and at which point she should call for the surgeon or the Stadtaccoucheur: the crisp distinction be-

---

95 See report from 19 March 1756 of Tit. (F) XLIV.D.1, 190–91, 'Stadtaccoucheur reports (Breuer)', 19 March 1756.
96 Seidel, *Neue Kultur*, 343–44; StadtAL, Tit. (F) XLIV.D.6b, Bd. I, 'Acta, Die Einrichtung der Kindermütter und Beÿweiber de Anno 1757', 222–26, 'Letter of resignation from Stadtaccoucheur Johann Carl Gehler', 30 October 1781, 222.

tween 'natural' and 'unnatural' births facilitated this new division of labour between midwives and surgeons.

Throughout much of the eighteenth century the figure of the Accoucheur or *Geburtshelfer* (as male obstetric practitioners increasingly became known towards the end of the eighteenth century) had been a source of terror for both women and their families. Maternal and infant mortality was very high throughout the period and, appearing only in times of crisis, the Stadtaccoucheur was for many an omen of impending death.[97] The tension between the ordinance and the will of mothers and their families was no more apparent than in the use of the Stadtaccoucheur. Sworn midwives were instructed to call for the assistance of the Stadtaccoucheur if they were unable to deliver a woman successfully. Yet their authority (and perhaps also willingness) to override the wishes of their clients was limited. The midwife Rosina Willendorf told the Leipzig Court in 1717 that 'the women did not want to have a doctor, [they] would rather die'.[98] The sworn midwife Johanna Stranz found herself in such a position in 1759 when attending the wife of a soldier in the city regiment who died before the child could be delivered. After questioning the witnesses and autopsying the corpse, the Stadtaccoucheur Johann Gottfried Breuer accused Stranz of not seeking out his assistance. Stranz responded that she had been unable to convince either the family or the mother that Breuer's presence was necessary. The mother 'had not wanted to admit one bit' that it was time to fetch the Stadtaccoucheur, saying 'that she would rather die than want to do this, seeing that she already felt that she would not survive [this childbed]'.[99]

And yet, judging from the relative frequency with which the Stadtaccoucheur appears to have intervened in births, both mothers and midwives *did* suffer the Stadtaccoucheur's instruments or, at the very least, his advice and medications. Despite their association with death, the early male practitioners of midwifery appear to have been quite successful in saving mothers. Of the some eighty operative interventions Stadtaccoucheur Benjamin Benedict Petermann recorded for the period between 1715 and 1723, the mother survived her confinement in 84 per cent of deliveries. The infants, however, fared badly and Petermann could deliver only 8 per cent alive.[100] The bulk of

---

97 Stadtaccoucheur Christoph Adolph Hartwig noted that maternal mortality in Leipzig during the 1780s was high at 12 per 1,000 women. See Tit. (F) XLIV.D.6b, 'Acta, Die Einrichtung der Kindermütter und Beÿweiber betr. de Anno 1782', 76–97, 'Stadtaccoucheur reports (Christoph Adolph Hartwig)', c. 21 April 1788–28 March 1791, 92. As a comparison, in London maternal mortality stood at 14.5 (deaths per 1,000 women) for the period 1700–49, and 11.4 for the period 1750–99. For non-urban English parishes, maternal mortality ranged between 11 (1700–49) and 8 (1750–99). Roger Schofield, 'Did the mothers really die? Three centuries of maternal mortality in the "world we have lost"', in Lloyd Bonfield et al., eds, *The World We Have Gained: Histories of Population and Social Structure* (Oxford: Blackwell, 1986), 232 and 249–50.

98 II. Sekt. W (F) Nr. 319, 1–27, 'Beschwerden (Willendorf)', 8 May–14 August 1717, 26r.

99 StadtAL, II. Sekt. M (F) Nr. 670, Bd. II, 'Hebammen. Verschiedenes 1748–59', 63–71, 'Negligence Johanna Sophia Stranz', 4–24 February 1759, 66–68.

100 Data collected from Petermann's reports on 'difficult births'. See Tit. (F) XLIV.D.3, 1–33, 'Petermanns erstattete Berichte', 23 January 1715–19 October 1723.

Stadtaccoucheur Johann Valentin Hartrauff's deliveries appear to have also ended in the death of the child: of the twenty deliveries he carried out in a six-month period in 1732, seventeen cases (85 per cent) were resolved by opening the head or taking the foetus out in pieces.[101]

According to his reports, Petermann appears to have been resigned to such high levels of infant mortality, frequently praising the midwives that they 'had not spared their part of the work' and stressing the inevitability of an 'operation' to 'free' the women 'of their belly's fruit'.[102] Yet by the time Hartrauff was appointed Stadtaccoucheur in 1732, he was no longer content to equate difficult births with dead infants. He was also no longer content to perpetuate the image of the Stadtaccoucheur as a harbinger of death. Hartrauff commented that whilst he 'learnt [embryotomy] as [part of] the [art of] Accouchement, [he] believed he [would] exercise it either never or at the least very seldom'.[103] Unlike his predecessor, Hartrauff was greatly concerned about the 'so many *Laborieuse* Accouchement' that he considered disproportionate to the size of the city.[104] Berating the midwives for their 'slowness and acts of negligence', which left him no alternative other than to deliver a child 'piece by piece', Hartrauff was convinced of the possibility of 'keeping the life of many a child through [the use of] version'.[105]

In her study of two midwifery texts, authored by a female midwife and a physician-cum-man-midwife in the early eighteenth century, Lynne Tatlock has shown that on a discursive level, midwives generally privileged the life of the mother over the infant. Conversely, she argues that male obstetricians were increasingly concerned about the survival of the child and advocated visual procedures such as caesarean section and the speculum over the traditional tactile techniques deployed by midwives, such as version. She relates this discursive shift to the increasing importance of the child in a changing economic climate as 'a subject vital to the transmission of property and the authority of the father'.[106] The evidence from Leipzig suggests a different narrative. Hartrauff certainly demonstrated a keen interest in bringing healthy rather than mangled infants into the world, yet his success as a practitioner did not rest on the privileged use of instruments. His revulsion at the prospect of carrying out embryotomies and his clear preference for techniques such as version, which obviated the use of instruments altogether, is at odds with the

---

101 Tit. (F) XLIV.D.1, 132–60, 'Stadtaccoucheur reports (Hartrauff)', 29 November 1732–13 March 1737, 134–35.
102 Tit. (F) XLIV.D.3, 1–33, 'Petermanns erstattete Berichte', 23 January 1715–19 October 1723, 1r, 5v and 8r.
103 Tit. (F) XLIV.D.1, 132–60, 'Stadtaccoucheur reports (Hartrauff)', 29 November 1732–13 March 1737, 134–35.
104 Ibid., 135.
105 Ibid., 134–35.
106 Tatlock, 'Speculum Feminarum', 757. However, as Seidel points out neither male nor female obstetric practitioners used their eyes to examine pregnant and labouring women until the latter nineteenth century. See Seidel, *Neue Kultur*, 405–6.

the discursive dichotomy of 'instruments-eyes-male practitioner of midwifery' versus 'hands-touch-female midwife' prevalent in obstetric discourses.

Hartrauff was clearly trying to distance himself from the traditional trappings of his surgical trade – instruments – for which I put forward two reasons. Firstly, Hartrauff had few surgical novelties or techniques up his sleeve that could distinguish his midwifery services from those of the city's midwives, for it was not until the forceps found widespread deployment and achieved greater levels of live deliveries in the latter part of the eighteenth century that the male midwife's surgical instruments had greater *potential* for providing speedy delivery of a live infant.[107] Invented by the Chamberlen family in seventeenth-century England, the forceps remained a family secret until the early eighteenth century. Their use was hotly contested amongst man-midwives and the wider public both there and on the Continent into the early 1900s.[108] In France, for example, they were practically unheard of until the 1730s and only gained widespread popularity in the latter part of the century, with some seventeenth- and early eighteenth-century writers of obstetric treatises eschewing instruments in favour of the hand altogether.[109] Even in England their deployment was limited to complicated births, so that the forceps can hardly be considered the key to the birth chamber.[110] Secondly, Hartrauff had to contend with the expectations of mothers and their families about propriety and ritual in the birthing chamber. And it never occurred to Hartrauff, nor any of his predecessors, to violate this cultural and social ritual of childbirth and childbed that privileged the midwife and the female collective.[111]

Faced with these challenges, instead of capitalising on their ability to wield surgical instruments, Hartrauff and Co. associated their practice with live mothers and live babies. This was a novel goal and they did so by pleading for the use of techniques that mothers would find acceptable because these were already part of the arsenal of techniques that the few highly skilled midwives, such as Justine Siegemund, were supposed to master.[112] This preference for the hand over instruments persisted amongst many notable male practitioners of midwifery into the early nineteenth century. For example, the director of the Göttingen maternity hospital from 1751 onwards, Johann Georg Roederer, was adamant the male midwife use his 'soft hand' to clear obstructions, not his

---

107 What Wilson terms 'the horizon of male practice'. See Wilson, *Making*, 49–57.
108 Jordanova argues these debates hinged on contested notions of gender. See Ludmilla Jordanova, *Nature Displayed: Gender, Science and Medicine 1760–1820* (London: Longman, 1999), 23–47. On the debate between Tory forceps proponents and court Whig Deventarians in London, see Wilson, *Making*, 107–22.
109 McTavish, *Childbirth*, 12–13.
110 Wilson, *Making*, 99–101.
111 Wilson notes this, arguing that the 'hegemony of the ritual' of childbirth was so powerful that male medical writers endorsed and inscribed it into their writings as part of the natural order. See *Ritual*, 212–13.
112 Documented in detail by Justine Siegemund. Siegemund, *Court Midwife*, 89–121.

instruments.[113] Both he and Lukas Johann Boër (director of the Vienna maternity hospital c. 1800) were vocal opponents of the forceps and instruments more generally, championing the cause of 'nature' in childbirth.[114] Thus with this shift towards saving infants as well as mothers, these early male midwives developed a new approach to surgical midwifery that spurned instruments and traditional obstetric 'emergency' surgery and cultivated instead techniques using the hands that both emulated and 'outperformed' the work of the female midwife.

In 1758, some twenty years after Hartrauff, the Stadtaccoucheur Johann Gottfried Breuer similarly expounded the virtues of 'skilled manual techniques that should be promoted without loss of time' which would prevent 'mothers and children ... to be lost without delivery'.[115] Breuer proceeded to cite two recent deaths in the countryside, which he claimed could have been averted if the midwives had implemented an earlier version and positioned the mother correctly. Breuer did not deploy these arguments to make a case for replacing female midwives with male practitioners. Rather, he was attempting to convince the Leipzig Council that the lessons he provided to the city's midwives and Beifrauen should be expanded to include midwives working in the countryside and manorial estates belonging to Leipzig.[116] Although scathing of the ignorance he perceived in many midwives, Breuer argued that it was through his careful and arduous instruction that these women might learn to save the lives of both mother and child.

Although the aim of training midwives had a utilitarian tone, the Leipzig Stadtaccoucheurs, endorsed by the Leipzig Council, were intent on upholding the traditional status of the physician as a humanist scholar and learned gentleman.[117] Even in the middle of the eighteenth century, physicians were not trained as practitioners but as scholars. Their identity did not rest on technical expertise, nor did they consider their education as the 'transmission of a body of expert knowledge'.[118] Less intervention on the Stadtaccoucheur's part in the birthing chamber, not more, was the hallmark of success. Instructing Leip-

---

113 Jürgen Schlumbohm, '"Die edelste und nützlichste unter den Wissenschaften": Praxis der Geburtshilfe als Grundlegung der Wissenschaft, ca. 1750–1820', in Hans Erich Bödeker et al., eds, *Wissenschaft als kulturelle Praxis, 1750–1900* (Göttingen: Vandenhoeck & Ruprecht, 1999), 275–97, 284.

114 Ibid., 284 and 293–94.

115 StadtAL, II. Sekt. M (F) Nr. 670, Bd. III, 'Hebammen. Verschiedenes über die Kindermütter, Wehemütter und Beifrauen (1756–69)', 48–49, 'Letter from Stadtaccoucheur Johann Gottfried Breuer to Leipzig Council', 21 August 1758, 48.

116 Ibid., 49.

117 See Chapter 2 of Thomas Neville Bonner, *Becoming a Physician: Medical Education in Britain, France, Germany and the United States, 1750–1945* (Baltimore, MD: The Johns Hopkins University Press, 1995). On the professional identity of physicians, see Thomas Broman, 'Rethinking Professionalization: Theory, Practice and Professional Ideology in Eighteenth-Century German Medicine', *Journal of Modern History* 67: 4 (1995): 835–72, 841–48; 'University Reform in Medical Thought at the End of the Eighteenth Century', *Osiris (2nd series)* 5 (1989): 36–53, 37–39.

118 Broman, 'Rethinking', 848.

zig's midwives was the key to this success, and so it was the status of teacher rather than practitioner that conferred prestige and expertise onto the Stadtaccoucheur. The emphasis placed on teaching midwives reflected the difficulty the Stadtaccoucheurs encountered in reconciling the divide between the intellectual labour of the physician and the manual labour required of a Stadtaccoucheur. It was not until medicine was transformed into a clinical pursuit in the late eighteenth and nineteenth centuries that this dichotomy could be overcome.[119]

The preference for teaching rather than practising amongst the Leipzig Stadtaccoucheurs can be traced back to developments in both France and Sweden. The midwifery school in Strasbourg was a kind of Mecca for many of the later Leipzig Stadtaccoucheurs. But the Swedish system of training midwives was perhaps an equal source of influence over the way in which Leipzig tackled the problem of improving urban midwifery provision. The first Stadtaccoucheur, Johann Valentin Hartrauff, used Johan Hoorn's midwifery manual for a number of years following his appointment. It is uncertain whether or not his successor Breuer also used Hoorn, however, Breuer's description of what he was teaching the midwives in 1756 (anatomy followed by natural and finally unnatural births) matches the general format of Hoorn's manual.[120]

As we have seen, there was little attempt on the part of the Leipzig Stadtaccoucheurs to replace midwives by attending normal births. This underpinned the existing division of labour between the midwife and the Stadtaccoucheur, as espoused by Hoorn. Hoorn's attitude towards obstetric practice was circumspect. After training in obstetrics at the Hôtel Dieu in Paris, he claimed to have returned to Sweden *not* to become an Accoucheur but instead to teach untrained midwives in Stockholm. By his own account, Hoorn was a reluctant practitioner; after publishing his midwifery manual he was forced into 'using his own hands' because women experiencing difficult labours insisted on calling upon his services.[121] And yet, Hoorn remained steadfast in his plan to up-skill and multiply Swedish midwives rather than replace them. His original Swedish text contained many examples of deliveries using sharp instruments, which most Swedish midwives were authorised to use.[122] In the German version many of these were omitted and subsumed into the Stadtaccoucheur's areas of responsibility. The midwife, meanwhile, was to deal with any situations in which the 'skilled hand of a knowledgeable midwife' would suffice.[123]

119 In Germany clinical medical education was most keenly taken up by the universities in the late eighteenth century. See Bonner, *Becoming*, 34–37. Practical education in obstetrics for male students and practitioners, however, continued to contain very little actual practice. See Schlumbohm, 'Practice', 35–36.

120 Tit. (F) XLIV.D.1, 190–91, 'Stadtaccoucheur reports (Breuer)', 19 March 1756, 190–91.

121 Hoorn, *Siphra*, 2v.

122 Across much of Europe midwives were forbidden from using instruments. On Sweden's experience, see Romlid, 'Swedish Midwives'.

123 Hoorn, *Siphra*, 8r.

And it was precisely this division of labour expressed by Hoorn that dominated midwifery instruction and practice in Leipzig throughout the eighteenth
century. None of the Stadtaccoucheurs strove to augment their obstetric activities over and above what was absolutely necessary. Even Johann Karl Gehler,
who was academically active in the burgeoning field of obstetrics, had a relatively small pool of experience. And he was no proponent of midwifery lessons. He neglected these entirely during his time as Stadtaccoucheur, favour-
ing instead the establishment of a midwifery institute in which he might train
medical students as well as midwives.[124] Yet Gehler was an aberration. Most
of his predecessors and successors dutifully instructed the city's midwives how
to carry out and manage both 'natural' and 'difficult' births. In the 1790s
Stadtaccoucheur Hartwig taught all the city's seven Beifrauen twice a week on
the 'phantom', instructing them on 'all types of easy as well as difficult births,
inasmuch as these belong to the midwives, for example, version, etc. using an
artificial child'.[125] Similarly, Menz provided the midwives in 1796 with lessons
regarding 'difficult cases in obstetrics ... and the application of necessary advantages in difficult births'.[126]

Clearly Leipzig's Stadtaccoucheurs were equipping the city's midwives
with the types of skills that would permit them to carry out most types of delivery, with the exception of the really difficult cases requiring the application
of instruments. The reform of midwifery in Leipzig took, in effect, the line of
least resistance. The physicians who inhabited the offices of Stadtaccoucheur
had little interest in providing hands-on care to women during their childbirth
travails, preferring instead to pursue the role of midwife instructor more in
keeping with their academic medical status. Meanwhile, the breadth of a midwife's practice changed very little, even though the distinction between a 'difficult' and an 'easy' birth was sharpened. Midwives were still expected to handle most easy and difficult births without the intervention of a surgeon or the
Stadtaccoucheur. Thus, the reform of midwifery training actually worked to
underpin rather than dismantle the traditional distinction between the learned,
gentleman-physician Stadtaccoucheur and the 'artisan', practitioner-midwife.
In Leipzig the desire for a medical landscape that might be useful for society
found its expression within the prevailing structures of the estates, thus pre-

124 Tit. (F) XLIV.D.6b, Bd. I, 222–26, 'Resignation (Gehler)', 30 October 1781. In his report
     Pohl mentions that lessons had been neglected since Stadtaccoucheur Breuer's term of
     office (18 years previously) and that there had been several 'unhappy accidents'. See
     StadtAL, Tit. (F) XLIV.D.6b, Bd. I, 'Acta, Die Einrichtung der Kindermütter und Beÿwei-
     ber de anno 1757', 233–44, 'Leipzig Council minutes (excerpt) re: instruction of mid-
     wives', 15 April 1782.
125 The 'phantom' was a stuffed dummy used to simulate delivery for the purpose of training
     midwives and surgeon men-midwives. See Hartwig's report from 25 November 1790 in
     Tit. (F) XLIV.D.6b, 76–97, 'Stadtaccoucheur reports (Hartwig)', c. 21 April 1788–28 March
     1791, 94–95.
126 See Menz's report from 6 February 1796 in Tit. (F) XLIV.D.6b, Bd. II, 'Acta, Die Einrich-
     tung der Kindermütter und Beÿweiber de Anno 1782', 99–133, 'Stadtaccoucheur reports
     (Dr. Carl Christian Menz)', 13 August 1792–14 March 1805, 111.

serving as far as possible the occupational distinction between the learned medicine of the physician and the medical practice of the midwife.[127]

Turning point? Booking the Accoucheur

The traditional division of labour between the *Accoucheur* (male surgeon-midwife) and the midwife only began to shift in the first half of the nineteenth century as it became ever more common for mothers to pre-arrange the use of an Accoucheur. By this period it was already *de rigueur* amongst the urban elite to engage the services of an Accoucheur in addition to the midwife. Triggered by the use of male practitioners in courtly birthing chambers, the 'fashion' (as contemporaries described the practice of keeping an Accoucheur on stand-by and in-house during labour) was a means for women and families to demonstrate social prestige and served to purchase perceived safety.[128] Accoucheurs' activities were restricted to 'on call' until well into the latter nineteenth century.[129] The similarity of this narrative with the English experience around a century earlier is striking. According to Wilson, man-midwives were propelled into 'fashion' by the rise of a leisure and literature class in eighteenth-century England. Women of the new educated leisure class sought to differentiate themselves socially from their lower-class counterparts by rupturing the traditional 'social leveller' of childbirth through a differentiated consumption of medical services.[130] In England the practice of man-midwives did not stop at obstetric emergencies and, from the middle of the eighteenth century, man-midwives increasingly replaced female midwives during natural births.[131]

According to Seidel, however, the premeditated use of an Accoucheur amongst the middle and lower classes in the mid-nineteenth century appears to have been less about fashion and more about perceived medical efficacy. Generally speaking, only middle- and lower-class women with prior experience of several stillbirths or difficult deliveries would seek out the services of an Accoucheur, as a preventative measure, prior to the birth.[132] Whereas in eighteenth-century England the use of a man-midwife appears by all accounts to have been 'classed', in Leipzig and other German cities, both Accoucheurs and midwives appear to have sustained a broad social mix of clients through-

---

127 Late seventeenth- and early eighteenth-century English surgical-obstetric practitioners, such as Percival Willughby, also supported the training of midwives and strove to respect the traditional division of labour between surgery (use of instruments to deliver a dead child) and midwifery (use of the hands to deliver a live child). See Wilson, *Making*, 52–53.
128 Seidel, *Neue Kultur*, 399.
129 Ibid., 403.
130 Wilson, *Making*, 185–92.
131 Ibid., 161–73.
132 Seidel shows that this preventative trend amongst the lower classes began during the 1840s. Seidel, *Neue Kultur*, 403.

out the period. The Berlin obstetrician Johann Phillip Hagen, for example, delivered women from almost every part of the social spectrum, although the patrician elite disproportionately made up over 40 per cent of his clientele.[133]

The nascent demand for male obstetric practitioners around 1800 in Leipzig was fuelled largely by the choices made by mothers and their families. On the basis of previous birth experiences, women were actively self-diagnosing prospective difficult births and securing the additional services of an Accoucheur in advance of the first pains. However, as the case discussed below will show, midwives continued to play a leading role in the birthing chamber and remained the first port of call for women when their pains commenced. Accoucheurs, even those whose services were procured in advance, remained adjunct practitioners in childbirth.

On 15 October 1803 Dr Friedrich August Müller, a practising physician and Geburtshelfer in Leipzig, submitted an eighteen-page letter to the Leipzig Council accusing the sworn midwife Erdmuth Ulrich of 'rash, negligent and rough conduct' resulting in 'lethal injuries' to the child.[134] The tragedy had begun in the early afternoon of 29 September as Eleanora Bölle, thinking that she was going into labour after experiencing some sporadic 'cutting in the belly', called both midwife Ulrich and Dr Müller to her house. When he arrived he found the pregnant woman pacing the room together with midwife Ulrich, who assured him that in the absence of 'real pains', labour was a long way off. Midwife Ulrich then examined Mrs Bölle, and found that 'the cervix was slightly open [and] the child's head stood in place'.[135] Dr Müller then examined the woman and finding the same, Ulrich and Müller departed, certain that labour had not yet begun.[136] Both midwife and doctor stopped by separately that evening to check on the woman, and Dr Müller called again early the next morning.[137]

Later that afternoon when Mrs Bölle felt her waters break and felt the child's hand, the couple sent for midwife Ulrich. Upon her arrival Ulrich, who had been attending another woman at the time, informed the parents there was nothing she could do and advised them to send for a doctor. Yet sensing there was little time, Ulrich sent for her Beifrau and set about working on Mrs Bölle's belly. After much 'raking about in the birthing parts', the Beifrau heard 'a certain crack to the child', after which Dr Müller arrived and took over from the midwife.[138] Müller managed to deliver the child 'according to all the measures of the art'.[139] Yet the child died from its injuries shortly after birth.[140]

133 Ibid., 396–97.
134 StadtAL, Tit. (F) XLIV.D.1a, 'Verschiedenes über die Kindermütter oder Hebammen betr. 1680–1831', 10r–31v, 'Letter from Dr. Friedrich August Müller to Leipzig Council', 15 October 1803, 26v–27v.
135 Ibid., 13r–13v.
136 Ibid., 13v–14v.
137 Ibid., 14v–15v.
138 Ibid., 19v–20r.
139 Ibid., 22v.
140 Ibid., 26v–27r.

Dr Müller handed the child over to midwife Ulrich, who 'in vain made a great effort to resuscitate the child', and then turned his attentions to the mother and sought 'with the greatest care … to bring the uterus back into its place'.[141] Midwife Ulrich 'busied herself with dressing the child accompanied by loud din and all manner of excuses for the death of the child' and then returned to the first mother, leaving the Beifrau with the dead child.[142]

The Bölle case demonstrates that at the outset of the nineteenth century, access to male obstetric practitioners was not restricted to the well-heeled. Even the lowly and often destitute day-labouring classes, to which the Bölle family belonged, might plausibly seek out and pay for the services of a privately practising, academically trained physician or surgeon. Moreover, according to Dr Müller's letter, his presence at Eleanora Bölle's confinement was premeditated and pre-emptive. Mrs Bölle had 'suffered greatly' during her last confinement one year previously, an ordeal that resulted in 'a difficult forceps operation' at the hands of another practising Accoucheur by the name of Keller.[143] The success of Dr Keller's procedure, whereby Mrs Bölle bore a 'healthy live child', prompted Adam Bölle to engage the services of Dr Müller for his wife's next confinement. Müller had then come to the house to examine the pregnant Eleanora prior to the birth (both internally and externally), finding her to be in the tenth month of pregnancy and suffering from 'a high degree of weakness and exhaustion'.[144] Armed with memories of her previous birth and hampered by her present ill health, Mrs Bölle and her husband appear to have convinced themselves that this birth would not be easy. Instead of waiting until the confinement turned into an emergency requiring the assistance of the Stadtaccoucheur Menz, the Bölle family sought from the outset to engage the practitioner they believed to be capable of bringing Mrs Bölle most safely through her travails.

Yet the Bölle family did not merely choose the Geburtshelfer over the midwife. Midwife Ulrich appears to have been the family's midwife – she had attended Mrs Bölle's previous birth – and the fact that they sought her out again implies that they counted themselves as Ulrich's clients. Indeed the course of events, even in the highly partial narrative of Dr Müller, suggests that although the Bölles contracted the services of the obstetrician, they did not intend for him to replace the midwife. Rather their particular situation – the prospect of a difficult birth – rendered the customary roles of the midwife and the Accoucheur ambiguous. Thus, when Eleanora Bölle felt herself to be on the verge of giving birth on 29 September 1803, her husband sent for both the midwife Erdmuth Ulrich *and* the Accoucheur Dr Müller.[145] Over the course of the next few days both Ulrich and Müller visited Mrs Bölle independently of one another. However, when the waters broke and the hand was

141 Ibid., 24r–24v.
142 Ibid., 24v.
143 Ibid., 10r–10v.
144 Ibid., 11r–12r.
145 Ibid., 12v–13r.

born, it was midwife Ulrich who was called to the house.[146] Dr Müller, who arrived a little later, was only summoned after Ulrich had conceded that there was little she could do.[147] During the delivery Müller took the lead, performing his manual operation and taking care of the mother. Midwife Ulrich was relegated to tending the hopelessly injured child: this particular birth transcended her responsibility as a midwife.

During lying-in it was once again Mr and Mrs Bölle who steered the medical encounter, rebuking the midwife and preventing her from carrying out her usual tasks. Postnatal care was traditionally the preserve of the midwife, her Beifrau and sometimes other women employed by the family to tend the new mother, so it was midwife Ulrich who returned to the Bölle house the next day to check on her client. Whilst dressing the dead child, Adam Bölle confronted the midwife, reproaching her that his child might still be alive had she waited for Dr Müller. Ulrich replied angrily that she had not had time to wait 'because otherwise the child would have come under the pelvis!', adding that 'the *Doctores* shatter several arms and feet and she has brought more than 100 children [into the world] in this manner without *Doctores*'.[148] The couple nevertheless allowed the midwife to dress the dead infant, thereby acknowledging the contract of obligation between practitioner and client and the responsibility of the midwife for tending the newborn infant. However, when Ulrich attempted to bind the mother's belly, Mrs Bölle refused, stating that Dr Müller had given orders not to do so. Ulrich replied: 'Hm! This is yet another new fashion'.[149]

Throughout the entire ordeal, the Bölles played an autonomous role. They engaged the services of two practitioners, a sworn midwife and an Accoucheur, and switched between them as and when they saw fit. We have to read Müller's account very judiciously as no further records of this case could be found, suggesting that the family did not pursue the matter. Yet his narrative provides us with an insight into how much the authority of the midwife or the Accoucheur was bound up in the wishes of the client. The Bölle family was ambivalent about how much trust they wished to invest in midwife Ulrich. This trust had been shaken – before the child was born – because Ulrich failed to meet the family's expectations as an attentive and competent midwife. As argued in Chapter Five, the basis of trust was visual, and it was perpetuated by the midwife's performance in the birthing chamber. Mr Bölle complained to Dr Müller that during the pre-birth examinations, midwife Ulrich had behaved very 'hastily', examining Mrs Bölle perfunctorily or not at all and neglecting to ask any questions.[150] When Ulrich arrived after Mrs Bölle's waters had broken, she injured her credibility further by presenting a grumpy demeanour and complaining she could spare but little time on the

146 Ibid., 16r–17v.
147 Ibid., 20r.
148 Ibid., 25r–25v.
149 Ibid., 26r.
150 Ibid., 15r, 16r.

mother.[151] Yet the Bölles continued to use their midwife throughout lying-in –
although they circumscribed her activities.

Conclusions

As we have seen in Leipzig, and indeed in the Germanies as a whole, there
was a good deal of structural reticence about displacing the midwife in the
birthing chamber throughout the eighteenth and the early nineteenth centuries. Unlike London, where man-midwife practitioners quickly incorporated
natural births into their repertoire of practice, the impediments to such a development in Leipzig were both structural and medico-cultural. In the early
decades of the eighteenth century, some of the conditions that were conducive
to the English experience were certainly present. There was a strong culture
of client-led and domestic medical care, from which midwifery was not ex-
empt, as well as a growing number of male practitioners with an interest in
obstetrics. And it was increasingly the procedure of birth itself, rather than the
attendant non-mechanical aspects of midwifery that were becoming the stuff
of academic and non-academic obstetric discourse. However, the strong civic
organisation of midwifery meant that the Leipzig Council was interested in
protecting and nurturing the occupational interests of its midwives. Like many
other urban authorities across Germany, it opted for increased training as a
solution to the problems of maternal and infant mortality. This insistence on
training served to reinforce the existing organisational structure of midwifery
and the status of the midwife as the main (but no longer the sole) practitioner
of childbirth. It also encouraged a more rigid delineation of an older division
of labour between midwives and male surgeons based on the emergency to a
new one that revolved around natural and unnatural births.
    The newer division of labour fitted in very nicely with the traditional cor-
porate model of medical practice, which segregated the mind (physicians)
from the hands (midwives, surgeons and other irregular practitioners). The
Stadtaccoucheurs appointed to train the midwives, generally physicians with
an active interest in obstetrics, were largely reluctant practitioners of midwifery. They saw themselves first and foremost as teachers. They considered it
their task to equip the city's midwives with the skills to deal with easy and the
many difficult births and to train them to know when an operative intervention would be necessary. Thus in Leipzig the emphasis on instruction and its
formalisation served to delineate and embed the division of labour between
male and female practitioners in the birthing chamber in more concrete
terms. However, in so doing, it ensured a greater degree of continuity than
change. In effect, the midwife's status within the traditional medical model
was shored up, not depleted, by the reforms to midwifery in the eighteenth
century. Around 1800, we find evidence that women in Leipzig were beginning to engage male practitioners in parallel with midwives when they fore-

---

151 Ibid., 18r.

saw a difficult delivery. Yet even in major urban centres such as Leipzig, midwives would never resign their place in the birthing chamber to the same extent that they did in parts of England. This division of labour was disrupted (but not dismantled) in the latter nineteenth century when male practitioners began to incorporate normal births into their everyday practice.

Chapter Seven

The 'Difficult Birth' of Clinical Midwifery

In March 1764 the Leipzig Stadtaccoucheur Johann Karl Gehler submitted his proposal for a *Hebammeninstitut* (midwifery institute) to the Leipzig Council. Gehler's plans were not novel. Just prior to this, the lazarette surgeon Johann George Hebenstreit had tendered his own suggestions for improving conditions in the city's lazarette at the Rannstädter Tor. Amongst other things, Hebenstreit included suggestions for improving the 'Accouchement' (confinement) in the city. 'As has been custom until now', he explained, 'all whores give birth and lie in under the so-called Beifrauen and Gaßen Mägden in return for a fee'. As an alternative, Hebenstreit suggested that indigent pregnant women be admitted into the eight 'completely vacant' rooms in the lazarette quarantine house two or three weeks prior to delivery, paying their keep through spinning and sewing.[1]

Although he argued that such a set-up would provide medical students, surgeons and midwives with the opportunity for practical instruction in the art of midwifery, Hebenstreit was not only concerned with improving obstetric training.[2] The current arrangements meant that unwed women who delivered their children in the homes of the Beifrauen and Gassenmägde were hired out as wet nurses 'whether or not they are suited to this as long as those persons [the Beifrauen and Gassenmägde] find advantage therein'.[3] The 'institution' in question would 'be of never-ending benefit for the city' because it would combat the vagaries of finding a wet nurse 'without illness and having been found to be able in breastfeeding a child'. Such a move would also reap praise from the community, he explained, for 'how many families made unhappy by unhealthy and unclean wet nurses would admire Your Magnificence's fatherly provision and ordinances, and those who escape their unhappiness through this [measure] will thank those very same with the greatest of reverence.'[4] In spite of both Hebenstreit's and Gehler's efforts, it would be a further four decades before a designated maternity hospital was established in Leipzig – a 'prequel' to the maternity hospital narrative that has been largely ignored by histories of the Triersches Institut thus far.[5] This chapter will explore why it took so long in such an economically and intellectually important city such as Leipzig for this proposal to bear fruit. As I argue here, this delay reveals a great deal about the dynamics of the relationship between the territorial gov-

---

1   StadtAL, Stift. I. 3, 1–21, 'Acta, Die von dem Lazareth=Chirurgo Johann George Hebenstreiten gethanen Vorschläge, zu Verbesserung des hiesigen Lazareths betr. 1764', (c. March) 1764, 2r.
2   Ibid. Also discussed in Schlenkrich, *Von Leuten*, 117–18.
3   Stift. I. 3, 1–21, 'Hebenstreit Vorschläge Lazareth', (c. March) 1764, 2r.
4   Ibid., 2v.
5   Fahrenbach, 'Johann Gottfried'; Sabine Fahrenbach and Heiko Leske, 'Immer zum Wohle der Patientinnen … die Frauenklinik im Wandel der Zeiten', *Gesundheit und mehr* 9 (2007): 4–5.

ernment and Leipzig University, on the one hand, and the Leipzig Council, on the other. And it forces us to reassess the importance of maternity hospitals for the reform of midwifery during the eighteenth century for, as we will see, contemporaries did not all consider these institutions as deserving of a place within the structures of urban midwifery.

Maternity hospitals in Germany and Europe

The few studies that engage with the pre-history of the German maternity hospitals suggest that their foundation was often fraught with cultural and financial difficulties. The Jena maternity hospital, for example, took seven years to build because citizens, who were concerned that such an institution would destroy local customs, refused to provide the necessary funding.[6] Tight-pursed territorial rulers were also to blame. The director of the Marburg maternity hospital, for example, spent two years petitioning his patron for additional funds before finally being granted only half of the annual budget he requested.[7] Tracing the protracted and 'difficult' birth of the Leipzig maternity hospital not only exposes financial obstacles; it reveals the variant values the Leipzig Council, the Leipzig University and the Saxon government saw in such an institution. Although all were generally concerned about depopulation and the necessity of improving midwifery, they did not all agree on how this was to be achieved. As we shall see, where the University saw the opportunity to teach practical obstetrics, the Leipzig Council feared yet another expensive and unnecessary public institution that threatened to rival its own system of midwifery provision. The idea of ramping up midwife education was popular on a local and a territorial level as well as within academic and Enlightenment circles.[8] However, the maternity hospital was only one instrument – admittedly highly visible and prestigious – amongst many deployed by territorial and local governments alike to improve midwifery provision.[9] It is the rub between these various visions that I will explore in this chapter.

Maternity hospitals were one of the cutting-edge medical-institutional inventions of the mid-eighteenth century and have been variously credited with raising the prestige of obstetrics and creating an academic, male-dominated

6   Stefan Wolter, "'… zwinget mich nicht dahin zu gehen, wo ich aller Schamhaftigkeit vergeßen sein soll". Aus den Anfängen der Jenaer Entbindungsanstalt', in Loytved, ed., *Von der Wehemutter*, 83–84.

7   Metz-Becker, *Der verwaltete Körper*, 107–11.

8   On the international networks of obstetric reform, see Jürgen Schlumbohm, 'Mütter und Kinder retten: Geburtshilfe und Entbindungshospitäler im 18. und frühen 19. Jahrhundert – europäische Netze und lokale Vielfalt', in Hans Erich Bödeker and Martin Gierl, eds, *Jenseits der Diskurse. Aufklärungspraxis und Institutionenwelt in europäisch komparativer Perspektive* (Göttingen: Vandenhoeck & Ruprecht, 2007), 323–24.

9   As has been noted by ibid., 338.

discipline out of traditional midwifery.[10] There was some lag following the establishment of the first maternity hospital in Strasbourg in 1728, however, from 1750 onwards, midwifery schools began sprouting up all over the Germanies.[11] By 1836, all German universities could boast a maternity hospital.[12] The Strasbourg maternity hospital proved a seminal learning hub for later Accoucheurs throughout Europe, of which Johann Karl Gehler was one.[13] Unlike the Strasbourg maternity hospital, which opened as a private institution within one of the city's municipal hospitals, most of the German institutions belonged to university medical faculties. The earliest maternity hospitals were established in Göttingen (1751) and Berlin (1751). They were provisional, often consisting of little more than a few rooms and a very light throughput of women.[14] It was not until the 1770s and 1780s that the maternity hospital became more ubiquitous, with Bamberg (1773), Jena (1779), Hanover (1781), Munich (1791) and Marburg (1791) amongst the first cities to follow the trend.[15] Around the same time existing maternity wards, such as that in Göttingen, were enlarged or rebuilt to cater for greater numbers of patients and personnel.[16]

Maternity hospitals across Europe in the eighteenth and nineteenth centuries demonstrated great variation with respect to function and size. They often fulfilled a socio-moral function and were built to both combat illegitimacy and save the lives of children borne out of wedlock. Not infrequently, they were

---

10   Metz-Becker, *Der verwaltete Körper;* Jürgen Schlumbohm, 'Der Blick des Arztes oder: Wie Gebärende zu Patientinnen wurden. Das Entbindungshospital der Universität Göttingen um 1800', in Jürgen Schlumbohm et al., eds, *Rituale der Geburt. Eine Kulturgeschichte* (Munich: Verlag C. H. Beck, 1998).

11   For an overview, see Carl-Joseph Gauß and Bernhard Wilde, *Die Deutschen Geburtshelferschulen. Bausteine zur Geschichte der Geburtshilfe* (Munich-Gräfeling: Banaschewski, 1956); Schlumbohm, 'Mütter und Kinder retten', esp. 334–43; Axel Karenberg, 'Lernen am Bett der Schwangeren. Zur Typologie des Entbindungshauses in Deutschland (1728–1840)', *Zentralblatt für Gynäkologie* 113 (1991): 899–912. For a comprehensive history of the first German maternity hospital in Göttingen, see Schlumbohm, *Lebendige Phantome.* For Berlin, see Loytved, 'Zur Gründung'. On Jena, see Wolter, 'Jenaer Entbindungsanstalt'.

12   Schlumbohm, 'Mütter und Kinder retten', 335.

13   The maternity hospital in Strasbourg was under the direction of Johann Jacob Fried. See Karenberg, 'Lernen', 899–903.

14   The Göttingen maternity hospital was in fact two rooms located in the city's medieval hospice, which cared for elderly persons. The average number of deliveries per year ranged between ten and thirty. See Schlumbohm, '"The Pregnant Women"', 62.

15   Gauß and Wilde, *Geburtshelferschulen,* 22 and 45. Gauß differentiates between maternity hospitals established within universities and those set up specifically to teach midwives. This demarcation, however, is not particularly useful as midwives tended to be trained within both, and obstetricians were not always blocked from attending the midwifery schools.

16   The new Göttingen edifice was a designated and politically representative building, catering to fourteen mothers at a time as well as housing all staff and apprentice midwives. See Schlumbohm, 'Practice', 4. See also '"The Pregnant Women"'.

constructed within or adjunct to existing orphanages.[17] Some, such as the midwife-run hospital of the Port-Royal in Paris, were devoted entirely to the training of midwives.[18] Physicians and surgeons seeking practical instruction in obstetrics had been banned from the Port-Royal since the early eighteenth century on the grounds that their presence hindered the aim of the hospital, which was to provide poor pregnant women with obstetric assistance.[19] In the large Viennese maternity hospital, the care of mothers and babies had precedence over the training of both medical students and midwives. Only a small number of trainee midwives and medical students (in relation to the large facilities) was admitted to the three-month-long courses. Their practical-pedagogical activities on live female patients were strictly limited to the preliminary examination during a woman's admission.[20]

The English lying-in hospitals, founded in the mid-eighteenth century as charitable institutions for the sick and lame poor, were designed to cater for and support the honourable poor and had no such blatant medical-pedagogical intentions. Funded through charitable contributions from the community, they had to appeal to ideas about the importance of urban charity and the morality of the poor. Many, such as the Middlesex Lying-In Hospital (opened in 1747), did not admit unmarried women, even when the hospital introduced domiciliary obstetric assistance in 1765.[21] Although two male obstetricians ran the Middlesex Hospital, male medical students and surgical apprentices were banned from attending births. No female midwife training took place in the hospital until 1758, a move that contemporaries claimed would serve to inculcate the use of man-midwives amongst female midwives.[22]

The German maternity hospitals, in particular those located in the Protestant regions, grew out of very different goals and ideals. Most were intended as spaces for training midwives and obstetricians. The welfare of destitute women was often an afterthought. In Göttingen, for example, the professor of obstetrics and director of the University maternity hospital, Friedrich Benjamin Osiander (1759–1822), maintained in 1800 that the hospital was first and foremost an institution for training skilled obstetricians 'worthy of the name of *Geburtshelfer*' (obstetrician). Its secondary function, he continued, was to train

17   For the charitable and social emphasis, see Seidel, *Neue Kultur*, 232–39. Metz-Becker, on the other hand, emphasises their role as places in which knowledge of the female body was pursued and the hegemony of the medical profession strengthened. See Metz-Becker, *Der verwaltete Körper*, 73–89, esp. 73.

18   Scarlett Beauvalet-Boutouyrie, 'Die Chef-Hebamme: Herz und Seele Pariser Entbindungshospitals von Port-Royal im 19. Jahrhundert', in Jürgen Schlumbohm et al., eds, *Rituale der Geburt. Eine Kulturgeschichte* (Munich: Verlag C.H. Beck, 1998); Schlumbohm, '"The Pregnant Women"', 63.

19   Beauvalet-Boutouyrie, 'Die Chef-Hebamme', 232–33; Seidel, *Neue Kultur*, 234–35.

20   The director of the Viennese maternity hospital, J. M. Boër, was a strict anti-interventionist and proponent of letting nature take its course where possible. His intellectual nemesis was the director of the Göttingen maternity hospital. See *Neue Kultur*, 236.

21   Bronwyn Croxson, 'The Foundation and Evolution of the Middlesex Hospital's Lying-In Service, 1745–86', *Social History of Medicine* 14: 1 (2001): 27–57, 36–37 and 43.

22   Ibid., 37.

midwives 'who distinguish themselves by their knowledge and their skills, as compared to ordinary midwives'. Last (and least), the Göttingen maternity hospital was designed as a 'safe shelter' for both wed and unwed indigent pregnant women during childbirth and lying-in that would 'grant them every support and help that might be required to maintain them and their children'.[23]

The emphasis on training and research that made the German lying-in hospitals so unique in the European context was due in part to the fact that they were established by the medical faculties for the purposes of instructing their own students. Dissatisfaction amongst many students and graduates with the training on offer in the major maternity hospitals in Vienna and Paris, meant that the German maternity hospitals were also responding to the demands of students.[24] In fact there was little that was 'charitable' about the German lying-in hospitals. They were not designed to reinforce morality or reward the deserving poor. As a place of learning-by-doing, in which men and women practised on live material, the German maternity hospitals appealed to a very particular clientele – the 'whore' ('Hure') whose social value was low and moral propriety almost non-existent.[25] These institutions had no ambitions as mainstream childbirthing spaces serving the community and its poor.

The Stadtaccoucheur plans a 'Hebammeninstitut'

After hearing of Hebenstreit's plans for the lazarette, Stadtaccoucheur Gehler raged indignantly against 'this presumptuous and meddlesome interference in the office incumbent on [him]'.[26] Yet in terms of its content, his own proposal differed but little from that of his rival. Gehler envisioned a midwifery institute in Leipzig that functioned as a training ground in the art of midwifery for medical students and midwives, modelled closely on the Strasbourg maternity hospital. He did not see the future Leipzig midwifery institute as a charitable institution for assisting indigent women and reducing the rates of infanticide. For Gehler, these women were first and foremost learning material.[27] The 'whores', he reasoned, were to be lured into their beds and would gladly take up the offer of a warm room and 'good care' in return for 'submitting themselves to the discomforts, which these days … are unavoidable as even during the birth several persons must be present'.[28] The task of the midwives and Accoucheur was not to 'help the labouring women in the hours of their delivery' but much more so to learn, that is 'to know and recognise the three differ-

---

23 Jürgen Schlumbohm, '"The Pregnant Women"', 63.
24 Seidel touches only very briefly on this. See Seidel, *Neue Kultur*, 236.
25 On the patients of these maternity hospitals, see Metz-Becker, *Der verwaltete Körper*, 145–83; Schlumbohm, *Lebendige Phantome*, 269–315.
26 Tit. (F) XLIV.D.2a, 10–13, 'Gehler's proposal re: midwifery institute', 19 March 1764, 10r.
27 See Item 2 of ibid., 11r.
28 See Item 2 of ibid.

ent changes in the belly of a pregnant woman, in particular those of the inner cervix; in addition to assess the care of women lying in and the newborns'.[29]

The building was to consist of four to five rooms, one of which contained eight beds together with several chairs and tables, and another in which stood two delivery beds or stools. A third room was to accommodate the Accoucheur together with his instruments and medications, and a further room was to house the 'Kindbettwärterin' (confinement nurse), Beifrau or a woman from one of the villages who wished to learn the 'art of midwifery'.[30] A maximum of eight women, four pregnant and four post-parturient, were to be admitted. They were to arrive six weeks prior to the birth and be discharged, pending good health, three weeks postpartum.[31] Whereas for 'honourable' women, confinement marked a period in which household and occupational responsibilities were suspended, these women were to clean, heat, spin and knit all through their stay. The practice of rendering productive the inmates of seventeenth- and eighteenth-century penitentiary institutions, such as the workhouses, orphanages, and some hospices, has been construed elsewhere as a technique of 'social discipline'.[32] Gehler, however, had little interest in social disciplining and inculcating the bourgeois work ethic into his patients. His concerns were largely directed towards the financial stability of the enterprise, for if it were to find favour with the state, the Leipzig Council and the University, it was paramount that the midwifery institute be portrayed as a fiscally efficient unit. The women staying in the midwifery institute were part of the house's oeconomy and were to 'make advantage for the house, each according to her strength', not rest and recover in idleness.[33] Their labour was part of a transaction: food, board and a 'safe' delivery in return for access to their bodies.

Gehler was careful about the way he justified the need to set up such a maternity hospital, well aware that in the 1760s, the idea was comparatively new and only a few such institutions were in existence. Indeed, his proposal marked an attempt to revolutionise a system of midwifery training he found to be quite lacking in any kind of merit. Gehler was unconvinced by the practice established in the early eighteenth century whereby the midwives received weekly lessons in obstetric theory at the hands of the Stadtaccoucheur. So much so that he failed to hold lessons for the midwives during most of his

---

29 See Item 3 of ibid., 11v.
30 See Item 10 of ibid., 13v.
31 See Item 3 of ibid., 11v.
32 Such as the Waldheim workhouse in Saxony. See Falk Bretschneider, 'Fürsorge oder Disziplinierung? Die Armen und das Waldheimer Zuchthaus im 18. Jahrhundert', in Helmut Bräuer, ed., *Arme – ohne Chance? Protocoll der internationalen Tagung "Kommunale Armut und Armutsbekämpfung vom Spätmittelalter bis zur Gegenwart" vom 23. bis 25. Oktober 2003 in Leipzig* (Leipzig: Leipziger Universitätsverlag, 2004).
33 See Item 4 of Tit. (F) XLIV.D.2a, 10–13, 'Gehler's proposal re: midwifery institute', 19 March 1764, 11v.

time as Stadtaccoucheur.[34] However, he recognised that there was considerable reluctance to back such a plan within the Council and amongst the burghers, who regarded the 'usefulness that might grow out of a nursery for good and sensible Accoucheurs and midwives, not just in all of Saxony, but also in the other cities and localities in Germany ... [as] somewhat unnecessary'.[35] To make matters worse, the city had been all but financially ruined through the Seven Years War. The problem was to put forward his proposal for such a massive project without slurring his own employer and the current state of midwifery in the city. Gehler achieved this by feigning applause for the 'courses for instructing the local midwives in our city which have redounded to the greatest fame [of our city], and have been endorsed and praised by everyone as a so [very] convincing example of the patriotic sensibilities that aim to [nurture] the true welfare of the citizens'.[36] Then he played the rural card: How unfortunate it was, claimed Gehler, that this marvellous method of training midwives could not provide the nearby villages with the same benefits.[37]

Whilst Gehler's arguments appealed to contemporary concerns that rural midwifery was a veritable black hole of superstition and incompetence, (an idea that would give impetus to establishing the Sanitätskollegium a few years later), they were unable to move the Leipzig Council to agree to establish a maternity hospital in Leipzig. Meanwhile in Dresden, the Collegium Medico-Chirurgicum (College of Medical Surgeons, CM) succeeded in setting up a midwifery school and maternity hospital in 1774.[38] In 1781 the Landtag assumed control of the midwifery school and ennobled it to the status of 'Landesentbindungsschule' (territorial midwifery school) for surgeon men-midwives, students of surgery, midwives and military surgeons. It was officially merged into the Collegium Medico-Chirurgicum in 1785.[39]

The Dresden midwifery school, which in 1782 could accommodate twelve women, was first and foremost a teaching facility. Midwives and male medical students were taught midwifery techniques on the 'phantom'. Surgical procedures such as caesarean sections, however, were only carried out by male medical students.[40] Midwife candidates undertook a six-month course of training.[41] In spite of its location, the Dresden midwifery school remained a relatively parochial institution, serving the city of Dresden and the surrounding coun-

---

34 Several Beifrauen complained about this in the 1780s and it was also noted by Gehler's successor Pohl. See Tit. (F) XLIV.D.6b, Bd. I, 233–44, 'LC minutes re: instruction of midwives', 15 April 1782.

35 Tit. (F) XLIV.D.2a, 10–13, 'Gehler's proposal re: midwifery institute', 19 March 1764, 10r.

36 Ibid.

37 See Item 1 of ibid., 10v.

38 Klimpel, *Das Dresdner CM*, 100.

39 Ibid., 96–97.

40 The midwifery school had an average annual throughput of between 140 and 160 women. See ibid., 101.

41 Ibid., 98.

tryside. There is no evidence to suggest that Leipzig's midwives attended the Dresden midwifery school, nor did it occur to either the Leipzig Council or its medical officials to send its aspirant midwives to Dresden.

On the contrary, the Leipzig Council was generally satisfied with the status quo and saw no immediate need to establish a maternity hospital. Arguments against the establishment of such an institution revolved, not least, around funding. In Dresden, every Taler spent on the maternity hospital, despite its rather spartan facilities, had been hard fought.[42] With both the communal and private treasuries in a desolate condition following the financial plunder exacted by the Prussians during the Seven Years War, Leipzig was financially bereft. As we shall see, the Council was unwilling to add to the already considerable cost of a – in their eyes at least – fully functional, even exemplary, system of midwifery provision.

Midwifery in the lazarette

The idea of training midwives in a clinical setting was not unheard of in Leipzig. The sworn midwife at the Rannstädter Tor and her Beifrau were unofficially accorded responsibility for delivering pregnant women in the lazarette around 1725. The *Lazarettarzt* (lazarette doctor) Professor Michael Ernst Etmüller (simultaneously ordinary professor of pathology in the Leipzig Medical Faculty 1724–25) reported an incident to the Council: an 'unclean woman' had given birth in the lazarette but it had been impossible to enlist the assistance of any of the sworn midwives or Beifrauen, who all feared scaring off or infecting their clientele. The midwives, Etmüller conveyed, were uneasy about preparing clysters for 'unclean' female patients, but he added that it was not reasonable to expect apothecary or barber-surgeon apprentices to carry out a task that was beneath them. Hence he suggested that a Beifrau or midwife candidate be employed in the lazarette specifically for this purpose.[43] As no record of the Council's response to Ettmüller's suggestions could be found, it is difficult to ascertain whether his recommendation was heeded immediately. By the 1780s, however, the midwife at the Rannstädter Tor was also officially responsible for women in the lazarette.

Built by the Leipzig Council in the 1560s as a plague hospital, by the 1630s the lazarette (located just outside the Rannstädter Tor) had developed into a general all-purpose hospital funded by both the city's poor relief and charitable contributions.[44] In the early eighteenth century it was also a place of refuge for unwed, indigent and homeless pregnant women.[45] Some histori-

---

42 Ibid., 100–1.
43 Tit. (F) XLIV.D.1, 83–118, 'Appointments (Greger and Veiß)', 22 November 1724–4 September 1725, 117–18.
44 Schlenkrich, *Von Leuten*, 27–29.
45 Schlenkrich has documented two cases of women seeking assistance in the lazarette from 1721 and 1719. See ibid., 113–14.

ans have painted a picture of these lazarettes depicting them as places of destitution and suffering that the general public did its best to avoid.[46] According to Elke Schlenkrich, fear of 'unclean' women amongst both midwives and their clients turned the Leipzig lazarette into a repository for diseased, socially marginal pregnant women because midwives often refused such women a place to give birth and lie in within their own lodgings.[47] And yet the fact that the Council assigned the midwives and Beifrauen serving the general community to the lazarette suggests a less critical view of the hospital held by contemporaries. Whereas the Council had previously appointed a plague midwife whose duties entailed the exclusive care of women in plague households, it chose not to 'quarantine' its midwifery services in the same way for the purposes of the lazarette.[48] And whilst fear of contagion persisted within the community, the lazarette appears to have been viewed increasingly as a social and medical aid – at least from the point of view of medical officers and the Leipzig Council.[49] However, it is important to remember that this development was not some programmatic initiative on the part of the Council or the Saxon government, but instead a single solution to a particular and immediate problem: the incidence of pregnant women giving birth in the lazarette.

In 1785, soon after he took over Johann Karl Gehler's office as Stadtaccoucheur, Johann Ehrenfried Pohl set about formalising the position of the lazarette midwife and institutionalising the training of new Beifrauen within the lazarette. Although the duties in the lazarette had been informally added to the office of midwife and Beifrau at the Rannstädter Tor, Pohl remarked that the instructions for both offices had not been amended, leading to quarrelling and 'resistance' amongst the city's midwives about whose task it was to attend the women there.[50] Like his predecessor Gehler, Pohl was a professor of the Medical Faculty and, like his mentor, he was an adamant proponent of establishing a maternity hospital in Leipzig. 'As we unfortunately still lack such a practical, and for this science so indispensable institution', he lamented in 1785, the training of new Beifrauen in the lazarette presented 'the only way through which we may train skilled midwives'.[51] In order to effect change at

---

46 The argument goes that most early modern people treated illness within the home and hospitals were strongly linked to destitution and epidemics. See, for example, Elke Schlenkrich, 'Johann Gregor Gurtthoff. Vom Leben und von der Arbeit eines (Pest)barbiers im 17. Jahrhundert', *Medizin, Gesellschaft und Geschichte. Jahrbuch des Instituts für Geschichte der Medizin* 21 (2003): 23–62.

47 *Von Leuten*, 113–14.

48 In Dresden the local authorities had formalised the activities of the midwife who attended women incarcerated in the city's lazarette by creating the office of *Lazareth Wehmutter* (lazarette midwife) in 1743. A plague midwife, however, had been associated with the lazarette in Dresden since at least the sixteenth century. See ibid., 115.

49 This ties in with Brockliss' and Jones' argument, which challenged the Enlightenment's 'black legend' of the hospital as a place of insalubrity and posited it instead as a medical aid. See Brockliss and Jones, *Medical World*, 717–29.

50 See Pohl's report from 22 December 1785 in Tit. (F) XLIV.D.6b, Bd. II, 53–62, 'Appointment (Gentsch)', 12 November–9 December 1785, 59–61.

51 Ibid.

some small level, Pohl requested that the Council insert an additional paragraph into the instruction of the new sworn midwife at the Rannstädter Tor,
obliging her to take her Beifrau along to each pregnant and parturient woman
lodging in the lazarette. This way, the midwife would provide the new Beifrau
'with the opportunity to acquire knowledge of palpating or the examination of
pregnant women as well as in practical aspects of obstetrics in order to have
her remain a skilled midwife for the future'.[52] Although Pohl clearly saw the
lazarette as a means of 'providing them [the Beifrauen] with the opportunity
to put the theoretical instruction received from [him] into practice', the practical training of the city's Beifrauen in the lazarette continued to take place
within the midwife–apprentice relationship and Beifrauen remained under
the direct supervision of their allocated midwife within the lazarette.[53] The
service provided by the lazarette remained small-scale and by the end of the
eighteenth century, only around seventeen illegitimate children born in the
Leipzig lazarette were baptised each year (in the church of St Thomas).[54]

Pohl's 'reforms' created problems for his successor, Christian Adolph
Hartwig, who assumed the office of Stadtaccoucheur in Leipzig when Pohl
was called to Dresden as electoral court counsel and personal physician to the
Saxon Elector in 1788.[55] Hartwig had graduated from Leipzig University in
1783 and had since established himself as a surgeon man-midwife in the city.[56]
He had no other official ties to the University or the Medical Faculty as professor or otherwise. Unlike his predecessor Pohl, Hartwig was not particularly
interested in lobbying the Council for a maternity hospital. In 1789 he thought
it unnecessary to establish a 'Hebammenanstalt' (midwifery institution), as he
was generally satisfied with the progress he had been making with the midwives in his weekly lessons.[57] Whilst Hartwig admitted that the younger Beifrauen were 'fairly behind' – partly because Pohl had been unable to complete
his course of instruction prior to his departure for Dresden and partly because
these Beifrauen lacked 'the experience so necessary in this vocation' – he assured the Council that by resuming lessons and through greater experience,
these Beifrauen would become 'good and useable midwives'.[58] For the midwives 'in the middle years' he could 'notice the consequences of good instruc-

---

52 Ibid.
53 Ibid. The Council ratified Pohl's suggestions and amended the instructions for the mid-
    wife and the Beifrau at the Rannstädter Tor on 9 December 1785. See ibid., 61–62.
54 Schlenkrich bases this figure on the invoice for baptismal expenses presented to the
    Leipzig Council by the lazarette overseer Justus Heinrich Hansen in 1799. However, this
    number does not take into account stillbirths or premature births. Hence the number of
    actual deliveries is probably much higher than 17. See Schlenkrich, *Von Leuten*, 116.
55 See entry for Johann Ehrenfried Pohl in Ulrich von Hehl, *Professorenkatalog der Universität
    Leipzig*, available at <http://uni-leipzig.de/unigeschichte/professorenkatalog/>, accessed
    26 October 2016.
56 See entry for Hartwig in Hirsch, ed., *Biographisches Lexikon*, vol. 3, 73.
57 Tit. (F) XLIV.D.6b, 76–97, 'Stadtaccoucheur reports (Hartwig)', c. 21 April 1788–28 March
    1791, 76–79.
58 Ibid.

tion ... very clearly, so much so that there is likely no other city that is better provided for on this point'.[59] Hartwig was a committed supporter of the method of training midwives that had been in place in Leipzig for most of the century and he retained his viewpoint on theoretical instruction at the hands of the Stadtaccoucheur and practical training within the midwife–Beifrau relationship until his death in 1791.

Hartwig encountered only one problem: ensuring that the Beifrau apprenticed to the lazarette midwife actually attended his courses. As Hartwig explained to the Council in 1789, since Pohl had obliged the Beifrau at the Rannstädter Tor to attend every birth carried out by her midwife, this Beifrau's workload had increased beyond what was normal for the other Beifrauen in the city. Furthermore, because the midwife at the Rannstädter Tor was ailing, the Beifrau (Mrs Gentsch), was carrying out most, if not all, of the sickly midwife's work.[60] A few months later the underlying tension between using the lazarette as a training institution for new midwives and maintaining the established old order of midwifery became even more apparent – but not just because the lazarette was feared by the midwives. The practice of allocating the newest Beifrau to the midwife at the Rannstädter Tor and the lazarette for training had proved largely incompatible with the traditional relationship between a Beifrau and her midwife-teacher, in which the Beifrau functioned as both a servant/apprentice and, later on, as a 'pension fund'. Mrs Behnhold, the midwife at the Rannstädter Tor, 'complains about constantly having new Beifrauen, who she is always having to train up and then let go, whereby she is also always required to be present in person in the lazarette, which would be very burdensome for anyone'.[61]

Whilst midwife Behnhold was obviously unhappy about the workload as a result of her new responsibility as the dedicated teacher of new Beifrauen, the problem was principally financial. The new instruction had turned an economic and pedagogical relationship into a largely pedagogical one. As we have seen, the sworn midwives relied on their Beifrauen for part of their income. Especially in old age and illness they would rely utterly on their Beifrau for their entitled 'living'. When a midwife became incapacitated, her Beifrau would ideally take on the midwife's clientele as a 'vice midwife' and the ailing midwife would skim a livelihood off her Beifrau's earnings. As Chapter Four showed, these were the terms of livelihood that governed the office of midwife in the early modern period. Mrs Behnhold, for example, was 'always ill and even bed-bound' and 'could have no use for a yet completely inexperienced Beifrau'.[62]

As a solution to this conundrum, Hartwig proposed a compromise that would ease the pressure exerted by this new concept of midwife training on

---

59   Ibid.
60   Ibid.
61   See Hartwig's report from 13 June 1789 in Tit. (F) XLIV.D.6b, Bd. II, 79–84, 'Appointment (Mehmel and Ulrich)', 27 April–7 July 1789, 82–83.
62   Ibid.

the dependent relationship between the midwife and her Beifrau in the lazarette. Midwife Behnhold was to retain her trusted Beifrau Mrs Gentsch, but all
the newly appointed Beifrauen should be made to attend deliveries carried
out by both Behnhold *and* Gentsch. The new Beifrauen should 'practice examining and touching and also not just be present at the births whenever they
are not needed by their midwives, but bit by bit ... attend these [births] under
the supervision of Mrs Behnhold ... or also Mrs Gentsch ... and deliver on
their own'.[63] This, Hartwig concluded, would enable the Beifrauen 'to gradually put into practice that which I have but only been able to teach them in
theory'.[64] Hartwig's compromise attempted to accommodate practical 'clinical' education for new Beifrauen without dismantling the apprenticeship
structure of midwife training and the economic dependencies inherent within
the midwife–Beifrau relationship. Although he certainly recognised that not
all new Beifrauen had the opportunity of gaining practical experience at the
hand of their midwives (often, he remarked, because of personal grudges),
Hartwig did not deem it necessary to reform the system of training per se. He
was careful to preserve the structures of entitlement, livelihood and obligation
that characterised early modern work and early modern midwifery.[65]

Renewing plans for a 'Hebammeninstitut'

Prior to taking over the office of Stadtaccoucheur from his mentor Gehler in
1782, Johann Ehrenfried Pohl launched a renewed effort to put the idea of an
'institute designated for the training of aspiring midwives' back on the political agenda.[66] This time, however, the proposal was backed by the Medical
Faculty, in which Pohl had been professor of botany since 1773. Pohl's 'Hebammeninstitut' was designed to bear fruit exclusively for the Saxon state and
for science. Since his appointment as Amtsphysicus in 1780 and his subsequent activities as Stadtaccoucheur Gehler's assistant, Pohl professed to have
witnessed cases in which 'through the ignorance of midwives and due to their
lack of necessary assistance, mother and child, whose lives may have been
saved, lost their lives'.[67] 'According to my modest understanding', Pohl continued, 'this evil will be bowed [avoided] and skilled midwives and obstetricians
educated for the various regions in this Your Mighty Land, if instruction in
that necessary theoretical knowledge were to be combined with the practical

---

63   Ibid.
64   See Hartwig's report from 13 June 1789 in ibid.
65   Hartwig reported in 1789 that the youngest Beifrau had only actively delivered two or
     three times despite having held her office for one-and-a-half years. He then commented
     that there were so many 'private matters' between the midwives and Beifrauen that gave
     the midwives reason not to take their Beifrauen along with them to births. See ibid.
66   UAL, Med. Fak. A IIId, Bd. 01 (Film Nr. 1334), 'Rescripte der Regierung Dresden und
     diesbezügliche Berichte über das Hebammenwesen (1772–83)', 52r–53, 'Letter from Jo-
     hann Pohl to Saxon government', 25 April 1781.
67   Ibid., 52v.

instruction in obstetrics in a designated institute'.[68] By teaching the midwives 'important terms in the treatment of pregnant women and those in confinement', such an 'Institute' would have the 'most excellent use' of lowering mortality which caused the state 'unending damage'.[69] It was a matter of 'practical' education as an elixir for the ills of the Saxon state.

Pohl's proposal was embraced enthusiastically by the Saxon government in Dresden as 'so desirable as well as charitable for the common [good]' as it would train 'skilful obstetricians and midwives for the entire state and be of particular use for the rural man'.[70] Yet words were cheap. Although the volume of correspondence between the Saxon government, the Sanitätskollegium, the Leipzig Medical Faculty and the Leipzig Council grew over the following years, the midwifery institute remained little more than ink on paper. At the heart of the problem was the question of where to locate the midwifery institute. Whilst the Sanitätskollegium suggested integrating it into one of Leipzig's existing hospitals, as had been done successfully in Dresden, the Medical Faculty preferred to accommodate it in the Pleißenburg castle, which housed the headquarters of the Leipzig Amt. The Council refused to accept either proposal and pressed the Saxon government to agree to buy 'a somewhat roomier house in a healthy location' or to erect a brand new institute.[71] The details of the Leipzig Council's objections of 1781 are detailed in a later letter from the Council dated 1786. The Council opposed the hospital solution on the grounds that such institutions accommodated in part 'lunatics … many punishable criminals … military, sick men and women … so that we cannot see before us the possibility of combining such an institute with one of these hospitals'. As for the Pleißenburg, this was a security hazard as the tax office was housed there and the rest of the castle was used for storing grain.[72] As a result of the gridlock, nothing happened.

Five years later, in 1786, Dr Pohl and the Medical Faculty relaunched their offensive.[73] In light of the Leipzig Council's objection to both the Medical Faculty's and the Sanitätskollegium's proposed locations, the Saxon government requested both the Council and the Leipzig Amt find a suitable property.[74]

---

68   Ibid.
69   Ibid., 53r.
70   Med. Fak. A IIId, Bd. 01 (Film Nr. 1334), 'Rescripte der Regierung Dresden und diesbezügliche Berichte über das Hebammenwesen (1772–83)', 39–40, 'Report from Saxon government re: the midwifery institute in Leipzig', 18 December 1783, 40r.
71   The location conundrum was mentioned in the Saxon government's report from 18 December 1783. See ibid., 39r.
72   StadtAL, Tit. (F) XLIV.D.8a, Bd. I, 'Acta, die Einrichtung eines Hebammen-Instituts alhier betr. Anno 1786', 17–18, 'Letter from Leipzig council to Saxon government re: the midwifery institute (draft)', 30 October 1786, 17a and 18r.
73   The Saxon government sent the Leipzig Council a letter (including Pohl's plans) regarding the midwifery institute in Leipzig. See Tit. (F) XLIV.D.7, 'Acta, die Errichtung eines Hebammen-Instituts alhier betr.', 1–2, 'Letter from Saxon government to Leipzig Council re: the midwife institute', 14 September 1786, 1–2.
74   Tit. (F) XLIV.D.7, 'Acta, die Errichtung eines Hebammen-Instituts alhier betr.', 61–62, 'Letter from Saxon government to Leipzig Council', 6 September 1787; Tit. (F)

Neither responded to this letter. Four increasingly insistent inquiries on the part of the Saxon government in 1788, 1789, 1790 and 1791 faced the same fate.[75] Finally, in the summer of 1791, the Leipzig Council informed the Saxon government in Dresden that it had been unable to locate an appropriate house and hence, could not provide Dresden with a purchase price. The Council laid the blame for the situation squarely with Dr Pohl, who had assumed the offices of court counsel and royal physician in Dresden in 1788 and left his Leipzig municipal offices in the hands of deputies. According to the Council 'as long as he had been here, [Pohl had] been unable to hand over anything to us, so that now, should a comfortable house be found, he would hardly be able to deal with the matter'. As a gesture of good will, however, the Council had conferred with its own Stadtphysicus and lazarette surgeon (both of whom it considered experts in obstetrics) and provided estimates of the costs of building and running the planned midwifery institute.[76]

A paucity of available funds, due largely to the fact that there were no bequests from burghers until 1799, was certainly an issue.[77] However, the main reason for the very protracted process of planning lay with the Leipzig Council. In 1791 the Leipzig Council had been successfully stalling the plans of its own Stadtaccoucheurs Gehler and Pohl, the Medical Faculty and the Saxon government for some seventeen years. And it continued to stymie any further attempts for several years more because it was not in the Council's interests to agree to locate a midwifery institute of any sort in Leipzig. The plans to establish a midwifery institute were initiated by the Medical Faculty and backed by both the Saxon government and the Sanitätskollegium. And whilst both Gehler and Pohl, the two main protagonists in this story, were in the salary of the Leipzig Council as Stadtaccoucheurs, they were first and foremost members of the Medical Faculty.[78]

XLIV.D.8a, Bd. I, 'Acta, Die Errichtung eines Hebammen Instituts alhier betr. Anno 1786', 19–20, 'Letter from Saxon government to Amt Leipzig and Leipzig Council', 6 September 1787, 19r.

75 Tit. (F) XLIV.8a, Bd. I, 'Acta, Die Errichtung eines Hebammen Instituts alhier betr. Anno 1786', 21–28, 'Letters from the Saxon government to the Leipzig council re: the midwife institute', 17 March 1788–25 June 1791.

76 Their estimate for the build was 2,880 Taler. Running costs totalled 1,997 Taler per annum. See Tit. (F) XLIV.D.8a, Bd. I, 'Die Errichtung eines Hebammen Instituts alhier betr. anno 1786', 34–37, 'Letter from Leipzig Council to Saxon Government (draft)', 2 August 1791, 34v–35v.

77 In 1799 Johann Wilhelm Richter, court counsel and high judge, left 1,333 Taler to be spent on a midwifery institute and in 1803, the Leipzig burgher, book dealer and chamber commissioner Christian Andreas Leich bequeathed 20,000 Taler for the same purpose. Following this, the Landrat (in Dresden) authorised the building of a maternity hospital in 1803. See Fahrenbach and Leske, 'Immer zum Wohle der Patientinnen', 4.

78 Both men occupied various municipal and territorial medical offices in addition to their posts in the Leipzig Medical Faculty. Johann Karl Gehler was dean of the Medical Faculty from 1789 until his death in 1796 and Johann Ehrenfried Pohl reached the zenith of his university career as professor ordinarius of therapy in 1796. He died in 1800.

As far as the University was concerned, the proposed midwifery institute would assist the state in maximising its population. It would also serve to bolster the attractiveness of Leipzig University to foreign students for it 'is generally the subject of complaint that no such Institute has been erected, for example in Leipzig, where they [the students] would otherwise happily stay for the purpose of their studies'.[79] A maternity hospital or midwifery institute was a cutting-edge academic facility and a real drawcard for a university because, as Pohl claimed, 'there will never be a lack of people who would give so much if they receive the opportunity ... to deliver women, to which practice always belongs, wherever they are already pursuing their studies'.[80] The Medical Faculty dreamed of acquiring a reputation equal to the maternity hospitals of Paris and Strasbourg, to which medical students had flocked since the early eighteenth century.[81] In order to ensure the success and status of the midwifery institute, Pohl and the Medical Faculty suggested that those individuals appointed to municipal or district medical offices – including midwives – should be made to train in Leipzig: 'This would thus bind the people more, and even necessitate the magistrates of smaller districts and cities to send these people here or to any place where such an institute is established in order to take instruction'.[82]

Andre Wakefield has recently argued that cameralism and science were the 'ideology of a desperate fisc; not a tool for technical experts'. Eighteenth-century states supported and founded universities such as Göttingen and mining academies such as those in Saxony, he argues, because the establishment of a state-of-the-art university had the potential to transform a rundown, unprofitable town (such as Göttingen) into a fashionable location that attracted foreign investment and commercial activity.[83] In as much as the proponents of the midwifery school in Leipzig may have truly believed that practical instruction was an indispensable means of acquiring medical knowledge, this new science and its novel setting also brought fiscal advantages for both the University and the Saxon state. Following the disaster and destruction of the Seven Years War and in the spirit of the Saxon Rétablissement, which

---

79   StadtAL, Tit. (F) XLIV.D.7, 'Acta, Die Errichtung eines Hebammen-Instituts alhier betr.', 3–31, 'Johann Ehrenfried Pohl's report on the planned midwifery institute in Leipzig', 1787, 19r–19v.

80   Leipzig had a relatively large medical faculty consisting of between 50 and 60 medical students and 40 surgical students per annum. Pohl intended to train 'only half, which is very few' of all students in obstetrics. See ibid., 23r.

81   Competition was a major driving force in the establishment of maternity hospitals. The Marburg institute, opened in 1792, was part of a general investment in the facilities of the University's medical faculty, including an anatomical institute and a chemical laboratory, to make it competitive and draw greater student numbers. See Metz-Becker, *Der verwaltete Körper*, 104–7. Similarly, the Jena Medical Faculty built its maternity hospital to allow the university to compete with rival medical faculties in Göttingen, Vienna, Berlin and Strasbourg. See Wolter, 'Jenaer Entbindungsanstalt', 82.

82   Tit. (F) XLIV.D.7, 3–31, 'Pohl's report re: midwifery institute', 1787, 24r–24v.

83   Wakefield, *The Disordered Police State*, 48–80.

aimed to reform the territorial government from the ground up, this was just the kind of reinvigoration that Leipzig so much needed.[84]

The Leipzig Council, however, was less enthusiastic about the merits and benefits of a midwifery institute. In 1797 the Council was well aware that the proposed midwifery institute would 'in no way be erected for the city of Leipzig' but that it was entirely for the purposes of the University and, indirectly, the Saxon government. Furthermore, the Council had no particular need of such a training institution as it had 'long ago established the institution, whereby the sworn midwives in the city of Leipzig receive the necessary instruction through a doctor selected by it [the Leipzig Council], who practises obstetrics and who receives a not inconsiderable salary each year'.[85] Although both agreed on the need to improve midwifery, the Council perceived the midwifery institute as a rival, rather than complementary means of training midwives. It feared that the Medical Faculty's plans had the potential to downgrade the status of the city's Stadtaccoucheur Carl Christian Friedrich Menz, appointed in 1792, and the reputation of its midwives. The Council had good reason for airing these concerns; the Medical Faculty of the University in Jena had demanded its maternity hospital be completely separate from the office of the *Provinzaccoucheur* (district surgeon man-midwife). Not only did the Jena Medical Faculty argue that the Provinzaccoucheur's surgical-obstetrical practice would preclude him from holding regular lessons. It also argued that he lacked the 'knowledge' and 'scholarliness' required of a director of a maternity hospital.[86]

Like most other city authorities in eighteenth-century Europe, the Leipzig Council provided largely domiciliary or 'outdoor' medical care and poor relief. Although there were plague houses, hospices for the elderly and orphanages, aside from the ad-hoc accommodation of indigent women in the lazarette, there was no publicly accessible physical space designated for childbirth and lying-in. Midwifery was not just a domestic matter; the care the city's sworn midwives provided was de facto 'outdoor'. For many late Enlightenment medical reformers, indoor medical institutions – in particular those already in existence – were places of destitution and, as Mary Lindemann has shown for late eighteenth-century Hamburg, councils and states were often loath to entrust the health of their 'indispensable' population to the suppos-

---

84 Many Saxon cities were heavily in debt at the end of the war. Leipzig had been forced to borrow 3.5 million Taler. The Saxon government estimated that it would have to channel some 65% of its annual income through taxation into servicing the territory's debt. See Karl Czok and Reiner Gross, 'Das Kurfürstentum, die sächsisch-polnische Union und die Staatsreform (1547–1789)', in Karl Czok, ed., *Geschichte Sachsens* (Weimar: Hermann Böhlaus Nachfolger, 1989), 288.

85 StadtAL, Tit.XLIV.D.8a, Bd. I, 'Acta, Die Errichtung eines Hebammen Instituts alhier betr. anno 1786', 53, 'Memorandum from Leipzig Council to Amt Leipzig and Amt Magistrate Johann Gottfried Blümer', 12 January 1798.

86 The office of Provinzaccoucheur was introduced in 1771, around the same time that the Saxon government in Sachsen-Weimar-Eisenach began planning the maternity hospital. See Wolter, 'Jenaer Entbindungsanstalt', 82.

edly fetid, deathly wards of hospitals. The Hamburg Council, for example, shunned the hospital and the workhouse, choosing instead to encourage forms of increasingly prophylactic medical care that kept the sick in their homes.[87] And it is apparent that the poor record of these eighteenth-century maternity hospitals in both infant and maternal mortality was well known to the enlightened public and there was lively debate about whether or not these institutions were truly useful.[88] Certainly the Leipzig Council had no intention of introducing clinical childbirth for the sake of poor women, as had been the case in England. As we have seen, when the Council periodically questioned its salaried Stadtaccoucheurs as to whether or not they considered it necessary to establish a midwifery institute, many responded with arguments relating to the training and instruction of the midwives, not the health and well-being of women in the community. Giving birth in a hospital setting was not considered unhealthy per se. Indeed, for indigent, unwed mothers it was thought preferable to circumstances that might lead to the accidental death of the infant, or worse, infanticide. The connection that contemporaries made between hospitals and the health of mother and child, however, did not rest on the idea of the clinical institution as the best form of *medical care*. The goal of the maternity hospital in Leipzig, as elsewhere in the Germanies, was to provide training to midwives and obstetricians.[89] This political agenda ensured that midwifery in Leipzig continued to be a largely domiciliary activity.

Aside from the fact that the Council considered Leipzig well served by its sworn midwives, Beifrauen and Stadtaccoucheurs, there was a more mundane issue causing unease amongst the councillors – the problem of the itinerant poor. In a report to the University and the Council in 1803, the Leipzig Stadtphysicus Ernst Hebenstreit stated that:

> throughout the past negotiations regarding the erection of an institute for practical obstetrics in Leipzig ... Your Magnificent Council ... appears to have primarily harboured the concern that because this institute is determined for the whole territory, that through its existence in Leipzig a great multitude of foreign pregnant women from other Saxon regions will be drawn here and then, after their delivery, would remain here in the city together with their children and fall burden to the city.[90]

---

87 Lindemann, 'Urban Charity', 145–46.
88 Schlumbohm points out that there was widespread consensus amongst hospital directors that the low socio-economic circumstances of parturient patients was to blame for high mortality, which exonerated the institution. See Jürgen Schlumbohm, 'Saving Mothers' and Children's Lives?: The Performance of German Lying-In Hospitals in the Late Eighteenth and Early Nineteenth Centuries', *Bulletin of the History of Medicine* 87: 1 (2013): 1–31, 28–29.
89 Schlumbohm argues that the educational agenda of the maternity hospitals was the main reason why high levels of maternal and infant mortality were largely overlooked across the Germanies. See ibid., 30.
90 StadtAL, Tit. (F) XLIV.D.8a, Bd. I, 'Die Errichtung eines Hebammen Instituts alhier betr. anno 1786', 74–75, 'Report from Stadtphysicus Ernst B. G. Hebenstreit to Leipzig University and Leipzig Council re: midwifery institute', 5 November 1803, 74r.

As Hebenstreit's report suggests, illegitimacy was perceived as a major socio-economic problem in the cities. By the end of the eighteenth century, illegitimacy had increased across much of Europe and contemporaries were
aware of the burgeoning problem.[91] Around the same time, the central tenet
of cameralism, the multiplication of the population, was facing increasing
criticism as the problem of overpopulation (rather than depopulation) began
to emerge.[92] Leipzig, a commercial and manufacturing hub that acted as a
magnet for in-migration, would have felt the pressures of the 'wrong kind' of
population growth acutely. Whereas the consequence of extramarital sexuality
was less problematic for women who could rely on established familial and
social networks to provide financial and social assistance, 'foreign' women
who did not or could not return to their place of birth for their confinement
posed a financial liability to the civic purse. And this was one of the Council's
central concerns.

The proposed midwifery institute also threatened the micro-economy of
wet-nursing and lying-in. As Chapter Four demonstrated, a well-functioning
'industry' of lying-in residences and wet-nursing agents in Leipzig, some run
by midwives and Beifrauen, others by Gassenmägde or other lay women, ensured that the majority of the unwed women who found themselves in the city
at the time of their confinement could give birth in a quasi-domestic environment. Many such women would subsequently take up positions as wet nurses,
which meant that neither they nor their children would become candidates
for Council poor relief.[93] The Council was most concerned about women
from outside of Leipzig being attracted to the city, for these were the women
less likely to be able to pay for their confinement in one of the city's many
privately run lying-in residences. And it was these women who were the target
clients of the maternity hospitals.[94]

The ability of the Leipzig Council, as head of the cities represented in the
Landtag, to hinder the plans of the University and the Saxon government was

---

91 Ulbricht, 'The Debate about Foundling Hospitals', 250–51; W. R. Lee, 'Bastardy and the
    Socioeconomic Structure of South Germany', *Journal of Interdisciplinary History* 7: 3 (1977):
    403–25, 407–10.

92 This undermined the arguments cameralists had brought forward for institutions de-
    signed to increase the population, such as foundling hospitals. See Ulbricht, 'The Debate
    about Foundling Hospitals', 254–55.

93 On wet-nursing in Hamburg towards the end of the eighteenth century, see Mary Linde-
    mann, 'Love for Hire: The Regulation of the Wet-Nursing Business in Eighteenth-Cen-
    tury Hamburg', *Journal of Family History* 6: 4 (1981): 379–95.

94 If the experience of Marburg is typical, then this was a valid concern as the majority of
    women who sought out the services of the Marburg maternity hospital came from rural
    areas of electoral Essen, not from within the city of Marburg itself. The poorest of the
    poor (generally domestic or farm servants) often walked for hours or days on foot to give
    birth in Marburg. See Metz-Becker, *Der verwaltete Körper*, 150–51 and 159. At the Göttin-
    gen maternity hospital 98% of the children born there were illegitimate, and 90% of
    mothers were servants. See Schlumbohm, 'Saving Mothers' and Children's Lives?', 19.

considerable.[95] The tug-of-war between the Council, on the one hand, and the University and the Saxon government, on the other, over the building of the Leipzig midwifery institute was indeed characteristic of the general political relationship between the city and other political jurisdictions within Saxony.[96] At the Landtag of 1799 there was so much protest against the rights of Leipzig and Wittenberg (home to Saxony's other university) to oppose the establishment of midwifery institutes, that the estates felt compelled to promise 'to take caution when establishing the maternity hospitals [so] that the rights of the two cities do not suffer any truncation'.[97] The pressure the Leipzig Council brought to bear on the decision-making process resulted in an assurance that only 'native' Leipzig women would be granted admission as patients to any future midwifery institute, ensuring – as Stadtphysicus Hebenstreit pointed out in 1803 – that the Council would not be 'bothered by foreign women and their children'.[98]

This appeased the Council somewhat and it expressed its willingness to go ahead with the plans to build the midwifery institute in Leipzig. Yet it is apparent from the temporary arrangements made for providing instruction to trainee midwives on a territorial scale that the Council was in no hurry to dismantle its own long-standing tradition of midwifery training. Nor was it prepared to co-operate on the building of the midwifery institute before the necessary funds could be provided. Instructed by the Saxon government to provide provisional training for midwives in the Leipzig and Thüringen Ämter (districts), the Council agreed to engage its own Stadtaccoucheur Menz to instruct a certain number of 'female apprentices' on the condition that it be granted 400–500 Taler per annum from the bequests for the midwifery institute for this purpose.[99] The Medical Faculty protested these plans: 'our inner conviction of the necessity of a general midwifery institute for this country prevents us from approving something through which the same [midwifery institute] ... could be delayed even further, which most certainly would occur if one part of the interest from the Leich bequest were allocated to an interim provision'.[100] The Medical Fa-

95 The Saxon Diet consisted of three estates (Stände): Nine deputies from the high nobility and six from the cathedral chapters of Meißen and Merseburg made up the first estate. The second and third estates consisted of lower nobility and representatives of the largest Saxon towns, headed up by Leipzig. The Diet met every six to ten years to review tax issues. See Beachy, *Soul of Commerce*, 12.

96 See ibid., 56–63. On the dependent and simultaneously antagonistic relationship between Leipzig and the Saxon state in the eighteenth century, see Blaschke, 'Die kursächsische Politik'.

97 Tit. (F) XLIV.D.8a, Bd. I, 74–75, 'Hebenstreit report re: midwifery institute', 5 November 1803, 75v.

98 Ibid.

99 StadtAL, Tit. (F) XLIV.D.9, 'Die bis zur wircklicher Anlegung eines Hebammen Instituts alhier zu Leipzig, beabsichtige einstweilige Einrichtung, und was dem anhängig betr.', 11–12, 'Letter from Amtsmann Benjamin Gottwald Weidlich to Leipzig Council', 2 October 1804, 11–12.

100 Tit. (F) XLIV.D.9, 'Die bis zur wircklicher Anlegung eines Hebammen Instituts alhier zu Leipzig, beabsichtigte einstweilige Einrichtung, und was dem anhängig betr.', 13–16,

culty assured the Council that it would oppose any temporary provision and put forward a motion to speed up the establishment of its midwifery institute.[101] The Council's plans never came to fruition as shortly afterwards, in 1806, the University was bequeathed land on which to build its midwifery institute. Liberated from its reliance on the Leipzig Council in finding a suitable property, the University was able to put a stop to the planned 'interim measure' and get on with the business of building.[102]

The Triersches Institut

After four decades of failed attempts to establish a maternity hospital, the Leipzig Medical Faculty finally opened the Triersches Institut near the Peterstor on 7 October 1810. The institute, funded largely by private donations from wealthy Leipzig burghers, was to a great degree the fruit of the lobbying activities of the former Stadtaccoucheur and dean of the Medical Faculty Professor Johann Karl Gehler. In 1806 relatives of Gehler, the childless *Appellationsrat* Dr. Karl Friedrich Trier (†1794) and his wife Rahel Amelia Auguste (1731–1806), bequeathed the couple's circa eleven-hectare-large garden before the Peterstor with express instructions to erect a school for training 'skilful and diligent women … in all that is necessary for them to do in a naturally occurring birth and delivery'.[103] Ernst Platner (1744–1818), who had succeeded Gehler in 1796 as dean of the Medical Faculty, oversaw the planning of the new midwifery institute. Although he had no particular academic interest in obstetrics and midwifery, Platner was convinced of the necessity of training midwives and obstetricians in both natural and unnatural births. The main aim was to teach midwifery from both a practical and a theoretical perspective. Pregnant women admitted to the institute at all stages of gestation were to serve as live teaching material, backed up with exercises on the so-called 'phantom'. Theory was to be taught in courses given by the professor of obstetrics and his assistant.[104]

In conjunction with the opening of the Triersches Institut, the Medical Faculty created a new ordinary professorial chair of obstetrics. At the behest of Elector Friedrich August I, this professor was to also direct the new midwifery institute. The honour of the post was given to Johann Christian Gottfried Jörg (1779–1856). Jörg had read the natural sciences and medicine in Leipzig, during which time he had secured a position as assistant to the then Stadtaccoucheur Carl Christian Friedrich Menz in 1802. Although he gained

'Letter from Leipzig Medical Faculty to Leipzig Council re: midwifery institute', 14 December 1804, 14v–15r.
101 Ibid., 15r–16r.
102 Tit. (F) XLIV.D.8c, Bd. II, 'Acta, Das Hebammeninstitut alhier betr. (1805)', 66–67, 'Letter from Leipzig University Rector Carl Gottlob Kuhn to Leipzig Amtsmann Benjamin Gottwalt Weidlich ', 10 April 1810.
103 Quoted in Fahrenbach and Leske, 'Immer zum Wohle der Patientinnen', 4.
104 Ibid.

considerable experience in operative obstetrics, because the Stadtaccoucheur's involvement in midwifery still only extended to complicated deliveries, Jörg was unable to witness natural births.[105] To remedy the situation, Jörg spent six months of 1804 in Vienna studying under the obstetrician Johann Lukas Boër, known for his conservative, non-interventionist views on childbirth.[106] On his return to Leipzig, Jörg obtained his Doctor of Philosophy and, in 1805, earned a Doctor of Medicine and Surgery. He then published his obstetric textbook *Systematisches Handbuch der Geburtshilfe für Geburtshelfer, Ärzte und Wundärzte* (Leipzig 1807).[107] Jörg went on to turn the Triersches Institut into one of the most famous maternity hospitals in nineteenth-century Europe.

Meanwhile, the midwives employed by the Leipzig Council continued to be appointed and trained as they had been for most of the eighteenth century. Following Stadtaccoucheur Hartwig's death in 1791, Carl Christian Friedrich Menz was appointed Stadtaccoucheur. Menz, like his predecessor, was not associated with the Medical Faculty in Leipzig, but instead had made a name for himself as an Accoucheur in the city.[108] Like his predecessor, Menz did not actively agitate for the erection of a maternity hospital, but continued to instruct the midwives and Beifrauen twice a week and use the lazarette to train newly appointed Beifrauen well into the second decade of the nineteenth century.[109] Yet he was perhaps more inclined to support a maternity hospital than his predecessor. When the Council asked him for his recommendations on how to improve midwifery in the city in 1796, he reported that in the absence of a midwifery institute, he had no further suggestions other than continuing with his 'thorough and conscientious instruction' of the midwives and Beifrauen and the appointment of an additional Beifrau in the Vorstadt.[110]

In 1818 an electoral edict wrested control over municipal medical functionaries from the cities and communes. As well as divesting the Stadtphysici of the right to examine midwives, the edict ruled that only those midwives and obstetricians trained 'theoretically and practically' in a maternity hospital in Saxony or abroad were to be permitted to practise obstetrics.[111] It was only after this edict that the municipal system of training and appointing midwives and Stadtaccoucheurs in Leipzig *began* to lose currency. Prior to 1818, however, and almost certainly for a good many years thereafter, 'institute' mid-

---

105 Fahrenbach, 'Johann Gottfried', 126.
106 On Boër and the controversy between him and his rival Friedrich Benjamin Osiander (Göttingen) over the merits of operative intervention during childbirth, see Schlumbohm, "Die edelste"', esp. 291–97.
107 For biographical details on Jörg, see Hehl, *Professorenkatalog Leipzig*; Fahrenbach, 'Johann Gottfried'.
108 Menz is not listed in any of the major eighteenth-, nineteenth-, or twentieth-century general and medical biographical lexica, which suggests that he was a medical 'nobody' as far as the Republic of Letters was concerned.
109 Tit. (F) XLIV.D.6b, Bd. II, 99–133, 'Stadtaccoucheur reports (Menz)', 13 August 1792–14 March 1805, 99–100 and 106–7.
110 Ibid., 111–13.
111 See Item 1 of Tit. (F) XLIV.A.18a, 104–6, 'Mandat Geburtsülfe', 2 April 1818, 104–6.

wifery and the traditional sworn midwifery practised in the city of Leipzig remained two discrete spheres. In 1814, for example, Menz was notified by one of the city's sworn midwives that the midwife employed in the midwifery institute had delivered the wife of a Leipzig carriage driver. Menz reported the matter to the Leipzig Council, recalling that said woman had two years previously attended another woman outside of her occupational jurisdiction. The Council interrogated the institute midwife Henriette Prachtmann, who pleaded that she had acted 'out of desperation' because the city's midwives lured all the women who might be able to pay for their confinement into their homes and 'take away her earnings'.[112] Despite the apparent hardship she faced, Prachtmann was fined 10 Taler. The Council was careful to preserve the occupational integrity of its own sworn midwives, even in the face of competition from a 'new' generation of midwives trained in the midwifery institutes and maternity hospitals – if only because this was a means of flexing political muscle and ensuring the entitlements and livelihood of the members of the urban community.

Conclusions

Until the 1760s the Saxon territorial government had intervened in local governance on matters concerning midwifery only sporadically and with vague intent. When the Stadtaccoucheurs Karl Gehler, Johann Ehrenfried Pohl and the Medical Faculty first tabled their plans for a midwifery institute in Leipzig in 1764, this called for greater involvement on the part of the Saxon government in Dresden. The calls to equip Leipzig with such a 'progressive' medical-pedagogical infrastructure reflected ideas about the state's role in medical policy emerging in the medical-political discourse known as medical police in the 1760s. Yet, as we have seen, the almost forty-year delay in establishing clinical training for midwives in Leipzig strongly suggests that if we wish to understand urban medicine, health and midwifery in eighteenth-century Germany, we must be careful not to inflate the power of the 'state' and 'doctors'. As evidenced by the complex and fragmented balance of power in Electoral Saxony, these realpolitical restrictions on the state were reinforced by a lack of wide-reaching authority, not just over its subjects but also over the various autonomous and politically potent jurisdictions that made up the complicated political patchwork of eighteenth-century territories. The conundrum of governance arising out of this jumble of interests – in this case the conflict of interests between the Leipzig Council, the Leipzig University and the Saxon government – was tested over the question of whether or not a maternity hospital should be built in Leipzig.

---

112 StadtAL, II. Sekt. H (F) Nr. 1157, 'Acta, Die von der im Hebammen Institute alhier angestellten Hebamme beschehenen Beeinträchtigungen der verpflichteten Stadthebammen betr.', 25 January–3 February 1814, 1r–1v.

It is important to remember that the midwifery institute was the 'brain-child' of the University Medical Faculty and was initiated and planned by two of its prominent members: Professor Johann Karl Gehler and Professor Johann Ehrenfried Pohl. Although both Gehler and Pohl were simultaneously in the pay of the Leipzig Council as Stadtaccoucheur and Stadtphysicus, their proposals did not reflect the political will of the Council, which consistently rejected the idea both as superfluous and a danger to the civic coffer. It is no coincidence that those Stadtaccoucheurs and Stadtphysici affiliated to the Medical Faculty, such as Gehler and Pohl, were proponents of the proposed midwifery institute. Those without formal ties to academic medicine were more inclined to either sit on the fence or deny any need for such an institution. Although Petermann enjoyed some prominence in his day, his successors Lischwitz, Hartrauff, Breuer, Hartwig and Menz were all medically insignificant figures with no professional associations with either the University or the Saxon government. Not one of these medical officials was demonstrably enthusiastic about the plans for a midwifery institute. The Saxon government, which saw great benefits for rural medical provision, was sympathetic to the project and lent its support. However, it was unable and unwilling to cough up the necessary funds and its often half-hearted attempts to woo the Leipzig Council into co-operating on the project largely ended in failure. Whereas the Saxon state and the Leipzig Council demonstrated a certain affinity of ideas about how midwifery could be improved during the latter seventeenth and early eighteenth centuries, the matter of maternity hospitals highlighted a major division of interests.

The history of the Triersches Institut in Leipzig is thus a story about political conflict in a political melee. This chapter has focused on the sources of institutional political power at play in efforts to reform midwifery during the latter eighteenth century, a period in which the state became a more vocal – if only mildly more effective – actor. Until the early nineteenth century the Leipzig Council managed to protect its political sovereignty and largely resist attempts to disturb the integrity of its own governance. The history of urban midwifery in eighteenth-century Leipzig is thus intimately tied to the fortune and the policy of the Leipzig Council.[113] The Council and its medical officials were intensely preoccupied with improving midwifery provision through better training and education. However, the Council was not prepared to sacrifice its local system of midwifery. The reforms implemented by the Council in the early eighteenth century aimed to improve midwifery without rendering defunct the 'traditional' economic and social nature of the relationship between midwife and apprentice or the sovereignty of the city's midwives over most normal births. The Council pursued this policy of preservation well into the nineteenth century. If far-reaching change were to come, it would have to wait until the collapse of municipal authority in the 1830s.

---

113 Loytved also stresses the localness of midwifery in Lübeck. See Loytved, *Hebammen*,
   281–82.

Conclusion

On 14 March 1831, following over four centuries of rule, the Leipzig Council ceased to exist. Changing patterns of international trade coupled with the loss of 60 per cent of Saxon territory to the Prussians following the defeat of Napoleon in 1814 had led to a steep decline in the competitiveness of the Leipzig fairs and the city's status as a commercial and financial powerhouse.[1] In the wake of the 'September unrest' of 1830, Leipzig burghers and merchants called for a new elected body to replace the Leipzig Council because of its 'antiquated relationship to the citizenry and its administration of the city treasury'.[2] With the support of the Saxon government, the new City Parliament (*Stadtverordneten*) was inaugurated and began negotiating the demise of the old Leipzig Council.[3] On 9 September 1831 the Saxon state sanctioned the new constitutional monarchy, leading to widespread reform of municipal and local governments throughout Saxony. It was only after this point that the state was able and willing to *begin* to directly exercise any far-reaching and systematic influence over Leipzig's municipal politics and structures.[4] The era of the corporatist, conservative, traditionalist and paternalistic Leipzig Council had come to an end.

As this study has shown, midwifery in early modern Leipzig was tied to the social, economic, political and cultural values of the Ständegesellschaft, to which concepts of livelihood, entitlement and obligation were central. The Leipzig Council embodied these values and the Saxon territorial state respected to a large degree the city's sovereignty over its own midwifery infrastructure, not least because it looked to midwifery provision in Leipzig as a shining example of how things ought to be done. The 'state', it could be said, was perhaps less innovative and strategic than hindsight would have us believe. Corporatism flourished as the dominant form of social, economic and occupational organisation and continued to shape both the structure of midwifery and the way in which midwives defined their occupation in moral-economic terms into the early nineteenth century.

The aim of this study was to re-examine the nature of and changes to urban midwifery provision and the profession of midwife during the late seventeenth and 'long' eighteenth centuries, a period that has been earmarked as a watershed moment in the history of midwifery and childbirth more generally by historians of all persuasions. My study has acknowledged the significance of this epoch but presents a more differentiated picture of the impact and aims of reforms, of midwifery regulation and of the *entrée* of the surgeon man-midwife. Most early modern cities and the emerging territorial states acknowledged midwifery as a worthwhile and necessary institution, yet they

---

1   Beachy, *Soul of Commerce*, 182–89.
2   According to a subsequent petition from the merchant and burgher group. Quoted in ibid., 206.
3   Ibid., 197–98.
4   Ibid., 207–9.

went about promoting their midwives in different ways. Faced with a largely poor and rural population, the Swedish Crown embarked on a mission of centralising midwifery training early in the eighteenth century and extending midwives' authority to cover surgical intervention – a move that for political reasons would have enjoyed considerably less success in Saxony during the same period.[5] In France the *tour de force* undertaken by the King's Midwife Mme du Coudray in the mid-eighteenth century, although fraught by local opposition, conveys a similarly spectacular attempt on the part of the state to up-skill its midwives for the benefit of the nation.[6] Leipzig, on the other hand, faced relatively little 'interference' from the Saxon state on matters relating to midwifery and clung fast to its own tried and tested brand of municipal midwifery provision and midwifery training, tweaking and tinkering with reforms wherever the Council saw fit. The strong culture of the community and the civic unit ensured that any novelties wove themselves relatively neatly into existing terms of social and economic provision upon which urban life and livelihood in the *ancien régime* at the level of the city were based. As Mary Lindemann's pioneering studies of poor relief reform in Hamburg and medical provision in the Duchy of Braunschweig-Wolfenbüttel have demonstrated, this pattern of change that was compatible with established value systems was not peculiar to Leipzig, but was something that characterised eighteenth-century communities both large and small, local and territorial throughout the northern German states.[7]

The reforms instituted by the Leipzig Council in the late seventeenth and early eighteenth centuries targeted maternal and, to a lesser degree, infant mortality and thus reflected both early cameralist anxieties about depopulation and religious concerns about correct baptism and the need to uphold the Protestant ideal of family and procreation as the cornerstone of a Godly life. As a central element of urban poor relief, the reform of midwifery also echoed wider developments in the care of the poor and the reformation of poor relief at the beginning of the eighteenth century. Yet in paternalistic Leipzig, improving urban midwifery provision was also about demonstrating civic pride and civic power; the marker of a great city was not merely its commercial or cultural importance but also the presence of a well-conceived and efficient network of welfare and medical provision (in theory at least!), in which midwifery played a central role. Above all, we have to remember that these reforms were largely local/municipal initiatives, not ones imposed from the state above. There were certainly many points of contact and concurrence between the Leipzig Council and the territorial government in Dresden, not least through the fluid exchange of medical personnel from Leipzig municipal office to state office. However, despite the territorial government's nascent interest in midwifery, in particular in the area of establishing standards, in Leip-

5   Romlid, 'Swedish Midwives', 54.
6   Rattner Gelbart, *The King's Midwife.*
7   Mary Lindemann, *Patriots and Paupers: Hamburg, 1712–1830* (New York & Oxford: Oxford University Press, 1990). See also *Health.*

zig midwifery was a matter for local government into the early nineteenth century. These findings have implications for our understanding of early modern society more generally. Throughout the eighteenth century it was first and foremost local units of governance, rather than the emerging absolute enlightened states, who steered political, social and economic life in the cities. In Leipzig the major reformation of municipal midwifery provision took place before 1732 – long before the discourse of medical Policey – under the hand of the Leipzig Council. And when the state and the University attempted to intervene in midwifery provision in Leipzig with the maternity hospital, the Leipzig Council pulled out all the stops to protect the interests of the city's community.

This study also suggests that norm-setting in the early modern city was a collective process. Drawing upon the concept of Policey as a communicative process between the governing and the governed, I found that Leipzig midwives played a productive role in the development and refinement of midwifery oaths and instructions because they so vigorously pursued those women who encroached upon their livelihood. They were instrumental in maintaining informal modes of midwifery by engaging unofficial apprentices and Wickelweiber. As this study has shown, by defending their moral-economic territory through petitions and supplications, midwives thus actively sharpened the contours of both their office and their occupation more generally. Consequently, these women were implicated in the formal mechanisms of political norm-setting in the early modern city, if only in a less visible and at times querulous manner.

By closely reading the administrative sources on midwifery, I have been able to reconstruct the occupational parameters and terms of practice that shaped midwifery in Leipzig, which has in turn enabled me to measure the reach of the late seventeenth- and early eighteenth-century reforms. Through this study I have shown how a very eclectic midwifery landscape could exist in a major urban centre *within and alongside* the framework of municipal regulation. Although many cities maintained sworn midwives and upheld midwifery ordinances, these urban 'midwifery landscapes' were diverse, depending on the micro-political, economic and social circumstances in each space. As this study has shown, the highly organised and 'bureaucratised' system of midwifery provision in Leipzig hid an entire 'grey' landscape of midwifery that was at certain points in time at odds with yet simultaneously integrally part of official midwifery, indicating that we need to qualify the 'regulated/unregulated' dichotomy. There is, therefore, greater scope for considering the position of midwives in German towns and cities within the context of community – as I have sought to do here by tracing client networks and patterns together with the lived parameters of midwifery practice – rather than just within the context of their municipal office.

Compared to other German and European cities, Leipzig appears to have carved its own little niche. Unlike some smaller cities, such as Göttingen, or larger royal residences such as Dresden or Berlin where midwife training took

place in a clinical setting from the middle of the eighteenth century, the road
to becoming a midwife in Leipzig continued along traditional 'apprenticeship'
lines within a domestic setting.[8] Despite the relatively early intervention of
Leipzig's Stadtaccoucheur in the selection and theoretical instruction of the
city's midwives (from the 1730s onwards), the underlying structure and organisational occupation of midwifery remained intact. Lübeck, a still powerful
Hanseatic city in the north of Germany, provides both parallels and contrasts
to Leipzig. The Lübecker Council appointed a Hebammenlehrer in the same
year as Leipzig but, as Christine Loytved argues, the new constellation had
little impact on midwifery in the city until this office assumed control over the
selection and instruction of apprentice midwives in the early nineteenth century.[9] In Leipzig, as we have seen, the Stadtaccoucheur had slightly more influence early on over the selection of both Beifrauen and midwives in his capacity to make recommendations. Nevertheless, this did little to alter the organisation and function of the midwifery landscape. From a European perspective
there are strong parallels between the official organisation and development
of midwifery in Leipzig (and similar German cities) and in Dutch towns and
cities, where medical and midwifery provision tended to be run by secular,
local authorities.[10]

As we have seen here, late seventeenth- and early eighteenth-century midwifery reforms in Leipzig – the formalisation of the midwife–apprentice relationship, the appointment of a designated physician to supervise the city's
midwives, and the introduction of regular formal instruction in anatomy and
obstetrics – impacted but little on the underlying structure and occupational
culture of urban midwifery. It was a matter of change *within* the confines of
continuity. Indeed, reforms often served to reinforce existing occupational
structures and cultures. The midwife–apprentice relationship persisted as the
primary form of knowledge transmission, enhanced but not replaced by lessons given by the Stadtaccoucheur. Indeed even Stadtaccoucheur Johann Karl
Gehler, who hankered after unspoilt Beifrauen that he might mould himself,
paradoxically neglected midwife instruction, ensuring (inadvertently perhaps)
that the flow of skills and training continued to emanate from older, established midwives. Similarly, unofficial midwifery constituted a structural component of the midwifery landscape, only to cause disruption when the activities of unsworn midwives encroached on the livelihoods of sworn midwives or
Beifrauen. The selection of midwives remained to a great extent in the hands
of both the lay public and midwives, even though formal mechanisms such as
consultations or elections amongst the city's 'honourable wives' appear to
have ceased in the early eighteenth century. Midwives also continued to establish and maintain their client networks as they had done before, through the
medium of trust. And, last but not least, the number of midwives and Beifrauen employed by the Leipzig Council remained static for most of the eigh-

8   On Berlin, see Loytved, 'Zur Gründung'. On Göttingen, see Hampe, *Zwischen Tradition.*
9   Loytved, *Hebammen,* 281–85.
10   Marland, '"Stately and dignified"'.

teenth century, despite an ever expanding population and the growth of urban poverty.

The division of births into 'natural' and 'unnatural' altered the existing division of labour between midwives and surgeons based on the emergency, but this new epistemological division did little to alter everyday practice in the city until the turn of the century. Midwives, both sworn and unsworn, continued to attend the overwhelming majority of women in Leipzig during childbirth. The Stadtaccoucheurs persisted as 'emergency' practitioners in the birthing chamber throughout the eighteenth century and well into the nineteenth, not merely due to their expense, as has been noted by Henrike Hampe, but because these scholars and gentleman physician-surgeons did not want to practice in any other capacity.[11] Although it was impossible for them to avoid manual medical labour altogether, the Stadtaccoucheurs attempted to limit their obstetric activities as much as possible by emphasising their role as teachers and advisors. For these men, practice and knowledge derived from performing everyday, hum-drum obstetrics was not what made them experts, and this insight underscores the relative scarcity of practical education for male obstetric students in the late eighteenth-century maternity hospitals.[12]

The apparent lack of competition between midwives and male practitioners in Leipzig during this period is quite striking, given that the 'battle' between the sexes in the domain of obstetrics and the medicalisation (and masculinisation) of childbirth and obstetric knowledge has been the subject of countless historical and cultural-sociological studies since the 1970s. This lack of competition has also been noted for eighteenth-century Lübeck by Loytved, who argues that trouble only began in the late 1780s and 1790s when male practitioners started to co-opt apprentice midwives as assistants in the birthing chamber, thereby bypassing the city's sworn midwives altogether.[13] I have sought to account for this lack of competition throughout most of the century from a less market-oriented perspective. As this study has shown, midwives in Leipzig did not perceive the Stadtaccoucheur as competition per se because his activities did not endanger midwives' livelihoods; not merely in terms of the number of births he attended, but also because of the contemporary understanding of what it meant to be a physician and the culture of medicine, health and healing in early modern Leipzig. General reluctance amongst Leipzig's Stadtaccoucheurs to actually practise emergency or non-emergency obstetrics and the emphasis placed on teaching midwives how to manage both 'natural' and 'difficult' births goes some way to explaining the situation in Leipzig.[14] A client-centric culture of medical care, as discussed in Chapter Six, which encouraged women and their families to dictate the terms of medical intervention and choice of practitioner, was another important factor.

11   Hampe, Zwischen Tradition, 134.
12   Schlumbohm, 'Practice', 35–36.
13   Ibid., 283.
14   There are parallels between this penchant for teaching rather than 'doing' amongst late seventeenth-century English male midwives. See Wilson, Making, 47–62.

This study has concentrated on the activities of the Stadtaccoucheur, although there were certainly other medical practitioners who gained a reputation as particularly knowledgeable or skilled in midwifery in Leipzig. Owing in part to the paucity of sources, there is still little known about the obstetric practices of surgeons and surgeon-physicians without municipal offices in Germany prior to the very end of the eighteenth century. A lack of disputes between midwives and such practitioners noted both here and elsewhere suggests, however, that privately practising obstetricians did not transcend the traditional division of labour between normal and emergency births, or at least not in any measure that proved injurious to the livelihoods of the city's sworn midwives and Beifrauen.[15]

What did change decisively towards the end of the eighteenth century in Leipzig were attitudes towards maturity, traditionally one of the key aspects of a midwife's identity – a trend also observable in Lübeck.[16] The sometimes fraught encounter between Stadtaccoucheur and sworn midwife in the context of anatomical lessons rendered female maturity unstable as 'teachability' became aligned with younger, 'unspoilt' women, and maturity associated with 'unreceptiveness'. Yet the practice of appointing younger women did not take effect until the 1770s and 1780s and, although new Beifrau recruits were supposed to be younger than thirty, motherhood and wifehood remained central qualifications for office. As this study has shown, midwifery was not per se tied to maturity; women often began learning midwifery at a young age and youth was no deterrent for women working unofficially within the midwifery landscape. Women appointed to the office of midwife, however, tended to be past their childbearing years at appointment until the 1770s, when the Stadtaccoucheur began to systematically appoint younger women. From this time onwards the office of sworn midwife (but not midwifery *per se*) ceased to be associated with the mature part of the life-cycle and thus began to assume the character of a long-term occupation.

With regards to the history of women's work, this study suggests that the opportunity for women to work outside the home and independently of their husbands actually increased during the eighteenth century. Leipzig, much like the great global commercial metropolis of Hamburg (if on a smaller scale), experienced high rates of population growth and thrived on an economy increasingly dependent upon trade and commercial transactions rather than the indigenous production of goods.[17] Similarly, the eighteenth century saw a general decline in the power of the guilds as a civic-political unit across Germany and increasing restrictions on guild membership. This had a knock-on effect for the occupational status of midwifery because, as we have seen, midwives were most closely associated with the artisan milieu throughout the eighteenth century. The changing economic conditions and modes of production meant that households were increasingly reliant on wage labour

15   Hampe, *Zwischen Tradition*, 134; Lindemann, 'Professionals?', 176.
16   Loytved, *Hebammen*, 283–84.
17   On Hamburg, see Lindemann, *Patriots*, 93–99.

and women, unable to earn a living within the economic unit of the household, sought extra-domestic work. When the Council began to lower the age of the city's sworn midwives and Beifrauen, there was no lack of applications from younger women dependent on a long-term, secure source of household income. Cruciger's comment in 1799 that midwives were no longer recruited from the 'middle estates' thus proves a red herring: it was the notion of which occupational and social groups constituted the 'middle estates' and a negative change in the fortunes of journeymen wanting to establish a workshop, *not* the socio-economic background of midwives that appears to have changed. It is clear that by the early eighteenth century, women belonging to the upper estates were no longer involved in commercial midwifery, even in an advisory capacity. The evidence suggests, however, that women from across the social spectrum sought out the services of Leipzig's sworn midwives and Beifrauen. The exodus of upper-estate women from the urban midwifery infrastructure suggests that 'class' was beginning to determine whether or not a woman worked outside of the household for money. In Leipzig, however, it does not yet seem to have been a factor influencing the choice of practitioner, whether midwife or Stadtaccoucheur.

Appendices

Appendix 1 Stadtphysici and Stadtaccoucheurs involved in midwifery in Leipzig 1659–1810: appointments, biographical data (in chronological order of office)

WELSCH, Gottfried W.

* 12 November 1618 (Leipzig), † 5 September 1690 (Leipzig)

1659–90   Stadtphysicus

Welsch studied medicine in Leipzig and, after gaining his Doctor of Philosophy in 1639, pursued further medical studies in Italy, France, Holland and England. On his return to Leipzig he worked as a Swedish military doctor during the Thirty Years War. After becoming a Doctor of Medicine in 1644 he was appointed extraordinary professor of anatomy and assessor in the Medical Faculty in Leipzig. He worked his way up through the professorial ranks within the Medical Faculty until he became professor of therapy and dean of the Faculty in 1664. The Leipzig Council appointed Welsch as Stadtphysicus in 1659, an office he retained until his death in 1690. In addition to various works on legal medicine and infant nutrition, Welsch was well known for publishing a German translation of Scipione Mercurio's midwifery manual *La Commare dell Scipione Mercurio, Kindermutter- oder Hebammen-Buch* (1653, 1671).

Sources: Julius Leopold Pagel, 'Welsch, Gottfried', in *Allgemeine Deutsche Biographie* (1896), available at <https://www.deutsche-biographie.de/gnd117345814.html#adbcontent>, accessed 6 September 2016, vol. 41, 681.

PETERMANN, Andreas

* 7 March 1649 (Werblin, near Danzig), † 3 April 1703 (Leipzig)

1680–1703   Stadtphysicus

Andreas Petermann studied medicine, theology and philosophy in both Halle and Leipzig. He received his doctoral title in Altdorf in 1673 and subsequently worked as a Stadtarzt (municipal doctor) in Torgau and Delitzsch (near Leipzig). Following his purportedly heroic deeds as Stadtarzt during the 1680 plague epidemic, the Leipzig Council appointed him Stadtphysicus. Once in Leipzig, A. Petermann established himself as a practical physician and became particularly well known as an expert in the area of obstetrics. In 1688 he was named extraordinary and in 1691 ordinary professor of anatomy and surgery in the Medical Faculty in Leipzig. Petermann is perhaps best known for his academic battle with the midwife to the court of Brandenburg Justine

Siegemund, who published her midwifery manual *Die Königl.-preußische und chur-brandenburgische Hof-Wehmutter* in 1691. Petermann published a criticism of the midwife's manual entitled *Gründliche Deduction vieler Handgriffe, die in dem Buche die Chur-Brandenb. Hoff-Wehe-Mutter genannt gerühmt werden* (Leipzig, 1692), which provoked Siegemund to defend herself by publishing a response of her own. The matter then turned into a battle between Andreas Petermann and the Medical Faculty at Frankfurt/Oder, which had vetted and conferred public approval onto Siegemund's work. His son Benjamin Benedict Petermann published his forensic work *Casuum medico-legalium decas I* and *II* posthumously in 1707–8.

Sources: See entry for 'Andreas Petermann' in August Hirsch, ed., *Biographisches Lexikon hervorragender Ärzte aller Zeiten und aller Völker vor 1880* (6 vols, Vienna: Urban & Schwarzenberg, 1886), vol. 4, 566; Justine Siegemund, *The Court Midwife. Justina Siegemund*, trans. Lynne Tatlock (Chicago, IL: The University of Chicago Press, 2005), 8–11; Maren Lorenz, *Kriminelle Körper, gestörte Gemüter. Die Normierung des Individuums in Gerichtsmedizin und Psychiatrie der Aufklärung* (Hamburg: Hamburger Edition, 1999), 543.

PETERMANN, Benjamin Benedict

* 1680 (Leipzig), † 17 April 1724 (Leipzig)

1708–19   **Amtsphysicus (Amt Leipzig)**

1715–24   **Physician in charge of midwives and pregnant women**

1719–24   **Stadtphysicus**

Petermann was the youngest son of Leipzig Stadtphysicus Andreas Petermann. Two of his three older brothers were also physicians to the Saxon Elector and in the city of Rostock. Petermann studied medicine in Halle and, after graduating in 1703, moved to Leipzig to set up a medical practice. In 1708 he was appointed Amtsphysicus to the Amt Leipzig by the Saxon Elector. In 1715 the Leipzig Council appointed him to provide particular care to the pregnant women in the city. The Council promoted him to Stadtphysicus in 1719 on condition that he resign his office as Amtsphysicus. Petermann married Sabine Feller and had three daughters and two sons. He published only one medical work, the *Observationum medicarum Dec. I–III*, which was appended to the 1707 edition of his father's work *Brevissima manuductio*, also edited by himself.

Sources: Jakob Christoff Beck and August Johann Buxtorf, *Supplement zu dem Baselischen allgemein historischen Lexico* (Basel: Johannes Christ sel. Wittib, 1744), 640. See entries for 'Benjamin Benedict Petermann' in Hirsch, ed., *Biographisches Lexikon*, vol. 4, 566; Johann Heinrich Zedler, *Grosses vollständiges Universal-Lexicon aller Wissenschaften und Künste* (online version) (64 vols, Bayerische Staatsbibliothek: 1731–54), available at <http://www.zedler-lexikon.de/index.html>, accessed 26 October 2016, vol. 27, 0525.

ETTMÜLLER, Michael Ernst E.

* 26 August 1673 (Leipzig), † 25 September 1732 (Leipzig)

1699–1732?   Lazarettarzt

Michael Etmüller was the son of Michael Etmüller, professor of botany in the Leipzig Medical Faculty, and Margaret Bose, daughter of one of Leipzig's most powerful and wealthy families. Ettmüller Jr. studied medicine in Leipzig before undertaking further medical studies in Holland and England. He obtained his Doctor of Medicine in 1699 and simultaneously took on the office of Lazarettarzt in Leipzig (although the entry in the *Protokoll zum Drey Rathen* of the Leipzig Council mentions he was appointed in 1706 to this post). In 1702 he was made extraordinary professor in the Medical Faculty in Leipzig and in 1709 he was appointed to the Chair of Physiology. He became professor of pathology in 1724, an office he held until his death in 1732.

Sources: StadtAL, Tit. (F) VIII Nr. 53, 'Protokoll zum Drey Rathen', 18 August 1704–7 September 1753, 18; Hirsch, ed., *Biographisches Lexikon*, vol. 5, 401; Zedler, *Grosses vollständiges Universal-Lexicon*, vol. 8, 1053.

LISCHWITZ, Johann Christoph

* 6 February 1693 (Lauban), † 27 August 1743 (Kiel)

1724–31   Stadtphysicus

Johann Christoph Lischwitz was the son of Joseph Lischwitz, clothmaker, burgher and senior taxation officer for the Saxon Elector in Lauban. Lischwitz studied in Lauban and then in Leipzig, where he obtained his Doctor of Medicine in 1720. In 1724 he was appointed extraordinary professor of botany and simultaneously succeeded the deceased Benjamin Benedict Petermann as Stadtphysicus. In 1731 the Leipzig Council divested him of his office. The following year (1732) Lischwitz moved to Kiel to become personal physician to the Herzog of Holstein and second professor of medicine at the University in Kiel. He later became counsel to the chancellor in 1736, justice counsel in 1740 and, finally, first professor of medicine at the Kiel University. He died in 1743.

Sources: 'Lischwitz, Johann Christoph' in *Biographisches Lexikon der Oberlausitz*, available online at <http://wiki.olgdw.de/index.php?title=*Lischwitz*_Johann_Christoph>, accessed 1 March 2011.

HARTRAUFF, Johann Valentin

Birth and death dates unknown

1731–Unknown (probably 1755)   Stadtaccoucheur

Johann Valentin Hartrauff was Leipzig's first formally named Stadtaccoucheur, appointed on 24 August 1731 by the Leipzig Council at a salary of 100 Taler. Uncharacteristically, Hartrauff appears not to have been a physician upon his appointment; he had probably learnt surgery with a master surgeon. He 're-placed' the former Stadtphysicus Johann Christoph Lischwitz in matters relating to obstetrics and midwifery in the city. It appears that he had already established a name for himself as a privately practising Accoucheur in Leipzig prior to this point, and even the city's sworn midwives and Beifrauen called upon his services. No records of publications could be found for Hartrauff.

Sources: Tit. (F) VIII Nr. 53, 'Protokoll zum Drey Rathen', 18 August 1704–7 September 1753, 173–74.

BREUER, Johann Gottfried

* Unknown, † 1763/64

1755–63/64   Stadtaccoucheur

The surgeon Johann Gottfried Breuer was appointed Stadtaccoucheur by the Leipzig Council in 1755. He also appears to have worked in the lazarette as by 1763, he was known as the Rats- und Lazarettchirurg. Breuer had enlisted the assistance of his brother and apprentice and, when his health was ailing in 1763, attempted unsuccessfully to have the brother appointed to his post. Breuer left no record of publications.

Sources: StadtAL, Tit. (F) XLIV.D.1, 'Kindermütter bey hiesiger Stadt betr. ingl. die angenommene Bey Weiber betr. 1673–1756', 190–91, 'Stadtaccoucheur reports (Johann Gottfried Breuer)', 19 March 1756; II. Sektion B (F) Nr. 1149, 'Acta Die von hiesigen Barbiern: Accoucheur Johann Gottfried Breuer gesuchte Erlaubniß …', 1763.

HEBENSTREIT, Johann George

No biographical information available.

c. 1763/64   Lazarette Surgeon

GEHLER, Johann Karl

* 17 May 1732 (Görlitz), † 6 May 1796 (Leipzig)

1759–81/82   Stadtaccoucheur

Johann Karl Gehler was born into the Görlitz patriciate. His grandfather, mayor of Görlitz Bartholomäus Gehler, and had been ennobled in the seventeenth century. Gehler studied medicine in Leipzig 1751–58 and published his thesis on mineralogy *De characteribus fossilium externis* in 1757. After receiving his Doctor of Medicine in 1758, Gehler undertook an extensive study tour through Switzerland and Germany, spending time in Strasbourg to attend lessons in obstetrics at the famous municipal maternity hospital with Johann Jakob Fried. On his return to Leipzig Gehler produced his *Habilitation* (postdoctoral thesis) work on mineralogy and turned his hand to medical practice, in particular obstetrics. In 1759 he was appointed Stadtaccoucheur by the Leipzig Council and simultaneously began lecturing in mineralogy at the Medical Faculty in Leipzig. Gehler was appointed extraordinary professor of botany in 1763 and was promoted to ordinary professor of physiology in 1773. Until his death in 1796 he worked his way up through the ranks of professorships from anatomy and surgery (1781–84), pathology (1784–89) and finally to therapy and dean of the Medical Faculty (1789–96). He published a handful of minor works on mineralogy and experimental chemistry whilst still alive. His two-volume *Kleine Schriften, die Entbindungskunst betreffend*, a collection of obstetric essays and smaller works written between 1760 and 1792, was published posthumously by Prof. Karl Gottlob Kühn in 1798.

Sources: See entry for 'Johann Karl Gehler' in Ulrich von Hehl, *Professorenkatalog der Universität Leipzig*, available at <http://uni-leipzig.de/unigeschichte/professorenkatalog/>, accessed 26 October 2016; August Hirsch, 'Gehler, Johann Karl', in *Allgemeine Deutsche Biographie* 8 (1878), 498–99, available online at <http://www.deutsche-biographie.de/pnd117530476.html>, accessed 22.02.2011.

POHL, Johann Ehrenfried

* 12 September 1746 (Leipzig), † 15 October 1800 (Dresden)

1780–82   Amtsphysicus

1781/82   Stadtaccoucheur

1788–1800   Electoral Counsel and Personal Physician in Dresden

Johann Ehrenfried Pohl was the son of Johann Christoph Pohl (*1706, †1780, professor of pathology in the Leipzig Medical Faculty and Amtsphysicus in Leipzig; later also Kreis- und Landphysicus). Pohl studied medicine in Leipzig 1763–69 before obtaining his Doctor of Medicine at Leipzig University in

1772. He then undertook a tour of the medical faculties in Strasbourg, Paris, Rouen and the Netherlands. (Strasbourg and Paris were famed for their maternity hospitals.) On his return in 1773 he was named extraordinary professor of botany in the Medical Faculty in Leipzig. Pohl Jr. succeeded his father as Amtsphysicus in 1780. In 1781 Johann Karl Gehler, Stadtaccoucheur in Leipzig, resigned his office and nominated Pohl as his successor. Pohl held this office until he was called to the court in Dresden as the Elector's counsel and personal physician in 1788. He retained his chair on the Medical Faculty, the day-to-day business of which he left to his substitutes/deputies, until his death in 1800. In 1789 he was appointed professor of pathology and in 1796 professor of therapy at the University in Leipzig. Amongst his published works was *Einige ohnmasgebliche und wohlgemeinte Vorschläge zu einer höchstnöthigen Verbesserung des Medicinalwesens in Sachsen* (Jena, 1791) and various Latin medical treatises on largely non-obstetric matters.

Sources: StadtAL, Tit. (F) XLIV.D.6b, Bd. I, 'Acta, Die Einrichtung der Kindermütter und Beÿweiber de Anno 1757', 222–26, 'Letter of resignation from Stadtaccoucheur Johann Carl Gehler', 30 October 1781. See entries for 'Johann Ehrenfried Pohl' and 'Johann Christoph Pohl' in Hehl, *Professorenkatalog Leipzig*.

HARTWIG, Christian Adolph

* 1755 (Meißen), † 18.11.1791 (Leipzig)

1789–91/92   Stadtaccoucheur

Hartwig studied medicine in Leipzig. After obtaining his Doctor of Medicine in 1783, he set up medical practice and quickly developed a reputation as a particularly skilled Accoucheur. The Leipzig Council appointed him Stadtaccoucheur in 1789 and he remained in this office until his death in 1791/92.

Sources: StadtAL, Tit. (F) X 23b, Bd. X, 'Instruktionen (1676–nach 1800)', 5–7, 'Instruktion für den Accoucheur', 1788–92. See entry for 'Hartwig, Christian Adolph H.' in Hirsch, ed., *Biographisches Lexikon*, vol. 3, 77.

MENZ, Carl Christian Friedrich

* 1757, † 1826

1792–min. 1814 Stadtaccoucheur

Little is known about Carl Christian Friedrich Menz. He published his medical dissertation *Dissertatio de varice interno morborum quorundam* at the University of Leipzig in 1789, but probably gained his qualification in 1785. The chief examiner (*präses*) at his *rigorosum* was Stadtaccoucheur Professor Johann Ehrenfried Pohl. Menz was appointed Stadtaccoucheur by the Leipzig Council in 1792 to succeed Christian Adolph Hartwig and remained in this office until at least 1814. He published only one other work on rheumatism in children in 1788.

Sources: Identity tag for 'Carl Christian Friedrich Menz' in Gemeinsamer Verbundkatalog (GVK), available online at <http://gso.gbv.de/DB=2.1/PPNSET?PPN=333199499>, accessed on 5 March 2011; StadtAL, Tit. (F) XLIV.D.6b, Bd. II, 'Acta, Die Einrichtung der Kindermütter und Beÿweiber de Anno 1782', 99–133, 'Stadtaccoucheur reports (Dr. Carl Christian Menz)', 13 August 1792–14 March 1805.

JÖRG, Johann Christian Gottfried

* 24 December 1779 (Predel bei Zeitz), † 20 September 1856 (Leipzig)

1809–56   Professor of Obstetrics and Director of the Triersches Institut, Leipzig

Jörg read the natural sciences and medicine in Leipzig, gaining his Doctor of Philosophy in 1804. During the course of his studies he assisted the Leipzig Stadtaccoucheur Christian Friedrich Menz and developed a keen interest in obstetrics. In 1804 he travelled to Vienna to attend practical lessons in obstetrics at the famous maternity hospital under the direction of Johann Lukas Boër. In 1805 he produced his Habilitation in obstetrics and obtained his Doctor of Medicine in the same year. Until 1809 he worked as a *Privatdozent* (private lecturer) in the Medical Faculty, Leipzig. He became the University's first ordinary professor of obstetrics in 1809, a position he held until his death in 1856. A condition of his promotion to professor was the right to establish a maternity hospital for teaching midwives and medical students the art of obstetrics; the Triersches Institut was inaugurated in 1810. His publications focused on largely obstetric and paediatric topics.

Sources: 'Johann Christian Gottfried Jörg' in Hehl, *Professorenkatalog Leipzig*, Hans G. Sohni, 'Jörg, Johann Christian Gottfried', in *Neue Deutsche Bibliographie* 10 (1974), 462–63, available online at <http://www.deutsche-biographie.de/NDB117148814.html>, accessed 22.04.2011; Sabine Fahrenbach, 'Johann Christian Gottfried Jörg und das "Triersche Institut". Zum 150. Todestag am 20. September 2006 und zum 200. Jubiläum der Trierschen Stiftung', *Jubiläen 2006. Personen/Ereignisse* (Leipzig: Universitätsarchiv Leipzig, 2006).

Bibliography

Manuscript sources

Sächsisches Hauptstaatsarchiv Dresden (SächsHSADD)

10115 Sanitätskollegium, Loc. 11609, vol. I, (1769–1782)

Sächsisches Staatsarchiv Leipzig (SächsSAL)

Loc. 20009, Amt Leipzig, Nr. 3891

Stadtarchiv Leipzig (StadtAL)

II. Sektion (II. Sekt.)
 H (F) Nr. 1157; K (F) Nr. 255; M (F) Nr. 670, Bd. II, III; M (F) Nr. 760; P (F) Nr. 175b;
 R (F) Nr. 91; R (F) Nr. 442; S (F) Nr. 1023; S (F) Nr. 2013; S (F) Nr. 2068; W (F) Nr. 319;
 W (F) Nr. 332
Leichenschreiberei
 Ratsleichenbücher (1595–1875)
Ratsstube
 Eidbücher 1590, 1613, 1689
Richterstube/Stadtgericht
 Akten Teil 1   Nr. 185
 Strafakten (Straf.) Nr. 67; 236; 624; 654; 674; 693; 708; 709; 715; 718; 735
 Testamente Rep. V, Paket 216, Nr. 3; Rep. V, Paket 236, Nr. 3
Stiftungsakten (Stift.)
 I   Jakobs-Hospital
       Nr. 3
Titelakten (Tit.)
 VIII   Ratswahlen, -protokolle und -beschlüsse sowie andere
       Angelegenheiten des Rates
       Nr. 53; 61
 X   Ratsbeamte
       23a; 23a Bd. III; 23b Bd. V, VIII, X; 23c Bd. I
 XLIV.A   Ärzte und Wundärzte, Anstalten
       1a; 18a
 XLIV.D   Hebammen
       Nr. 1, Bd. I, II; 1a; 2a; 3; 4; 5; 6; 6b, Bd. I, II; 6c; 7; 8a, Bd. I; 8c,
       Bd. II; 9
 LX.A   Kaiserliche und landesherrliche Gesetze
       Nr. 18a
 LX.B   Verordnungen und Patente des Rates
       Nr. 7–8

Kirchenarchiv Leipzig (KAL)

Taufbücher, Traubücher

Universitätsarchiv Leipzig (UAL)

Medizinische Fakultät (Med. Fak.)
    A01/52, Bd. 01–03   Medizinal Polizei (Film Nr. 1285)
    A IIId, Bd. 01   (Film Nr. 1334)
Gerichtsamt (GA)
    IV 205   Schwängerungsacta

Maps

Karte von Leipzig inner der Stadtmauer, gestochen von W. Engelmann in *Von Reillyschen Land-karten und Kunstwerke Verschliess-Kontor in Wien* (Vienna, ca. 1800), reproduced in Pro Leipzig / Thomas Nabert, ed., *Leipziger Stadtpläne: Verzeichnis der in Leipziger Institutionen verfügbaren Karten und Pläne* (2nd edn, Leipzig: Passage-Verlag, 1994).

Leipzig, eine florisante, auch befestigte Handels-Stadt und weitberühmte Universitaet in dem Ober-Saexischen Craiß (M. Seutter: Augsburg, 1723), reproduced in Pro Leipzig / Thomas Nabert, ed., *Leipziger Stadtpläne: Verzeichnis der in Leipziger Institutionen verfügbaren Karten und Pläne* (2nd edn, Leipzig: Passage-Verlag, 1994).

Neuster Plan der Stadt Leipzig, nach den besten Quellen bearbeitet (Leipzig: F. Krätschmer, 1840), reproduced in Pro Leipzig/Thomas Nabert, ed., *Leipziger Stadtpläne: Verzeichnis der in Leipziger Institutionen verfügbaren Karten und Pläne* (2nd edn, Leipzig: Passage-Verlag, 1994).

Müller, Ernst, *Häuserbuch zum Nienborgschen Atlas* (Berlin: Akademie-Verlag, 1997).

Nienborg, Hans August, *Description über die Grund-Legung und in richtigen Abriß gebrachte berühmte Handels-Stadt Leipzig* [Nienborgscher Atlas] (Leipzig, 1710), facsimile of the original (Berlin: Akademie-Verlag, 1997).

Printed primary sources

Agenda, das ist: Kirchenordnung / Wie sich die Pfarrherrn vnd Seelsorger in ihren Ampten und Diensten halten sollen / Für die Diener der Kirchen in Hertzog Heinrichen zu Sachsen V. G. H. Fürstenthumb gestellet, (Leipzig: Henning Großen des Altern, 1624).

'Leipziger Almosenordnung. 1704', transcribed in Helmut Bräuer, ed., *Der Leipziger Rat und die Bettler: Quellen und Analysen zu Bettlern und Bettelwesen in der Messestadt bis ins 18. Jahrhundert* (Leipzig: Universitätsverlag, 1997), 133–44.

'Mandat wegen Errichtung eines Sanitäts=Collegii zur Verbesserung des Medicinalwesens vom 13. September 1768', *Handbuch der im Königreich Sachsen geltenden Medicinal=Polizei-gesetze, sämmtliche Gesetze enthaltend, welche der unterm 30. Juli 1836 erschienene, allgemeinen Instruction der Bezirksärzte, Gerichtsärzte und Amtschirurgen zum Grunde liegen* (Leipzig: Ch. S. Kayser'sche Buchhandlung (F. Beyer), 1837), 1–5.

Beck, Jakob Christoff and August Johann Buxtorf, *Supplement zu dem Baselischen allgemein historischen Lexico* (Basel: Johannes Christ sel. Wittib, 1744).

Bourgeois, Louise, *Hebammen Buch,* trans. Severin Pineau (4 vols, Frankfurt am Main: Matthaei Merian, c. 1644), vol. 1.

Cruciger, Moritz, *Leipzig im Profil. Ein Taschenwörterbuch* (Solothurn: Krüger und Weber, 1799).

Ettner von Eiteritz, Johann Christoph, *Des getreuen Eckharts Unvorsichige Heb-Amme* (Leipzig: Braun, 1715).

Hoorn, Johan von, *Die zwo um Ihrer Gottesfurcht und Treue willen von Gott wohl belohnte Weh=Mutter, Siphra und Pua* (Stockholm and Leipzig: Johann Heinrich Rußworm, 1726).

Horenburg, Anna Elizabeth, *Wohlmeynender und nöhtiger Unterricht der Heeb=Ammen* (Hannover and Wolfenbüttel: Gottfried Freytag, 1700).

Joerdens, Peter Gottfried, *Von den Eigenschaften des aechten Geburtshelfers: eine Skizze; zur besonderen Berherzigung für meine Landesleute* (Leipzig: Dykische Buchhandlung, 1789).

Leonhardi, Friedrich Gottlieb, *Geschichte und Beschreibung der Kreis- und Handelsstadt Leipzig nebst der umliegenden Gegend* (Leipzig: Beygang, 1799).

Petermann, Andreas, *Casuum medico-legalium decas II* (2 vols, Leipzig: Benjamin B. Petermann, 1709), vol. 2.

Rau, Wolfgang Thomas, *Gedanken von dem Nutzen und der Nothwendigkeit einer medizinischen Policeyordnung in einem Staat* (2nd edn, Ulm: Gaum, 1764).

Rößlin, Eucharius d. Ä., *Der Swangern Frauwen vnd hebamen Rosengarten* (Straßburg: Martin Flach, 1513).

Sachs, Hans, *Eygentliche Beschreibung Aller Stände auff Erden* (Frankfurt am Main, 1568).

Scipione, Mercurio, *La Commare dell Scipione Mercurio. Kindermutter. Oder Hebammen Buch*, trans. Gottfried Welsch (Leipzig: Timothei Ritzschens, 1652).

Siegemund, Justine, *The Court Midwife. Justina Siegemund*, trans. Lynne Tatlock (Chicago, IL: The University of Chicago Press, 2005).

Siegemundin, Justine, *Die Chur=Brandenburgische Hoff=Wehe=Mutter* (Cölln an der Spree: Ulrich Liebperten, Churfl. Brandenb. Hofbuchdrucker, 1690).

Vogel, Johann Jakob, *Leipzigisches Geschichts-Buch oder Annales, das ist: Jahr- und Tagebücher der weltberühmten Königl. und Churfürstlichen Sächsischen Kauff= und Handels=Stadt Leipzig ... von Anno 1661 ... bis in das 1714 Jahr* (Leipzig: Friedrich Lanckischens sel. Erben, 1714).

Von Schröder, Wilhelm, *Fürstliche Schatz- und Rentenkammer* (edition unknown, Königsberg: 1752).

Printed secondary sources

Abreu-Ferreira, Darlene, 'Work and Identity in Early Modern Portugal: What Did Gender Have to Do with It?', *Journal of Social History* 35: 4 (2002): 1–31.

Ackerknecht, Erwin, 'Midwives as Experts in Court', *Bulletin of the New York Academy of Medicine* 52: 10 (1976): 1224–28.

Aurig, Rainer, 'Betrachtungen zur wirtschaftlich-sozialen Situation in Sachsen im Gefolge des Dreißigjährigen Krieges', *Sächsische Heimatblätter* 6 (1995): 343–51.

Barth-Scalmani, Gunda, '"Freundschaftlicher Zuruf eines Arztes an das Salzburgische Landvolk". Staatliche Hebammenausbildung und medizinische Volksaufklärung am Ende des 18. Jahrhunderts', in Jürgen Schlumbohm, Barbara Duden, Jacques Gélis and Patrice Veit, eds, *Rituale der Geburt. Eine Kulturgeschichte* (Munich: Verlag C. H. Beck, 1998), 102–18.

Bártori, Ingrid, 'Frauen in Handel und Handwerk in der Reichsstadt Nördlingen im 15. und 16. Jahrhundert', in Barbara Vogel and Ulrike Weckel, eds, *Frauen in der Ständegesellschaft. Leben und Arbeiten in der Stadt vom späten Mittelalter bis zur Neuzeit* (Hamburg: Kramer, 1991), 27–48.

Beachy, Robert, *The Soul of Commerce: Credit, Property and Politics in Leipzig, 1750–1840* (Leiden: Brill, 2005).

Beauvalet-Boutouyrie, Scarlett, 'Die Chef-Hebamme: Herz und Seele Pariser Entbindungshospitals von Port-Royal im 19. Jahrhundert', in Jürgen Schlumbohm, Barbara Duden,

Jacques Gélis and Patrice Veit, eds, *Rituale der Geburt. Eine Kulturgeschichte* (Munich: Verlag C.H. Beck, 1998), 221–41.

Berger, Beate, Bodo Gronemann and Jakuf Pacer, *Vom Aderlass zum Gesundheitspass. Zeittafel zur Geschichte des öffentlichen Gesundheitswesens in Leipzig* (Leipzig: Leipziger Universitätsverlag, 2000).

Bergfeld, Ingolf, *Leipzig. Eine kleine Stadtgeschichte* (Erfurt: Sutton, 2002).

Birkelbach, Dagmar and Sabine Luecken, 'Zur Entwicklung des Hebammenwesens vom 14. bis zum 16. Jahrhundert am Beispiel der Regensburger Hebammenordnungen', *Beiträge zur feministischen Theorie und Praxis* 5 (1981): 83–98.

Blaschke, Karlheinz, 'Zur Behördengeschichte der kursächsischen Lokalverwaltung', in Staatliche Archivverwaltung im Staatssekretariat für innere Angelegenheiten, ed., *Archivar und Historiker. Studien zur Archiv- und Geschichtswissenschaft* (Berlin: Rütten & Loening, 1956), 343–64.

—, *Bevölkerungsgeschichte von Sachsen bis zur industriellen Revolution* (Weimar: Hermann Böhlaus Nachfolger, 1967).

—, 'Die kursächsische Politik und Leipzig im 18. Jahrhundert', in Wolfgang Martens, ed., *Leipzig. Aufklärung und Bürgerlichkeit* (Heidelberg: Verlag Lambert Schneider, 1990), 23–38.

Blickle, Renate, 'Nahrung und Eigentum als Kategorien in der ständischen Gesellschaft', in Winifried Schulze and Helmut Gabel, eds, *Ständische Gesellschaft und soziale Mobilität* (Munich: Oldenbourg Verlag GmbH, 1988), 73–93.

Blumenfeld-Kosinski, Renate, *Not of Woman Born: Representations of Caesarean Birth in Medieval and Renaissance Culture* (Ithaca, NY: Cornell University Press, 1990).

Bonner, Thomas Neville, *Becoming a Physician: Medical Education in Britain, France, Germany and the United States, 1750–1945* (Baltimore, MD: The Johns Hopkins University Press, 1995).

Botelho, Lynn, 'Old Age and Menopause in Rural Women of Early Modern Suffolk', in Lynn Botelho and Pat Thane, eds, *Women and Ageing in British Society since 1500* (Harlow: Longman, 2001), 43–65.

Bräuer, Helmut, 'Das zünftige Handwerk in Sachsen und die "Landes-Oeconomie-Manufactur- und Commercien-Deputation" im 18. Jahrhundert', in Karl Czok and Helmut Bräuer, eds, *Studien zur älteren sächsischen Handwerksgeschichte* (Berlin: Akademie-Verlag, 1990), 50–84.

—, 'Arme Leute in Sachsen im 18. Jahrhundert', in Stadtarchiv Leipzig, ed., *Räume voll Leipzig 94. Arbeitsberichte des Stadtarchivs Leipzig* (Leipzig: Tangent Verlag, 1994), 72–87.

—, *Der Leipziger Rat und die Bettler: Quellen und Analysen zu Bettlern und Bettelwesen in der Messestadt bis ins 18. Jahrhundert* (Leipzig: Universitätsverlag, 1997).

—, 'Leipzigs Messen und die armen Leute während der frühen Neuzeit', in Günter Bentele, Thomas Topfstedt and Hartmut Zwahr, eds, *Leipzigs Messen 1497–1997. Gestaltwandel – Umbrüche – Neubeginn, Teilband 1: 1497–1914* (2 vols, Cologne: Böhlau, 1999), vol. 1, 317–28.

—, *Stadtchronistik und städtische Gesellschaft. Über die Widerspiegelung sozialer Strukturen in der obersächsisch-lausitzischen Stadtchronistik der frühen Neuzeit* (Leipzig: Leipziger Universitätsverlag GmbH, 2009).

Bretschneider, Falk, 'Fürsorge oder Disziplinierung? Die Armen und das Waldheimer Zuchthaus im 18. Jahrhundert', in Helmut Bräuer, ed., *Arme – ohne Chance? Protocoll der internationalen Tagung "Kommunale Armut und Armutsbekämpfung vom Spätmittelalter bis zur Gegenwart" vom 23. bis 25. Oktober 2003 in Leipzig* (Leipzig: Leipziger Universitätsverlag, 2004), 135–57.

Breuer, Stefan, 'Sozialdisziplinierung. Probleme und Problemverlagerungen eines Konzepts bei Max Weber, Gerhard Oestreich und Michel Foucault', in Christoph Sachße and Florian Tennstedt, eds, *Soziale Sicherheit und soziale Disziplinierung. Beiträge zu einer historischen Theorie der Sozialpolitik* (Frankfurt am Main: Suhrkamp, 1986), 45–69.

Brockliss, Laurence and Colin Jones, *The Medical World of Early Modern France* (Oxford: Clarendon Press, 1997).

Broman, Thomas, 'University Reform in Medical Thought at the End of the Eighteenth Century', *Osiris (2nd series)* 5 (1989): 36–53.

—, 'Rethinking Professionalization: Theory, Practice and Professional Ideology in Eighteenth-Century German Medicine', *Journal of Modern History* 67: 4 (1995): 835–72.

—, 'Zwischen Staat und Konsumgesellschaft: Aufklärung und die Entwicklung des deutschen Medizinalwesens im 18. Jahrhundert', in Bettina Wahrig-Schmidt and Werner Sohn, eds, *Zwischen Aufklärung, Policey und Verwaltung. Zur Genese des Medizinalwesens 1750–1850* (Wiesbaden: Harrossowitz Verlag, 2003), 91–107.

Burkhard, Georg, *Die deutschen Hebammenordnungen von ihren ersten Anfängen bis auf die Neuzeit* (Leipzig, 1912).

Capp, Bernard, 'Separate Domains? Women and Authority in Early Modern England', in Paul Griffiths, Adam Fox and Steve Hindle, eds, *The Experience of Authority in Early Modern England* (Basingstoke: Macmillan Press, 1996), 117–45.

—, *When Gossips Meet: Women, Family, and Neighbourhood in Early Modern England* (Oxford: Oxford University Press, 2003).

Cavallo, Sandra, *Artisans of the Body in Early Modern Italy*, trans. Liz Heron and Sandra Cavallo (Manchester: Manchester University Press, 2007).

Cody, Lisa Forman, *Birthing the Nation: Sex, Science, and the Conception of Eighteenth-Century Britons* (Oxford: Oxford University Press, 2005).

—, 'The Body in Birth and Death', in Carol Reeves, ed., *A Cultural History of the Human Body in the Age of the Enlightenment* (6 vols, Oxford: Berg, 2010), vol. 4, 13–32.

Cook, Harold J., 'Good Advice and Little Medicine. The Professional Authority of Early Modern English Physicians', *Journal of British Studies* 33 (1994): 1–31.

Cressy, David, 'Purification, Thanksgiving and the Churching of Women in Post-Reformation England', *Past and Present* 141 (1993): 106–46.

—, *Birth, Marriage and Death: Ritual, Religion, and the Life-Cycle in Tudor and Stuart England* (Oxford: Oxford University Press, 1997).

Crowther-Heyck, Kathleen, '"Be Fruitful and Multiply": Genesis and Generation in Reformation Germany', *Renaissance Quarterly* 55: 3 (2002): 904–35.

Croxson, Bronwyn, 'The Foundation and Evolution of the Middlesex Hospital's Lying-In Service, 1745–86', *Social History of Medicine* 14: 1 (2001): 27–57.

Cunningham, Andrew, 'Introduction: "Where there are three physicians, there are two atheists"', in Ole Peter Grell and Andrew Cunningham, eds, *Medicine and Religion in Enlightenment Europe* (Aldershot and Burlington, VT: Ashgate, 2007), 1–4.

Cunningham, Andrew and Ole Peter Grell, *The Four Horsemen of the Apocalypse: Religion, War, Famine, and Death in Reformation Europe* (Cambridge and New York, NY: Cambridge University Press, 2000).

Czok, Karl, *Leipzig. Geschichte der Stadt in Wort und Bild* (Berlin GDR: VEB Deutscher Verlag der Wissenschaften, 1978).

—, *Vorstädte. Zu ihrer Entstehung, Wirtschaft und Sozialentwicklung in der älteren deutschen Stadtgeschichte* (Berlin: Akademie-Verlag 1979).

Czok, Karl and Reiner Gross, 'Das Kurfürstentum, die sächsisch-polnische Union und die Staatsreform (1547–1789)', in Karl Czok, ed., *Geschichte Sachsens* (Weimar: Hermann Böhlaus Nachfolger, 1989), 208–96.

Darnton, Robert, *The Great Cat Massacre and Other Episodes in French Cultural History* (New York, NY: First Vintage Books, 1985).

Davis, Natalie Zemon, *Fiction in the Archives: Pardon Tales and Their Tellers in Sixteenth-Century France* (Cambridge: Polity Press, 1987).

Dawson, Ruth, 'The Search for Women's Experience of Pregnancy and Birth: Eighteenth-Century Accounts', in Katherine M. Faull, ed., *Anthropology and the German Enlightenment: Perspectives on Humanity* (Lewisburg, PA: Bucknell University Press, 1995), 101–25.

De Renzi, Silvia, .'Medical Expertise, Bodies, and the Law in Early Modern Courts', *Isis* 98: 2 (2007): 315–22.

—, 'The Risks of Childbirth. Physicians, Finance, and Women's Deaths in the Law Courts of Seventeenth-Century Rome', *Bulletin of the History of Medicine* 84: 4 (2010): 549–77.

Dietzmann, Elisabeth, *Die Leipziger Einrichtungen der Armenpflege bis zur Übernahme der Armenverwaltung durch die Stadt 1881* (Leipzig: Steiger, 1932).

Dinges, Martin, 'The Reception of Michel Foucault's Ideas on Social Discipline, Mental Asylums, Hospitals and the Medical Profession in German Historiography', in Colin Jones and Roy Porter, eds, *Reassessing Foucault: Power, medicine, and the body* (London: Routledge, 1994), 181–212.

—, 'Medicinische Policey zwischen Heilkundigen und "Patienten" (1750–1830)', in Karl Härter, ed., *Policey und frühneuzeitliche Gesellschaft* (Frankfurt am Main: Vittorio Klostermann, 2000), 261–95.

—, '"Policeyforschung" statt "Sozialdisziplinierung"?', *Zeitschrift für Neuere Rechtsgeschichte* 24: 3/4 (2002): 327–44.

—, 'Medical Pluralism – Past and Present: Towards a more precise concept', in Robert Jütte, ed., *Medical Pluralism – Past – Present – Future* (Stuttgart: Franz Steiner Verlag, 2013), 195–205.

Donnison, Jean, *Midwives and Medical Men: A History of Inter-Professional Rivalries and Women's Rights* (2nd edn, London: Heinemann Educational, 1988).

Duden, Barbara, *Geschichte unter der Haut. Ein Eisenacher Arzt und seine Patientinnen um 1730* (Stuttgart: Klett-Cotta, 1987).

—, 'Medicine and the History of the Body: The Lady of the Court', in Jens Lachmund and Gunnar Stollberg, eds, *The Social Construction of Illness: Illness and Medical Knowledge in Past and Present* (Stuttgart: F. Steiner, 1992), 23–28.

Dülmen, Richard van, *Frauen vor Gericht. Kindsmord in der frühen Neuzeit* (Frankfurt am Main: Fischer Taschenbuch Verlag, 1991).

—, *Kultur und Alltag in der Frühen Neuzeit. Zweiter Band. Dorf und Stadt 16.–18. Jahrhundert* (3 vols, Munich: Verlag C. H. Beck, 1992), vol. 2.

—, *Kultur und Alltag in der Frühen Neuzeit. Erster Band. Das Haus und seine Menschen 16.–18. Jahrhundert* (2nd edn, 3 vols, Munich: Verlag C. H. Beck, 1995), vol. 1.

Earle, Peter, 'The Female Labour Market in London in the Late Seventeenth and Early Eighteenth Centuries', *Economic History Review*, ser. 2, 42: 3 (1989): 328–53.

Ehmer, Josef and Peter Gutschner, 'Befreiung und Verkrümmung durch Arbeit', in Richard van Dülmen, ed., *Erfindung des Menschen. Schöpfungsträume und Körperbilder 1500–2000* (Vienna: Böhlau, 1998), 283–303.

—, 'Probleme und Deutungsmuster der "Arbeitsgesellschaft" in der Gegenwart und in der frühen Neuzeit', in Gerhard Ammerer, Christian Rohr and Alfred Stefan Weiss, eds, *Tradition und Wandel. Beiträge zur Kirchen-, Gesellschafts- und Kulturgeschichte. Festschrift für Heinz Dopsch* (Vienna: Verlag für Geschichte und Politik, 2001), 305–20.

Ehmer, Josef and Catharina Lis, *The Idea of Work in Europe from Antiquity to Modern Times* (Farnham and Burlington: Ashgate, 2009).

—, 'Introduction: Historical Studies in Perceptions of Work', in Josef Ehmer and Catharina Lis, eds, *The Idea of Work in Europe from Antiquity to Modern Times* (Farnham and Burlington: Ashgate, 2009), 1–32.

Ehrenreich, Barbara and Deirdre English, *Witches, Midwives and Nurses: A History of Women Healers* (2nd edn, Old Westbury, NY: The Feminist Press, 1973).

Engelsing, Rolf, *Analphabetentum und Lektüre. Zur Sozialgeschichte des Lesens in Deutschland zwischen feudaler und industrieller Gesellschaft* (Stuttgart: J. B. Metzler, 1973).

Evenden, Doreen, 'Mothers and their midwives in seventeenth-century London', in Hilary Marland, ed., *The Art of Midwifery: Early Modern Midwives in Europe* (London: Routledge, 1993), 9–26.

—, *The Midwives of Seventeenth-Century London* (Cambridge: Cambridge University Press, 2000).

Fahrenbach, Sabine, 'Johann Christian Gottfried Jörg und das "Triersche Institut". Zum 150. Todestag am 20. September 2006 und zum 200. Jubiläum der Trierschen Stiftung', *Jubiläen 2006. Personen/Ereignisse* (Leipzig: Universitätsarchiv Leipzig, 2006), 125–30.

Fahrenbach, Sabine and Heiko Leske, 'Immer zum Wohle der Patientinnen … die Frauenklinik im Wandel der Zeiten', *Gesundheit und mehr* 9 (2007): 4–5.

Fischer-Homberger, Esther, *Medizin vor Gericht. Gerichtsmedizin von der Renaissance bis zur Aufklärung* (Bern: H. Huber, 1983).

Fissell, Mary, *Patients, Power and the Poor in Eighteenth-Century Bristol* (Cambridge: Cambridge University Press, 1991).

—, 'Introduction: Women, Health and Healing in Early Modern Europe', *Bulletin for the History of Medicine* 82 (2008): 1–17.

—, *Vernacular Bodies: The Politics of Reproduction in Early Modern England* (Oxford: Oxford University Press, 2004).

Flügge, Sibylla, 'Die gute Ordnung der Geburtshilfe. Recht und Realität am Beispiel des Hebammenrechts der Frühneuzeit', in Ute Gerhard, ed., *Frauen in der Geschichte des Rechts. Von der Frühen Neuzeit bis zur Gegenwart* (Munich: Verlag C. H. Beck, 1997), 140–50.

—, *Hebammen und heilkundige Frauen. Recht und Rechtswirklichkeit im 15. und 16. Jahrhundert* (Frankfurt am Main: Stroemfeld, 1998).

Forbes, Thomas Rogers, *The Midwife and the Witch* (New Haven, CT: Yale University Press, 1966).

Frevert, Ute, *Krankheit als politisches Problem 1770–1880: Soziale Unterschichten in Preußen zwischen medizinischer Polizei und staatlicher Sozialversicherung* (Göttingen: Vandenhoeck & Ruprecht, 1984).

Frey, Axel, 'Der "Leipziger Platz". Buch- und Verlagswesen', in Axel Frey and Bernd Weinkauf, eds, *Leipzig als ein Pleißathen. Eine geistesgeschichtliche Ortsbestimmung* (Leipzig: Reclam Verlag, 1995), 127–71.

Fuhrmann, Martin, *Volksvermehrung als Staatsaufgabe? Bevölkerungs- und Ehepolitik in der deutschen politischen und ökonomischen Theorie des 18. und 19. Jahrhunderts* (Paderborn: Ferdinand Schöningh, 2002).

Fuhrmann, Rosi, Beat Kümin and Andreas Würgler, 'Supplizierende Gemeinden. Aspekte einer vergleichenden Quellenbetrachtung', in Peter Blickle, ed., *Gemeinde und Staat im alten Europa* (Munich: R. Oldenbourg Verlag, 1998), 267–323.

Gauß, Carl-Joseph and Bernhard Wilde, *Die Deutschen Geburtshelferschulen. Bausteine zur Geschichte der Geburtshilfe* (Munich-Gräfeling: Banaschewski, 1956).

Gélis, Jacques, *La sage-femme ou le médecin: une nouvelle conception de la vie* (Paris: Fayard, 1988).

—, *Die Geburt: Volksglaube, Rituale und Praktiken von 1500–1900*, trans. Clemens Wilhelm (Munich: Diederichs, 1989).

—, *History of Childbirth: Fertility, Pregnancy and Birth in Early Modern Europe*, trans. Rosemary Morris (Cambridge: Polity Press, 1991).

Gentilcore, David, 'Medical Pluralism and the Medical Marketplace in Early Modern Italy', in Robert Jütte, ed., *Medical Pluralism – Past – Present – Future* (Stuttgart: Franz Steiner Verlag, 2013), 45–55.

Gleixner, Ulrike, 'Die "Gute" und die "Böse". Hebammen als Amtsfrauen auf dem Land (Altmark/Brandenburg, 18. Jahrhundert)', in Heide Wunder and Christina Vanja, eds, *Weiber, Menscher, Frauenzimmer. Frauen in der ländlichen Gesellschaft 1500–1800* (Göttingen: Vandenhoeck & Ruprecht, 1996), 96–112.

Gottschalk, Karin, 'Wissen über Land und Leute. Administrative Praktiken und Staatsbildungsprozesse im 18. Jahrhundert', in Peter Collin and Thomas Horstmann, eds, *Das Wissen des Staates: Geschichte, Theorie und Praxis* (Baden-Baden: Nomos, 2004), 149–74.

Gowing, Laura, *Common Bodies: Women, Touch and Power in Seventeenth-Century England* (New Haven, CT: Yale University Press, 2003).

Gray, Marion W., 'Kameralismus: Die säkuläre Ökonomie und die getrennten Geschlechter-sphären', *WerkstattGeschichte* 19 (1998): 41–57.

Green, Monica, *Making Women's Medicine Masculine: The Rise of Male Authority in Premodern Gynaecology* (Oxford and New York, NY: Oxford University Press, 2008).

Greilshammer, Myriam, 'The Midwife, the Priest, and the Physician: The Subjugation of Midwives in the Low Countries at the End of the Middle Ages', *Journal of Medieval and Renaissance Studies* 21: 2 (1991): 285–329.

Grell, Ole Peter and Andrew Cunningham, *Medicine and Religion in Enlightenment Europe* (Aldershot and Burlington, VT: Ashgate, 2007).

Gross, Reiner, *Geschichte Sachsens* (Leipzig: Edition Leipzig, 2001).

Grundy, Isobel, 'Sarah Stone: Enlightenment Midwife', *Clio Medica* 29 (1995): 128–44.

Haberling, Elseluise, *Beiträge zur Geschichte des Hebammenstandes I. Der Hebammenstand bis zum Dreißigjährigen Krieg* (Berlin, 1940).

Hackenberg, Michael R., 'Books in Artisan Homes of Sixteenth-Century Germany', *Journal of Library History* 21 (1986): 72–91.

Hammerstein, Notker, 'Die Universität Leipzig im Zeichen der frühen Aufklärung', in Wolfgang Martens, ed., *Zentren der Aufklärung III: Leipzig. Aufklärung und Bürgerlichkeit* (Heidelberg: Verlag Lambert Schneider, 1990), 125–40.

Hampe, Henrike, *Zwischen Tradition und Instruktion. Hebammen im 18. und 19. Jahrhundert in der Universitätstadt Göttingen* (Göttingen: Schmerse, 1998).

—, 'Hebammen und Geburtshelfer im Göttingen des 18. Jahrhunderts. Das Jahr 1751 und seine Folgen', in Christine Loytved, ed., *Von der Wehemutter zur Hebamme: Die Gründung von Hebammenschulen mit Blick auf ihren politischen Stellenwert und praktischen Nutzen* (Osnabrück: Universitäts-Verlag Rasch, 2001), 53–62.

Harkness, Deborah E., 'A View from the Streets: Women and Medical Work in Elizabethan London', *Bulletin of the History of Medicine* 82: 1 (2008): 52–85.

Harley, David, 'Historians as Demonologists: The Myth of the Midwife-Witch', *Society for the History of Medicine* 3 (1990): 1–26.

Harrington, Joel F., *The Unwanted Child: The Fate of Foundlings, Orphans, and Juvenile Criminals in Early Modern Germany* (Chicago, IL and London: The University of Chicago Press, 2009).

Härter, Karl, ed., *Policey und frühneuzeitliche Gesellschaft* (Frankfurt am Main: Vittorio Klostermann, 2000).

Hatcher, John, 'Labour, Leisure and Economic Thought before the Nineteenth Century', *Past and Present* 160 (1988): 64–115.

Hausen, Karin, 'Family and Role-Division: The Polarisation of Sexual Stereotypes in the Nineteenth Century – an Aspect of the Dissociation of Work and Family Life', in Richard J. Evans and W. Robert Lee, eds, *The German Family: Essays on the Social History of the Family in Nineteenth- and Twentieth-Century Germany* (London and Totowa, NJ: Croom Helm; Barnes & Noble, 1981), 51–83.

Heinsohn, Gunnar and Otto Steiger, *Die Vernichtung der weisen Frauen. Beiträge zur Theorie und Geschichte von Bevölkerung und Kindheit* (2nd edn, Herbstein: März-Verlag, 1985).

Helbig, Herbert with Joachim Gontard, *Die Vertrauten, 1680–1980: eine Vereinigung Leipziger Kaufleute: Beiträge zur Sozialfürsorge und zum bürgerlichen Gemeinsinn einer kaufmännischen Führungsschicht* (Stuttgart: Anton Hiersemann Verlag, 1980).

Hess, Ann Giardina, 'Midwifery Practice Among the Quakers in Southern Rural England in the Late Seventeenth Century', in Hilary Marland, ed., *The Art of Midwifery: Early Modern Midwives in Europe* (London: Routledge, 1993), 49–76.

Hilpert, Claudia, *Wehemütter. Amtshebammen, Accoucheure und die Akademisierung der Geburtshilfe im kurfürstlichen Mainz, 1550–1800* (Frankfurt am Main: Peter Lang, 2000).

Hirsch, August, ed., *Biographisches Lexikon hervorragender Ärzte aller Zeiten und aller Völker vor 1880* (6 vols, Vienna: Urban & Schwarzenberg, 1886).

Holenstein, André, 'Bittgesuch, Gesetze und Verwaltung. Zur Praxis "guter Policey" in Gemeinde und Staat des Ancien Regime am Beispiel der Markgrafschaft Baden(-Durlach)', in Peter Blickle, ed., *Gemeinde und Staat im alten Europa* (Munich: R. Oldenbourg Verlag, 1998), 325–57.

—, 'Die Umstände der Normen – die Normen der Umstände. Policeyordnungen im kommunikativen Handeln von Verwaltung und lokaler Gesellschaft im Ancien Regime', in Karl Härter, ed., *Policey und frühneuzeitliche Gesellschaft* (Frankfurt am Main: Vittorio Klostermann, 2000), 2–46.

Hudson, Pat and W.R. Lee, *Women's Work and the Family Economy in Historical Perspective* (Manchester: Manchester University Press, 1990).

Huerkamp, Claudia, *Der Aufstieg der Ärzte im 19. Jahrhundert: Vom gelehrten Stand zum professionellen Experten. Das Beispiel Preußens* (Göttingen: Vandenhoeck & Ruprecht, 1985).

Hunter, Lynette, 'Sisters of the Royal Society: The Circle of Katherine Jones, Lady Ranelagh', in Lynette Hunter and Sarah Hutton, eds, *Women, Science and Medicine 1500–1700: Mothers and Sisters of the Royal Society* (Stroud: Sutton Publishing, 1997), 178–97.

—, 'Women and Domestic Medicine: Lady Experimenters, 1570–1620', in Lynette Hunter and Sarah Hutton, eds, *Women, Science and Medicine 1500–1700: Mothers and Sisters of the Royal Society* (Stroud: Sutton Publishing, 1997), 89–107.

Jackson, Mark, 'Developing Medical Expertise: Medical Practitioners and the Suspected Murders of New-Born Children', in Roy Porter, ed., *Medicine in the Enlightenment* (Amsterdam: Rodopi, 1995), 145–65.

—, ed., *Infanticide: Historical Perspectives on Child Murder and Concealment, 1550–2000* (Ashgate: Aldershot, 2002).

Jarzebowski, Claudia, 'Loss and Emotion in Funeral Works on Children in Seventeenth-Century Germany', in Lynne Tatlock, ed., *Enduring Loss in Early Modern Germany: Cross Disciplinary Perspectives* (Leiden: Brill, 2010), 187–214.

Jenner, Mark S.R. and Patrick Wallis, 'The Medical Marketplace', in Mark S.R. Jenner and Patrick Wallis, eds, *Medicine and the Market in England and Its Colonies, c.1450–c.1850* (Basingstoke: Palgrave Macmillan, 2007), 1–23.

—, eds, *Medicine and the Market in England and Its Colonies c.1450–c.1850* (Basingstoke: Palgrave Macmillan, 2007).

Jones, Colin, 'The Great Chain of Buying. Medical Advertisement, the Bourgeois Public Sphere, and the Origins of the French Revolution', *The American Historical Review* 101: 1 (1996): 13–40.

Jones, Colin and Roy Porter, 'Introduction', in Colin Jones and Roy Porter, eds, *Reassessing Foucault: Power, medicine, and the body* (London: Routledge, 1994), 1–16.

Jones, Peter Murray and Lea T. Olsan, 'Performative Rituals for Conception and Childbirth in England, 900–1500', *Bulletin of the History of Medicine* 89: 3 (2015): 406–33.

Jordanova, Ludmilla, *Nature Displayed: Gender, Science and Medicine 1760–1820* (London: Longman, 1999).

Jütte, Robert, *Obrigkeitliche Armenfürsorge in deutschen Reichsstädten der frühen Neuzeit. Städtisches Armenwesen in Frankfurt am Main und Köln* (Cologne: Böhlau, 1984).

—, '"Wo kein Weib ist, da seufzet der Kranke" – Familie und Krankheit im 16. Jahrhundert', in Robert Jütte, ed., *Medizin, Gesellschaft und Geschichte. Jahrbuch des Instituts für Geschichte der Medizin der Robert Bosch Stiftung 7* (Stuttgart: Hippokrates-Verlag, 1989), 7–24.

—, 'Health care provision and poor relief in early modern Hanseatic towns: Hamburg, Bremen and Lübeck', in Andrew Cunningham and Ole Peter Grell, eds, *Health Care and Poor Relief in Protestant Europe, 1500–1700* (London: Routledge, 1997), 108–28.

—, ed., *Medical Pluralism – Past – Present – Future* (Stuttgart: Franz Steiner Verlag, 2013).

—, 'Medical Pluralism in Early Modern Germany', in Robert Jütte, ed., *Medical Pluralism – Past – Present – Future* (Stuttgart: Franz Steiner Verlag, 2013), 11–44.

Karant-Nunn, Susan C., 'Babies, Baptism, Bodies, Burials, and Bliss: Ghost Stories and their Rejection in the Late Sixteenth Century', in Marion Kobelt-Groch and Cornelia Niekus

Moore, eds, *Tod und Jenseits in der Schriftkultur der Frühen Neuzeit* (Wiesbaden: Harrasso-witz Verlag, 2008), 10–22.

Karenberg, Axel, 'Lernen am Bett der Schwangeren. Zur Typologie des Entbindungshauses in Deutschland (1728–1840)', *Zentralblatt für Gynäkologie* 113 (1991): 899–912.

Kassell, Lauren, 'Magic, Alchemy and the Medical Economy in Early Modern England: The Case of Robert Fludd's Magnetical Medicine', in Mark S. R. Jenner and Patrick Wallis, eds, *Medicine and the Market in England and Its Colonies, c.1450–c.1850* (Basingstoke: Pal-grave Macmillan, 2007), 88–107.

Keller, Katrin, '"Gemeinschaft des hantwergs weiber und kinder". Zunft und Familie im Leip-ziger Handwerk des 16. Jahrhunderts', *Sächsische Heimatblätter* 36: 2 (1990): 74–79.

—, 'Handwerkeralltag im 16. Jahrhundert', in Karl Czok and Helmut Bräuer, eds, *Studien zur älteren Sächsischen Handwerksgeschichte* (Berlin: Akademie-Verlag, 1990), 7–49.

—, 'Kursachsen am Ende des 17. Jahrhunderts – Beobachtungen zur regionalen und wirtschaftlichen Struktur der sächsischen Städtelandschaft', in Uwe Schirmer, ed., *Sachsen im 17. Jahrhundert. Krise, Krieg und Neubeginn* (Beucha: Sax-Verlag, 1998), 131–60.

Kervorkian, Tanya, 'Laien und die Leipziger religiöse Öffentlichkeit 1685–1725', *Leipziger Kalender* (1996), 86–97.

—, 'Clerics and their Career Paths in Early Modern Leipzig', in Heide Wunder, ed., *Jedem das Seine. Abgrenzungen und Grenüberschreitungen im Leipzig des 17. und 18. Jahrhunderts* (Frankfurt am Main: Klostermann, 2000), 291–306.

—, 'The Rise of the Poor, Weak, and Wicked: Poor Care, Punishment, and Religion in Leip-zig, 1700–1730', *Journal of Social History* 34 (2000): 163–81.

King, Helen, *Midwifery, Obstetrics and the Rise of Gynaecology. The Uses of a Sixteenth-Century Compendium* (Aldershot: Ashgate, 2007).

Kinzelbach, Annemarie, 'Heilkundige und Gesellschaft in der frühneuzeitlichen Reichsstadt Überlingen', *Medizin, Gesellschaft und Geschichte* 8 (1989): 119–49.

—, 'Konstruktion und konkretes Handeln. Heilkundige Frauen im oberdeutschen Raum, 1450–1700', *Historische Anthropologie: Kultur, Gesellschaft, Alltag* 7: 2 (1999): 165–90.

Klairmont Lingo, Alison, 'Empirics and Charlatans in Early Modern France: The Genesis of the Classification of the "Other" in Medical Practice', *Journal of Social History* 19: 4 (1986): 583–603.

Kleemann, W. J., 'Die gerichtliche Medizin an der medizinischen Fakultät vor der Gründung des Institutes', in A. Graefe, R. K. Müller and W. J. Kleemann, eds, *100 Jahre forensische Toxikologie im Institut für Rechtsmedizin in Leipzig* (Leipzig: MOLINApress, 2004).

Klimpel, Volker, *Das Dresdner Collegium Medico-Chirurgicum* (Frankfurt am Main: Peter Lang, 1995).

Kobelt-Groch, Marion, 'Selig auch ohne Taufe? Gedruckte lutherische Leichenpredigten für ungetauft verstorbene Kinder des 16. und 17. Jahrhunderts', in Marion Kobelt-Groch and Cornelia Niekus Moore, eds, *Tod und Jenseits in der Schriftkultur der Frühen Neuzeit* (Wiesbaden: Harrassowitz Verlag, 2008), 63–78.

Koslofsky, Craig, 'Suicide and the Secularization of the Body in Early Modern Saxony', *Continuity and Change* 16 (2001): 45–70.

Krauss, H., 'Zur Geschichte des Hebammenwesens im Fürstentum Ansbach', *Archive für Geschichte der Medizin* 6 (1913): 64–71.

Kruse, Britta-Juliane, *Verborgene Heilkünste: Geschichte der Frauenmedizin im Spätmittelalter* (Ber-lin: W. de Gruyter, 1996).

Künnemann, Otto and Martina Güldemann, *Geschichte der Stadt Leipzig* (Gudensberg-Gleichen: Wartberg Verlag, 2000).

Labouvie, Eva, 'Selbstverwaltete Geburt. Landhebammen zwischen Macht und Reglemen-tierung (17.–19. Jahrhundert)', *Geschichte und Gesellschaft* 18 (1992): 477–506.

—, 'Frauenberuf ohne Vorbildung? Hebammen in den Städten und auf dem Land', in Elke Kleinau and Claudia Opitz, eds, *Geschichte der Mädchen- und Frauenbildung: Bd. 1 Vom*

Mittelalter bis zur Aufklärung (2 vols, Frankfurt am Main: Campus Verlag, 1996), vol. 1, 218–33.

—, 'Sofia Weinranck, Hebamme von St. Johann. Städtische Geburtshilfe und die Entrechtung der Bürgerinnen im 18. Jahrhundert', in Annette Keinhorst and Petra Messinger, eds, *Die Saarbrückerinnen. Beiträge zur Stadtgeschichte* (St Ingbert: Röhrig Universitätsverlag, 1998), 225–48.

—, *Beistand in Kindsnöten. Hebammen und weibliche Kultur auf dem Land, 1550–1910* (Frankfurt am Main: Campus Verlag, 1999).

—, *Andere Umstände: Eine Kulturgeschichte der Geburt* (Cologne: Böhlau, 2000).

—, '"Sanctuaires à répit". Zur Wiedererweckung toter Neugeborener, zur Erinnerungskultur und zur Jenseitsvorstellung im katholischen Milieu', in Marion Kobelt-Groch and Cornelia Niekus Moore, eds, *Tod und Jenseits in der Schriftkultur der Frühen Neuzeit* (Wiesbaden: Harrassowitz Verlag, 2008), 79–96.

Landwehr, Achim, 'Policey vor Ort. Die Implementation von Policeyordnungen in der ländlichen Gesellschaft der frühen Neuzeit', in Peter Landau and R. H. Helmholz, eds, *Grundlagen des Rechts: Festschrift für Peter Landau zum 65. Geburtstag* (Paderborn: F. Schöningh, 2000), 46–70.

Langbein, John H., *Prosecuting Crime in the Renaissance: England, Germany, France* (Cambridge, MA: Harvard University Press, 1974).

Lee, W. R., 'Bastardy and the Socioeconomic Structure of South Germany', *Journal of Interdisciplinary History* 7: 3 (1977): 403–25.

Leong, Elaine, 'Making Medicines in the Early Modern Household', *Bulletin of the History of Medicine* 82: 1 (2008): 145–68.

Leong, Elaine and Sara Pennell, 'Recipe Collections and the Currency of Medical Knowledge in the Early Modern "Medical Marketplace"', in Mark S. R. Jenner and Patrick Wallis, eds, *Medicine and the Market in England and Its Colonies, c.1450–c.1850* (Basingstoke: Palgrave Macmillan, 2007), 133–52.

Lewis, Margaret Brannan, *Infanticide and Abortion in Early Modern Germany* (London: Routledge, 2016).

Lindemann, Mary, 'Love for Hire: The Regulation of the Wet-Nursing Business in Eighteenth-Century Hamburg', *Journal of Family History* 6: 4 (1981): 379–95.

—, *Patriots and Paupers: Hamburg, 1712–1830* (New York & Oxford: Oxford University Press, 1990).

—, 'Professionals? Sisters? Rivals? Midwives in Braunschweig 1750–1800', in Hilary Marland, ed., *The Art of Midwifery. Early Modern Midwives in Europe* (London: Routledge, 1993), 176–92.

—, 'The Enlightenment Encountered: The German Physicus and His World', in Roy Porter, ed., *Medicine in the Enlightenment* (Amsterdam: Rodopi, 1995), 181–97.

—, *Health and Healing in Eighteenth-Century Germany* (Baltimore, MD: Johns Hopkins University Press, 1996).

—, 'Urban Charity and the Relief of the Sick Poor in Northern Germany, 1750–1850', in Ole Peter Grell and Andrew Cunningham, eds, *Health Care and Poor Relief in Eighteenth- and Nineteenth-Century Northern Europe* (Aldershot: Ashgate Publishing Limited, 2002), 136–56.

Loetz, Francisca, *Vom Kranken zum Patienten: 'Medikalisierung' und medizinische Vergesellschaftung am Beispiel Badens 1750–1850* (Stuttgart: Franz Steiner, 1993).

Lorenz, Maren, '"… als ob ihr ein Stein aus dem Leibe kollerte …". Schwangerschaftswahrnehmungen und Geburtserfahrungen von Frauen im 18. Jahrhundert', in Richard van Dülmen, ed., *Körper-Geschichten* (Frankfurt am Main: Fischer Taschenbuch Verlag, 1996), 99–121.

Loytved, Christine, ed., *Von der Wehemutter zur Hebamme. Die Gründung von Hebammenschulen mit Blick auf ihren politischen Stellenwert und ihren praktischen Nutzen* (Osnabrück: Universitäts-Verlag Rasch, 2001).

—, 'Zur Gründung der Hebammenschule an der Berliner Charité 1751', in Christine Loytved, ed., *Von der Wehemutter zur Hebamme: Die Gründung von Hebammenschulen mit Blick auf ihren politischen Stellenwert und praktischen Nutzen* (Osnabrück: Universitäts-Verlag Rasch, 2001), 63–78.

—, *Hebammen und ihre Lehrer. Wendepunkte in Ausbildung und Amt Lübecker Hebammen (1730–1850)* (Osnabrück: Universitäts-Verlag Rasch, 2002).

—, 'Einmischung wider Willen und gezielte Übernahme: Geschichte der Lübecker Hebammenausbildung im 18. und Anfang des 19. Jahrhunderts', in Bettina Wahrig and Werner Sohn, eds, *Zwischen Aufklärung, Policey und Verwaltung. Zur Genese des Medizinalwesens 1750–1850* (Wiesbaden: Harrassowitz Verlag, 2003), 131–46.

Marland, Hilary, 'The "*burgerlijke*" midwife: the *stadsvroedvrouw* of eighteenth-century Holland', in Hilary Marland, ed., *The Art of Midwifery: Early Modern Midwives in Europe* (London: Routledge, 1993), 192–213.

—, '"Stately and dignified, kindly and God-fearing": midwives, age and status in the Netherlands in the eighteenth century', in Hilary Marland and Margaret Pelling, eds, *The Task of Healing: Medicine, Religion and Gender in England and the Netherlands, 1450–1800* (Rotterdam: Erasmus Publications, 1996), 271–306.

McClive, Cathy, 'The Hidden Truths of the Belly: The Uncertainties of Pregnancy in Early Modern Europe', *Social History of Medicine* 15: 2 (2002): 209–27.

—, 'Blood and Expertise. The Trials of the Female Medical Expert in the Ancien-Régime Courtroom', *Bulletin of the History of Medicine* 82: 1 (2008): 86–108.

—, *Menstruation and Procreation in Early Modern France* (Farnham, Surrey and Burlington, VT: Ashgate, 2015).

McTavish, Lianne, *Childbirth and the Display of Authority in Early Modern France* (Aldershot: Ashgate, 2005).

Metz-Becker, Marita, *Der verwaltete Körper. Die Medikalisierung schwangerer Frauen in den Gebärhäusern des frühen 19. Jahrhunderts* (Frankfurt am Main: Campus Verlag, 1997).

Metzke, Hermann, *Lexikon der historischen Krankheitsbezeichnungen* (Neustadt an der Aisch: Verlag Degener & Co., 2005).

Middell, Katharina, 'Leipziger Sozietäten im 18. Jahrhundert. Die Bedeutung der Soziabilität für die kulturelle Integration von Minderheiten', *Neues Archiv für sächsische Geschichte* 69 (1998): 126–57.

Mitterauer, Michael, *Grundtypen alteuropäischer Sozialformen: Haus und Gemeinde in vorindustriellen Gesellschaften* (Stuttgart: Frommann-Holzboog, 1979).

Möller, Caren, *Medizinalpolizei. Die Theorie des staatlichen Gesundheitswesens im 18. und 19. Jahrhundert* (Frankfurt am Main: Vittorio Klostermann, 2005).

Mutschler, Ben, 'Illness in the "Social Credit" and "Money" Economies of Eighteenth-Century New England', in Mark S. R. Jenner and Patrick Wallis, eds, *Medicine and the Market in England and Its Colonies, c.1450–c.1850* (Basingstoke: Palgrave Macmillan, 2007), 175–95.

Ogilvie, Sheilagh, 'Consumption, Social Capital, and the "Industrious Revolution" in Early Modern Germany', *The Journal of Economic History* 70: 2 (2010): 287–325.

Ogilvie, Sheilagh C., *A Bitter Living: Women, Markets and Social Capital in Early Modern Germany* (Oxford: Oxford University Press, 2003).

Park, Katharine, 'The Death of Isabella Della Volpe. Four Eyewitness Accounts of a Postmortem Caesarean Section in 1545', *Bulletin of the History of Medicine* 82: 1 (2008): 169–87.

Pelling, Margaret, 'Thoroughly Resented? Older Women and the Medical Role in Early Modern London', in Lynette Hunter and Sarah Hutton, eds, *Women, Science and Medicine 1500–1700: Mothers and Sisters of the Royal Society* (Stroud: Sutton Publishing, 1997), 63–88.

—, *Medical Conflicts in Early Modern London: Patronage, Physicians and Irregular Practitioners 1540–1640* (Oxford: Oxford University Press, 2003).

Perkins, Wendy, *Midwifery and Medicine in Early Modern France: Louise Bourgeois* (Exeter: University of Exeter Press, 1996).

Pomata, Gianna, '"Practising between Earth and Heaven": Women Healers in Early Modern Bologna', *Dynamis* 19 (1999): 119–43.

—, 'Menstruating Men: Similarity and Difference of the Sexes in Early Modern Medicine', in Valeria Finucci and Kevin Brownlee, eds, *Generation and Degeneration: Tropes of Reproduction in Literature and History from Antiquity to Early Modern Europe* (Durham, NC: Duke University Press, 2001), 109–52.

Porter, Roy, 'The Patient's View: Doing Medical History from Below', *Theory and Society* 14 (1985): 175–98.

—, *Health for Sale: Quackery in England, 1660–1850* (Manchester: Manchester University Press, 1986).

—, 'William Hunter: a surgeon and gentleman', in W. F. Bynum and Roy Porter, eds, *William Hunter and the Eighteenth-Century Medical World* (Cambridge & London: Cambridge University Press, 2002), 7–34.

Pulz, Waltraud, *"Nicht alles nach der Gelahrten Sinn geschrieben": Das Hebammenanleitungsbuch von Justina Siegemund. Zur Rekonstruktion geburtshilflichen Überlieferungswissens frühneuzeitlicher Hebammen und seiner Bedeutung bei der Herausbildung der modernen Geburtshilfe* (Munich: Münchner Vereinigung für Volkskunde, 1994).

—, 'Gewaltsame Hilfsbereitschaft? Die Arbeit der Hebamme im Spiegel eines Gerichtskonflikts (1680–1685)', in Jürgen Schlumbohm, Barbara Duden, Jacques Gélis and Patrice Veit, eds, *Rituale der Geburt. Eine Kulturgeschichte* (Munich: Verlag C. H. Beck, 1998).

—, 'Zur Erforschung geburtshilflichen Überlieferungswissens von Frauen in der frühen Neuzeit', in Christine Loytved, ed., *Von der Wehemutter zur Hebamme. Die Gründung von Hebammenschulen mit Blick auf ihren politischen Stellenwert und ihren praktischen Nutzen* (Osnabrück: Universitäts-Verlag Rasch, 2001), 11–18.

Rabin, Dana, 'Bodies of Evidence, States of Mind: Infanticide, Emotion and Sensibility in Eighteenth-Century England', in Mark Jackson, ed., *Infanticide: Historical Perspectives on Child Murder and Concealment, 1550–2000* (Ashgate: Aldershot, 2002), 73–92.

Rachel, Walther, *Verwaltungsorganisation und Ämterwesen der Stadt Leipzig bis 1627* (Leipzig: B. G. Teuber, 1902).

Raeff, Marc, *The Well-Ordered Police State: Social and Institutional Change through Law in the Germanies and Russia 1600–1800* (New Haven, CT: Yale University Press, 1983).

Ramsey, Matthew, 'Medical Pluralism in Early Modern France', in Robert Jütte, ed., *Medical Pluralism – Past – Present – Future* (Stuttgart: Franz Steiner Verlag, 2013), 57–80.

Rattner Gelbart, Nina, *The King's Midwife: A History and Mystery of Madame du Coudray* (Berkeley and Los Angeles: University of California Press, 1998).

Reith, Reinhold, *Arbeits- und Lebensweise im städtischen Handwerk. Zur Sozialgeschichte Augsburger Handwerksgesellen im 18. Jahrhundert, 1700–1806* (Göttingen: Verlag Otto Schwartz & Co., 1988).

Richter, Joachim, 'Zur Geschichte des Öffentlichen Gesundheitsdienstes in Sachsen', *Ärzteblatt Sachsen* 11 (2001): 518–21.

Ritzmann, Iris, 'Der Faktor Nachfrage bei der Ausformung des modernen Medizinalwesens', in Bettina Wahrig-Schmidt and Werner Sohn, eds, *Aufklärung, Policey und Verwaltung. Zur Genese des Medizinalwesens 1750–1850* (Wiesbaden: Harrossowitz Verlag, 2003), 163–78.

Romlid, Christina, 'Swedish midwives and their instruments in the eighteenth and nineteenth centuries', in Hilary Marland and Anne Marie Rafferty, eds, *Midwives, Society and Childbirth: Debates and Controversies in the Modern Period* (London: Routledge, 1997), 38–60.

Ronnefeldt, Christian, 'Zur Gewerbe- und Sozialtopographie in der Grimmaischen Vorstadt in Leipzig vom 15. Jahrhundert bis zur 1. Hälfte des 17. Jahrhunderts', *Leipziger Kalender* (2004): 73–94.

Roper, Lyndal, *The Holy Household: Women and Morals in Reformation Augsburg* (Oxford: Oxford University Press, 1989).

—, *Witch Craze. Terror and Fantasy in Baroque Germany* (New Haven and London: Yale University Press, 2004).

Rosenstrauch, Hazel, 'Leipzig als "Centralplatz" des deutschen Buchhandels', in Wolfgang Martens, ed., *Zentren der Aufklärung III: Leipzig. Aufklärung und Bürgerlichkeit* (Heidelberg: Verlag Lambert Schneider, 1990), 103–24.

Rublack, Ulinka, 'Pregnancy, Childbirth and the Female Body in Early Modern Germany', *Past and Present* 150 (1996): 84–110.

—, 'The Public Body: Policing Abortion in Early Modern Germany', in Lynn Abrams and Elizabeth Harvey, eds, *Gender Relations in German History: Power, Agency and Experience from the Sixteenth to the Twentieth Century* (London: UCL Press, 1996), 57–80.

—, *The Crimes of Women in Early Modern Germany* (Oxford: Clarendon Press, 2001).

—, 'Erzählungen vom Geblüt und vom Herzen. Zu einer historischen Anthropologie des frühneuzeitlichen Körpers', *Historische Anthropologie* 9 (2001): 214–32.

Rule, John, 'Industrial Disputes, Wage Bargaining and the Moral Economy', in Adrian Randall and Andrew Charlesworth, eds, *Moral Economy and Popular Protest: Crowds, Conflict and Authority* (Basingstoke: Macmillan Press, 2000), 166–86.

Sander, Sabine, 'Die Bürokratisierung des Gesundheitswesens. Zur Problematik der "Modernisierung"', *Jahrbuch des Instituts für Geschichte der Medizin der Robert Bosch Stiftung* 6 (1987): 185–218.

Schilling, Heinz, *Die Stadt in der frühen Neuzeit* (2nd edn, Munich: R. Oldenbourg Verlag, 2004).

Schirmer, Uwe, 'Wirtschaftspolitik und Bevölkerungsentwicklung in Kursachsen (1648–1756)', *Neues Archiv für sächsische Geschichte* 68 (1997): 125–55.

Schlenkrich, Elke, *Von Leuten auf dem Sterbestroh. Sozialgeschichte obersächsischer Lazarette in der frühen Neuzeit* (Beucha: Sax-Verlag, 2002).

—, 'Johann Gregor Gurtthoff. Vom Leben und von der Arbeit eines (Pest)barbiers im 17. Jahrhundert', *Medizin, Gesellschaft und Geschichte. Jahrbuch des Instituts für Geschichte der Medizin* 21 (2003): 23–62.

Schlumbohm, Jürgen, 'Gesetze, die nicht durchgesetzt werden – ein Strukturmerkmal des frühneuzeitlichen Staates?', *Geschichte und Gesellschaft* 23 (1997): 647–63.

—, 'Der Blick des Arztes oder: Wie Gebärende zu Patientinnen wurden. Das Entbindungshospital der Universität Göttingen um 1800', in Jürgen Schlumbohm, Barbara Duden, Jacques Gélis and Patrice Veit, eds, *Rituale der Geburt. Eine Kulturgeschichte* (Munich: Verlag C.H. Beck, 1998), 170–91.

—, '"The Pregnant Women Are Here for the Sake of the Teaching Institution": The Lying-In Hospital of Göttingen University', *Social History of Medicine* 14: 1 (2001): 59–78.

—, 'The Practice of Practical Education: Male Students and Female Apprentices in the Lying-In Hospital of Göttingen University, 1792–1815', *Medical History* 51: 1 (2007): 3–36.

—, *Lebendige Phantome: ein Entbindungshospital und seine Patientinnen 1751–1830* (Göttingen: Wallstein Verlag, 2012).

—, 'Saving Mothers' and Children's Lives?: The Performance of German Lying-In Hospitals in the Late Eighteenth and Early Nineteenth Centuries', *Bulletin of the History of Medicine* 87: 1 (2013): 1–31.

—, '"Die edelste und nützlichste unter den Wissenschaften": Praxis der Geburtshilfe als Grundlegung der Wissenschaft, ca. 1750–1820', in Hans Erich Bödeker, Peter Hanns Reill and Jürgen Schlumbohm, eds, *Wissenschaft als kulturelle Praxis, 1750–1900* (Göttingen: Vandenhoeck & Ruprecht, 1999), 275–97.

—, ed., *Die Entstehung der Geburtsklinik in Deutschland 1751–1850: Göttingen, Kassel, Braunschweig* (Göttingen: Wallstein, 2004).

—, 'Mütter und Kinder retten: Geburtshilfe und Entbindungshospitäler im 18. und frühen 19. Jahrhundert – europäische Netze und lokale Vielfalt', in Hans Erich Bödeker and

Martin Gierl, eds, *Jenseits der Diskurse. Aufklärungspraxis und Institutionenwelt in europäisch komparativer Perspektive* (Göttingen: Vandenhoeck & Ruprecht, 2007), 323–44.

—, 'Als Mann in der Sphäre der Frauen: der schwierige Start einer geburtshilflichen Praxis im späten 18. Jahrhundert', in Michaela Fenske and Carola Lipp, eds, *Alltag als Politik, Politik im Alltag: Dimensionen des Politischen in Vergangenheit und Gegenwart: ein Lesebuch für Carola Lipp* (Berlin: LIT-Verlag, 2010), 227–46.

Schmitz, Britta, *Hebammen in Münster. Historische Entwicklung, Lebens- und Arbeitsumfeld, berufliches Selbstverständnis* (Münster: Waxmann, 1994).

Schofield, Roger, 'Did the mothers really die? Three centuries of maternal mortality in the "world we have lost"', in Lloyd Bonfield, Richard M. Smith and Keith Wrightson, eds, *The World We Have Gained: Histories of Population and Social Structure* (Oxford: Blackwell, 1986), 231–60.

Schötz, Susanne, 'Von Kauffrauen und Kuchenweibern. Weibliche Handelstätigkeit auf Leipzigs Messen im 18. und 19. Jahrhundert', in Günter Bentele, Thomas Topfstedt and Hartmut Zwahr, eds, *Leipzigs Messen 1497–1997. Gestaltwandel – Umbrüche – Neubeginn, Teilband 1: 1497–1914* (2 vols, Cologne: Böhlau, 1999), vol. 1, 377–401.

—, 'Zur Mitgliedschaft von Frauen in der Leipziger Kramerinnung im Spätmittelalter bzw. zu Beginn der frühen Neuzeit', in Henning Steinführer, Uwe Schirmer, Manfred Straube, Manfred Unger and Hartmut Zwahr, eds, *Leipzig, Mitteldeutschland und Europa. Festgabe für Manfred Straube und Manfred Unger zum 70. Geburtstag* (Beucha: Sax-Verlag, 2000), 57–67.

—, *Handelsfrauen in Leipzig. Zur Geschichte von Arbeit und Geschlecht in der Neuzeit* (Cologne: Böhlau, 2004).

Schrader, Catharina, *"Mother and Child were Saved". The Memoirs (1693–1740) of the Frisian Midwife Catharina Schrader*, trans. Hilary Marland (Amsterdam: Rodopi, 1987).

Schunka, Alexander, *Gäste, die bleiben: Zuwanderer in Kursachsen und der Oberlausitz im 17. und frühen 18. Jahrhundert* (Berlin: LIT-Verlag, 2006).

Scott, James C., 'The Moral Economy as an Argument and as a Fight', in Adrian Randall and Andrew Charlesworth, eds, *Moral Economy and Popular Protest: Crowds, Conflict, and Authority* (Basingstoke: Macmillan Press, 2000), 187–208.

Seidel, Hans-Christoph, *Eine neue Kultur des Gebärens. Die Medikalisierung von Geburt im 18. und 19. Jahrhundert in Deutschland* (Stuttgart: Steiner Verlag, 1998).

Sharpe, Pam, 'Disruption in the Well-Ordered Household: Age, Authority, and Possessed Young People', in Paul Griffiths, Adam Fox and Steve Hindle, eds, *The Experience of Authority in Early Modern England* (Basingstoke: Macmillan Press, 1996), 187–212.

Signori, Gabriela, 'Defensivgemeinschaften. Kreißende, Hebammen und "Mitweiber" im Spiegel spätmittelalterlicher Geburtswunder', *Das Mittelalter. Perspektiven mediävistischer Forschung* 1: 2 (1996): 113–34.

Simon-Muscheid, Katharina, ed., *"Was nützt die Schusterin dem Schmied?": Frauen und Handwerk vor der Industrialisierung* (Frankfurt am Main: Campus, 1998).

Stannek, Simone, 'Armut und Überlebensstrategien von Frauen im sächsischen Zunfthandwerk des 16.–18. Jahrhunderts', in Katharina Simon-Muscheid, ed., *"Was nützt die Schusterin dem Schmied?": Frauen und Handwerk vor der Industrialisierung* (Frankfurt am Main: Campus, 1998), 99–110.

Stolberg, Michael, 'The Monthly Malady: A History of Premenstrual Suffering', *Medical History* 44 (2000): 301–22.

—, 'Deutungen und Erfahrungen der Menstruation in der Frühen Neuzeit', in Barbara Mahlmann-Bauer, ed., *Scientiae et artes. Die Vermittlung alten und neuen Wissens in Literatur, Kunst und Musik* (2 vols, Wiesbaden: Harrassowitz in Kommission, 2004), vol. 2, 913–31.

—, 'Bedside Teaching and the Acquisition of Practical Skills in Mid-Sixteenth-Century Padua', *Journal for the History of Medicine and Allied Sciences* 69: 4 (2014): 633–61.

Stolleis, Michael, 'Was bedeutet "Normdurchsetzung" bei Policeyordnungen der frühen Neuzeit?', in Peter Landau and R. H. Helmholz, eds, *Grundlagen des Rechts: Festschrift für Peter Landau zum 65. Geburtstag* (Paderborn: F. Schöningh, 2000), 739–57.

Stuart, Kathy, *Defiled Trades and Social Outcasts: Honor and Ritual Pollution in Early Modern Germany* (Cambridge: Cambridge University Press, 1999).

Tatlock, Lynne, 'Speculum Feminarum: Gendered Perspectives on Obstetrics and Gynaecology in Early Modern Germany', *Signs* 17: 4 (1992): 725–60.

—, 'Volume Editor's Introduction', in Justine Siegemund, *The Court Midwife. Justina Siegemund,* trans. Lynne Tatlock (Chicago, IL: The University of Chicago Press, 2005), 1–26.

Tebeaux, Elizabeth, 'Women and Technical Writing, 1475–1700: Technology, Literacy, and Development of a Genre', in Lynette Hunter and Sarah Hutton, eds, *Women, Science and Medicine 1500–1700: Mothers and Sisters of the Royal Society* (Stroud: Sutton Publishing, 1997), 29–62.

Thane, Pat, *Old Age in English History: Past Experiences, Present Issues* (Oxford: Oxford University Press, 2000).

Thatcher-Ulrich, Laurel, *A Midwife's Tale: The Life of Martha Ballard, Based on Her Diary, 1785–1812* (New York, NY: Vintage Books, 1991).

Thieme, Horst and Sigrid Gerlach, eds, *Das Leipziger Eidbuch von 1590* (Leipzig: VEB Fachbuchverlag, 1986).

Thomas, Samuel, 'Midwifery and Society in Restoration York', *Social History of Medicine* 16: 1 (2003): 1–16.

Thompson, E. P., 'The Moral Economy of the English Crowd in the Eighteenth Century', *Past and Present* 50: 1 (1971): 76–136.

—, *Customs in Common* (New York: The New Press, 1991).

Töpfer, Thomas, *Die "Freyheit" der Kinder. Territoriale Politik, Schule und Bildungsvermittlung in der vormodernen Stadtgesellschaft. Das Kurfürstentum und Königreich Sachsen 1600–1815* (Stuttgart: Franz Steiner Verlag, 2012).

Toppe, Sabine, *Die Erziehung zur guten Mutter. Medizinisch-pädagogische Anleitungen zur Mutterschaft im 18. Jahrhundert* (Oldenburg: BIS Universität Oldenburg, 1993).

Tribe, Keith, *Governing Economy. The Reformation of German Economic Discourse 1750–1840* (Cambridge: Cambridge University Press, 1988).

Ulbricht, Otto, 'The Debate about Foundling Hospitals in Enlightenment Germany: Infanticide, Illegitimacy, and Infant Mortality Rates', *Central European History* 18: 3/4 (1985): 211–56.

—, *Kindsmord und Aufklärung in Deutschland* (Munich: R. Oldenbourg, 1990).

van Lieburg, M. J., 'Catharina Schrader (1656–1746) and Her Notebook', in Hilary Marland, ed., *"Mother and Child were Saved". The Memoirs (1693–1740) of the Frisian Midwife Catharina Schrader* (Amsterdam: Rodopi, 1987), 6–22.

Vann Sprecher, Tiffany D. and Ruth Mazo Karras, 'The Midwife and the Church. Ecclesiastical Regulation of Midwives in Brie, 1499–1504', *Bulletin of the History of Medicine* 85: 2 (2011): 171–92.

Waardt, Hans de, 'Chasing Demons and Curing Mortals: The Medical Practice of Clerics in the Netherlands', in Hilary Marland and Margaret Pelling, eds, *The Task of Healing: Medicine, Religion and Gender in England and the Netherlands, 1450–1800* (Rotterdam: Erasmus Publications, 1996), 171–204.

Wakefield, Andre, 'Books, Bureaus, and the Historiography of Cameralism', *European Journal of Law and Economics* 19 (2005): 311–20.

—, *The Disordered Police State: German Cameralism as Science and Practice* (Chicago, IL: University of Chicago Press, 2009).

Walker, Mack, *German Home Towns. Community, State and General Estate, 1648–1871* (Ithaca, NY: Cornell University Press, 1971).

Weiss, Volkmar, *Bevölkerung und soziale Mobilität. Sachsen 1550–1880* (Berlin: Akademie-Verlag, 1993).

—, 'Bevölkerungsentwicklung und Mobilität in Sachsen von 1550 bis 1880', *Neues Archiv für sächsische Geschichte* 64 (1993): 53–60.

Wermes, Martina, 'Die Analyse von Patenschaften und ihr Wert für sozialgeschichtliche Untersuchungen – dargestellt am Beispiel Leipziger Familien', *Genealogie. Deutsche Zeitschrift für Familienkunde* 24: 5–6 (1999): 592–601.

Wessling, Mary Nagle, 'Official Medicine and Customary Medicine in Early Modern Württemberg: The Career of Christoph Friedrich Pichler', *Medizin, Gesellschaft und Geschichte* 9 (1990): 21–44.

—, 'Infanticide Trials and Forensic Medicine: Württemberg 1757–1793', in Michael Clark and Catherine Crawford, eds, *Legal Medicine in History* (Cambridge: Cambridge University Press, 1994), 117–44.

Wiesner, Merry, 'Early Modern Midwifery: A Case Study', in Barbara A. Hanawalt, ed., *Women and Work in Preindustrial Europe* (Bloomington, IN: Indiana University Press, 1986), 94–114.

—, 'The Midwives of South Germany and the Public/Private Dichotomy', in Hilary Marland, ed., *The Art of Midwifery: Early Modern Midwives in Europe* (London: Routledge, 1993), 77–94.

—, 'Gender and the Worlds of Work', in Robert Scribner, ed., *Germany: A New Social and Economic History, 1450–1630* (2 vols, London: Edward Arnold, 1996), vol. 1, 209–32.

—, 'Spinning Out Capital: Women's Work in Preindustrial Europe 1350–1750', in Renate Bridenthal, Susan Mosher Stuard and Merry Wiesner, eds, *Becoming Visible: Women in European History* (3rd edn, Boston, MA: Houghton Mifflin, 1998), 203–32.

—, *Working Women in Renaissance Germany* (New Brunswick, NJ: Rutgers University Press, 1986).

Wiesner Wood, Merry, 'Paltry Peddlers or Essential Merchants? Women in the Distributive Trades in Early Modern Nuremberg', *Sixteenth Century Journal* 12: 2 (1981): 3–13.

Wille, Dr. F. C., 'Über Stand und Ausbildung der Hebammen im 17. und 18. Jahrhundert in Chur-Brandenburg', *Abhandlungen zur Geschichte der Medizin und der Naturwissenschaften* Heft 4 (1934).

Wilson, Adrian, *The Making of Man-Midwifery: Childbirth in England 1660–1770* (London: UCL Press, 1995).

—, 'A Memorial of Eleanor Willughby, a Seventeenth-Century Midwife', in Lynette Hunter and Sarah Hutton, eds, *Women, Science and Medicine 1500–1700: Mothers and Sisters of the Royal Society* (Sutton: Stroud, 1997), 138–77.

—, 'Participant or Patient? Seventeenth-Century Childbirth from the Mother's Point of View', in Roy Porter, ed., *Patients and Practitioners: Lay Perceptions of Medicine in Pre-Industrial Society* (Cambridge: Cambridge University Press, 2002), 129–44.

—, 'Midwifery in the "Medical Marketplace"', in Mark S. R. Jenner and Patrick Wallis, eds, *Medicine and the Market in England and Its Colonies, c. 1450–c.1850* (Basingstoke: Palgrave Macmillan, 2007), 153–74.

—, *Ritual and Conflict: The Social Relations of Childbirth in Early Modern England* (Farnham: Ashgate, 2013).

Wolff, Eberhard, 'Medikalisierung von Unten? Das Beispiel der jüdischen Krankenbesuchgesellschaften', in Bettina Wahrig-Schmidt and Werner Sohn, eds, *Aufklärung, Policey und Verwaltung. Zur Genese des Medizinalwesens 1750–1850* (Wiesbaden: Harrossowitz Verlag, 2003), 179–90.

Wolter, Stefan, '"… zwinget mich nicht dahin zu gehen, wo ich aller Schamhaftigkeit vergeßen sein soll". Aus den Anfängen der Jenaer Entbindungsanstalt', in Christine Loytved, ed., *Von der Wehemutter zur Hebamme: Die Gründung von Hebammenschulen mit Blick auf ihren politischen Stellenwert und praktischen Nutzen* (Osnabrück: Universitäts-Verlag Rasch, 2001), 79–96.

Wunder, Heide, 'Überlegungen zum Wandel der Geschlechterbeziehungen im 15. und 16. Jahrhundert aus sozialgeschichtlicher Sicht', in Heide Wunder and Christina Vanja, eds, *Wandel der Geschlechterbeziehungen zu Beginn der Neuzeit* (Frankfurt am Main: Suhrkamp, 1991), 13–26.

—, *"Er ist die Sonn', sie ist der Mond". Frauen in der frühen Neuzeit* (Munich: Verlag C. H. Beck, 1992).

Würgler, Andreas, 'Desideria und Landesordnungen. Kommunaler und landständischer Einfluß auf die fürstliche Gesetzgebung in Hessen-Kassel 1650–1800', in Peter Blickle, ed., *Gemeinde und Staat im alten Europa* (Munich: R. Oldenbourg Verlag, 1998), 149–208.

Zande, Johan van der, 'Statistik and History in the German Enlightenment', *Journal of the History of Ideas* 71: 3 (2010): 411–32.

Unpublished papers and theses

Baruch, Friedrich, 'Das Hebammenwesen im Reichsstädtischen Nürnberg' (Dissertation, Erlangen, 1955).

Feige, Wolfgang, 'Die Sozialstruktur der spätmittelalterlichen deutschen Stadt im Spiegel der historischen Statistik – mit besonderer Berücksichtigung der niederen Schichten der Bevölkerung und mit einem Exkurs in das Leipzig des 16. Jahrhunderts' (Dissertation, Karl-Marx-Universität Leipzig, 1965).

Gabler, Susanne, 'Das Hebammenwesen in Nördlingen des 16. Jahrhunderts' (Dissertation, Technical University Munich, 1985).

Hess, Ann Giardina, 'Community Case Studies of Midwives from England and New England c. 1650–1720' (PhD thesis, University of Cambridge, 1994).

Hub, Johann, 'Die Hebammenordnung des XVII. Jahrhunderts' (Dissertation, Würzburg, 1914).

McClive, Cathy, 'Bleeding Flowers and Waning Moons: A History of Menstruation in France c. 1495–1761' (PhD thesis, Warwick University, 2004).

Nöth, Alois, 'Die Hebammenordnungen des XVIII. Jahrhunderts' (Dissertation, Würzburg, 1931).

Robilliard, Gabrielle, 'Midwives in Early Modern Frankfurt am Main c. 1500–1700: Organisation, Socio-Economic Status and Work Identity' (MPhil thesis, University of Cambridge, 2004).

Steilen, Lena Irene, 'Zwischen Vertrauen und Kontrolle. Hebammen im Münden des 19. Jahrhunderts' (MA thesis, Göttingen, 2003).

Online sources

Deutsches Wörterbuch von Jacob und Wilhelm Grimm, (16 vols, S. Hirzel: 1854–1961), available at <http://dwb.uni-trier.de/de/>, accessed 21 October 2016.

Hehl, Ulrich von, *Professorenkatalog der Universität Leipzig*, available at <http://uni-leipzig.de/unigeschichte/professorenkatalog/>, accessed 26 October 2016.

Keil, Gundolf, *Neue Deutsche Biographie* (2003), available at <https://www.deutsche-biographie.de/gnd104156686.html#ndbcontent>, accessed 27 September 2016.

Kettler, Rolf, *Eine kurze Geschichte des Abfalls* (Bundesamt für Umwelt, Wald und Landschaft, Abteilung Abfall, Switzerland: 2000), available at <www.booze.ch/cm_data/muell.pdf >, accessed 26 October 2016.

Kirchhofer, Anton, Martin Mulsow and Olaf Simons, *Pierre Marteau webspace, entry on 'Holy Roman Empire: Money'* (3 April 2008 (last page update)), available at <http://pierre-marteau.com/wiki/index.php?title=Money_(Holy_Roman_Empire)#Sachsen.2FMei.C3.9Fen_.28Saxonia.29>, accessed 20 October 2016.

Krünitz, Dr Johann Georg, *Oekonomische Encyklopädie oder allgemeines System der Staats- Stadt- Haus- und Landwirthschaft* (242 vols, Joachim Pauli: 1773), available at <http://www.kruenitz1.uni-trier.de/>, accessed 26 October 2016.

Mielisch, Arlett, *Wie die Hebamme ihren Meister fand. Der lange Weg zur ersten Dresdner Hebammenordnung von 1764* (Technische Universität Dresden: 2014/15), available at <https://
tu-dresden.de/gsw/phil/ige/fnz/ressourcen/dateien/studium/dat_praes/plakmiel?lang
=de>, accessed 15 November 2016.

Pagel, Julius Leopold, *Deutsche Biographie* (1896), available at <https://www.deutsche-
biographie.de/gnd117345814.html#adbcontent>, accessed 6 September 2016.

Wagner, Siegfried and Ursula Dittrich-Wagner, *C-A-F-F-E-E, trink nicht soviel Caffe. Aus der
Frühzeit der Naumburger Kaffee-Häuser* (Museumsverein Naumberg: undated), available at
<http://mv-naumburg.de/kaffeegeschichte>, accessed 26 October 2016.

Zedler, Johann Heinrich, *Grosses vollständiges Universal-Lexicon aller Wissenschaften und Künste
(online version)* (68 vols, Bayerische Staatsbibliothek: 1731–54), available at <http://www.
zedler-lexikon.de/index.html>, accessed 26 October 2016.

Indices

General names and places

Women in Midwifery in Leipzig

MEDIZIN, GESELLSCHAFT UND GESCHICHTE — BEIHEFTE

Herausgegeben von Robert Jütte.

Franz Steiner Verlag   ISSN 0941–5033

18. Jens-Uwe Teichler
**„Der Charlatan strebt nicht
nach Wahrheit, er verlangt nur
nach Geld"**
Zur Auseinandersetzung zwischen natur-
wissenschaftlicher Medizin und Laienme-
dizin im deutschen Kaiserreich am Beispiel
von Hypnotismus und Heilmagnetismus
2002. 233 S. mit 16 Abb., kt.
ISBN 978-3-515-07976-1

19. Claudia Stein
**Die Behandlung der Franzosen-
krankheit in der Frühen Neuzeit
am Beispiel Augsburgs**
2003. 293 S., kt.
ISBN 978-3-515-08032-3

20. Jörg Melzer
Vollwerternährung
Diätetik, Naturheilkunde,
Nationalsozialismus, sozialer Anspruch
2003. 480 S., kt.
ISBN 978-3-515-08278-5

21. Thomas Gerst
**Ärztliche Standesorganisation
und Standespolitik in Deutschland
1945–1955**
2004. 270 S., kt.
ISBN 978-3-515-08056-9

22. Florian Steger
Asklepiosmedizin
Medizinischer Alltag in der römischen
Kaiserzeit
2004. 244 S. und 12 Taf. mit 17 Abb., kt.
ISBN 978-3-515-08415-4

23. Ulrike Thoms
**Anstaltskost im
Rationalisierungsprozeß**
Die Ernährung in Krankenhäusern und
Gefängnissen im 18. und 19. Jahrhundert
2005. 957 S. mit 84 Abb., kt.
ISBN 978-3-515-07935-8

24. Simone Moses
Alt und krank
Ältere Patienten in der Medizinischen
Klinik der Universität Tübingen zur Zeit
der Entstehung der Geriatrie 1880 bis 1914

2005. 277 S. mit 61 Tab. und 27 Diagr.
ISBN 978-3-515-08654-7

25. Sylvelyn Hähner-Rombach (Hg.)
„Ohne Wasser ist kein Heil"
Medizinische und kulturelle Aspekte
der Nutzung von Wasser
2005. 167 S., kt.
ISBN 978-3-515-08785-8

26. Heiner Fangerau / Karen Nolte (Hg.)
**„Moderne" Anstaltspsychiatrie
im 19. und 20. Jahrhundert**
Legitimation und Kritik
2006. 416 S., kt.
ISBN 978-3-515-08805-3

27. Martin Dinges (Hg.)
**Männlichkeit und Gesundheit
im historischen Wandel ca. 1800 –
ca. 2000**
2007. 398 S. mit 7 Abb., 22 Tab.
und 4 Diagr., kt.
ISBN 978-3-515-08920-3

28. Marion Maria Ruisinger
Patientenwege
Die Konsiliarkorrespondenz Lorenz
Heisters (1683–1758) in der Trew-
Sammlung Erlangen
2008. 308 S. mit 7 Abb. und 16 Diagr., kt.
ISBN 978-3-515-08806-0

29. Martin Dinges (Hg.)
**Krankheit in Briefen im deutschen
und französischen Sprachraum**
17.–21. Jahrhundert
2007. 267 S., kt.
ISBN 978-3-515-08949-4

30. Helen Bömelburg
Der Arzt und sein Modell
Porträtfotografien aus der deutschen Psy-
chiatrie 1880 bis 1933
2007. 239 S. mit 68 Abb. und 2 Diagr., kt.
ISBN 978-3-515-09096-8

31. Martin Krieger
Arme und Ärzte, Kranke und Kassen
Ländliche Gesundheitsversorgung und
kranke Arme in der südlichen Rheinprovinz
(1869 bis 1930)

2009. 452 S. mit 7 Abb., 16 Tab. und 5 Ktn.,
kt.
ISBN 978-3-515-09171-8

32. Sylvelyn Hähner-Rombach
**Alltag in der Krankenpflege /
Everyday Nursing Life**
Geschichte und Gegenwart /
Past and Present
2009. 309 S. mit 22 Tab., kt.
ISBN 978-3-515-09332-3

33. Nicole Schweig
Gesundheitsverhalten von Männern
Gesundheit und Krankheit in Briefen,
1800–1950
2009. 288 S. mit 4 Abb. und 8 Tab., kt.
ISBN 978-3-515-09362-0

34. Andreas Renner
**Russische Autokratie
und europäische Medizin**
Organisierter Wissenstransfer
im 18. Jahrhundert
2010. 373 S., kt.
ISBN 978-3-515-09640-9

35. Philipp Osten (Hg.)
Patientendokumente
Krankheit in Selbstzeugnissen
2010. 253 S. mit 3 Abb., kt.
ISBN 978-3-515-09717-8

36. Susanne Hoffmann
**Gesunder Alltag im
20. Jahrhundert?**
Geschlechterspezifische Diskurse und
gesundheitsrelevante Verhaltensstile
in deutschsprachigen Ländern
2010. 538 S. mit 7 Abb., kt.
ISBN 978-3-515-09681-2

37. Marion Baschin
**Wer lässt sich von einem
Homöopathen behandeln?**
Die Patienten des Clemens Maria Franz von
Bönninghausen (1785–1864)
2010. 495 S. mit 45 Abb., kt.
ISBN 978-3-515-09772-7

38. Ulrike Gaida
**Bildungskonzepte der
Krankenpflege in der
Weimarer Republik**
Die Schwesternschaft des Evangelischen
Diakonievereins e.V. Berlin-Zehlendorf
2011. 346 S. mit 12 Abb., kt.
ISBN 978-3-515-09783-3

39. Martin Dinges / Robert Jütte (ed.)
**The transmission of health
practices (c. 1500 to 2000)**

2011. 190 S. mit 4 Abb. und 1 Tab., kt.
ISBN 978-3-515-09897-7

40. Sylvelyn Hähner-Rombach
**Gesundheit und Krankheit im
Spiegel von Petitionen an den
Landtag von Baden-Württemberg
1946 bis 1980**
2011. 193 S. mit 27 Tab., kt.
ISBN 978-3-515-09914-1

41. Florian Mildenberger
**Medikale Subkulturen in der
Bundesrepublik Deutschland
und ihre Gegner (1950–1990)**
Die Zentrale zur Bekämpfung der
Unlauterkeit im Heilgewerbe
2011. 188 S. mit 15 Abb., kt.
ISBN 978-3-515-10041-0

42. Angela Schattner
**Zwischen Familie, Heilern und
Fürsorge**
Das Bewältigungsverhalten von
Epileptikern in deutschsprachigen
Gebieten des 16.–18. Jahrhunderts
2012. 299 S. mit 5 Abb. und 2 Tab., kt.
ISBN 978-3-515-09947-9

43. Susanne Rueß / Astrid Stölzle (Hg.)
**Das Tagebuch der jüdischen Kriegs-
krankenschwester Rosa Bendit,
1914 bis 1917**
2012. 175 S. mit 6 Abb., kt.
ISBN 978-3-515-10124-0

44. Sabine Herrmann
**Giacomo Casanova und die Medizin
des 18. Jahrhunderts**
2012. 214 S. mit 8 Abb., kt.
ISBN 978-3-515-10175-2

45. Florian Mildenberger
**Medizinische Belehrung
für das Bürgertum**
Medikale Kulturen in der Zeitschrift
„Die Gartenlaube" (1853–1944)
2012. 230 S. mit 11 Abb., kt.
ISBN 978-3-515-10232-2

46. Robert Jütte (Hg.)
Medical Pluralism
Past – Present – Future
2013. 205 S. mit 3 Abb., kt.
ISBN 978-3-515-10441-8

47. Annett Büttner
**Die konfessionelle Kriegskranken-
pflege im 19. Jahrhundert**
2013. 481 S. mit 22 Abb., kt.
ISBN 978-3-515-10462-3

48. Annika Hoffmann
Arzneimittelkonsum

und Geschlecht
Eine historische Analyse
zum 19. und 20. Jahrhundert
2014. XVI, 217 S. mit 11 Abb., 63 Graf.
und 32 Tab., kt.
ISBN 978-3-515-10455-5

49. Astrid Stölzle
**Kriegskrankenpflege im
Ersten Weltkrieg**
Das Pflegepersonal der freiwilligen
Krankenpflege in den Etappen
des Deutschen Kaiserreichs
2013. 227 S. mit 18 Abb., kt.
ISBN 978-3-515-10481-4

50. Martin Dinges (Hg.)
**Medical Pluralism and Homoeo-
pathy in India and Germany
(1810–2010)**
A Comparison of Practices
2014. 250 S. mit 30 Abb. und 12 Tab., kt.
ISBN 978-3-515-10484-5

51. Alois Unterkircher
**Jungen und Männer als Patienten
bei einem Südtiroler Landarzt
(1860–1900)**
2014. 392 S. mit 18 Abb., 29 Graf.
und 41 Tab., kt.
ISBN 978-3-515-10612-2

52. Marion Baschin
**Ärztliche Praxis im letzten Drittel
des 19. Jahrhunderts**
Der Homöopath Dr. Friedrich Paul von
Bönninghausen (1828–1910)
2014. 318 S. mit 5 Abb., 33 Graf.
und 61 Tab., kt.
ISBN 978-3-515-10782-2

53. Anja Faber
**Pflegealltag im stationären Bereich
zwischen 1880 und 1930**
2015. 251 S. mit 2 Abb. und 40 Graf., kt.
ISBN 978-3-515-10685-6

54. Sylvelyn Hähner-Rombach (Hg.)
Geschichte der Prävention
Akteure, Praktiken, Instrumente
2015. 256 S. mit 8 Abb., 8 Graf.
und 3 Tab., kt.
ISBN 978-3-515-10998-7

55. Melanie Ruff
Gesichter des Ersten Weltkrieges
Alltag, Biografien und Selbstdarstellungen
von gesichtsverletzten Soldaten
2015. 281 S. mit 44 Abb. und 3 Tab., kt.
ISBN 978-3-515-11058-7

56. Florian Mildenberger
Verschobene Wirbel –

verschwommene Traditionen
Chiropraktik, Chirotherapie
und Manuelle Medizin in Deutschland
2015. 344 S. mit 12 Abb., kt.
ISBN 978-3-515-11151-5

57. Nicole Schweig
Suizid und Männlichkeit
Selbsttötungen von Männern auf See,
in der Wehrmacht und im zivilen Bereich,
1893 – ca. 1986
2016. 126 S. mit 2 Tab., kt.
ISBN 978-3-515-11176-8

58. Martin Dinges / Andreas Weigl (Hg.)
**Gender-Specific Life Expectancy
in Europe 1850–2010**
2016. 217 S. mit 2 Abb., 63 Graf.
und 25 Tab., kt.
ISBN 978-3-515-11258-1

59. Jenny Linek
**Gesundheitsvorsorge in der DDR
zwischen Propaganda und Praxis**
2016. 242 S. mit 7 Abb. und 3 Tab., kt.
ISBN 978-3-515-11281-9

60. Philipp Eisele
**Pluralismus in der Medizin
aus der Patientenperspektive**
Briefe an eine Patientenorganisation
für alternative Behandlungsmethoden
(1992–2000)
2016. 497 S. mit 4 Abb., 43 Schaubildern
und 34 Tab., kt.
ISBN 978-3-515-11255-0

61. Nina Grabe
**Die stationäre Versorgung
alter Menschen in Niedersachsen
1945–1975**
2016. 425 S. mit 13 Abb., 30 Graf.
und 2 Tab., kt.
ISBN 978-3-515-11332-8

62. Susanne Kreutzer / Karen Nolte (Hg.)
Deaconesses in Nursing Care
International Transfer of a Female Model of
Life and Work in the 19th and 20th Century
2016. 230 S. mit 6 Abb. und 9 Tab., kt.
ISBN 978-3-515-11355-7

63. Pierre Pfütsch
**Das Geschlecht des „präventiven
Selbst"**
Prävention und Gesundheitsförderung
in der Bundesrepublik Deutschland aus
geschlechterspezifischer Perspektive
(1949–2010)
2017. 425 S. mit 24 s/w-Abb., 22 Farbabb.
und 64 Tab., kt.
ISBN 978-3-515-11638-1